Effective Patient Education
A Guide to Increased Adherence

Fourth Edition

Donna R. Falvo, PhD, RN, CRC
Clinical Professor
Allied Health Sciences
School of Medicine
University of North Carolina at Chapel Hill
Chapel Hill, North Carolina

JONES AND BARTLETT PUBLISHERS
Sudbury, Massachusetts
BOSTON   TORONTO   LONDON   SINGAPORE

World Headquarters
Jones and Bartlett Publishers
40 Tall Pine Drive
Sudbury, MA 01776
978-443-5000
info@jbpub.com
www.jbpub.com

Jones and Bartlett Publishers
Canada
6339 Ormindale Way
Mississauga, Ontario L5V 1J2
Canada

Jones and Bartlett Publishers
International
Barb House, Barb Mews
London W6 7PA
United Kingdom

Jones and Bartlett's books and products are available through most bookstores and online booksellers. To contact
Jones and Bartlett Publishers directly, call 800-832-0034, fax 978-443-8000, or visit our website, www.jbpub.com.

Substantial discounts on bulk quantities of Jones and Bartlett's publications are available to corporations,
professional associations, and other qualified organizations. For details and specific discount information,
contact the special sales department at Jones and Bartlett via the above contact information or send an email
to specialsales@jbpub.com.

The authors, editors, and publisher have made every effort to provide accurate information. However, they are
not responsible for errors, omissions, or for any outcomes related to the use of the contents of this book and take
no responsibility for the use of the products and procedures described. Treatments and side effects described
in this book may not be applicable to all people; likewise, some people may require a dose or experience a side
effect that is not described herein. Drugs and medical devices are discussed that may have limited availability
controlled by the Food and Drug Administration (FDA) for use only in a research study or clinical trial. Research,
clinical practice, and government regulations often change the accepted standard in this field. When consideration is being given to use of any drug in the clinical setting, the health care provider or reader is responsible for
determining FDA status of the drug, reading the package insert, and reviewing prescribing information for the
most up-to-date recommendations on dose, precautions, and contraindications, and determining the appropriate
usage for the product. This is especially important in the case of drugs that are new or seldom used.

Production Credits
Publisher: Kevin Sullivan
Acquisitions Editor: Amy Sibley
Associate Editor: Patricia Donnelly
Editorial Assistant: Rachel Shuster
Production Editor: Amanda Clerkin
Marketing Manager: Rebecca Wasley
V.P., Manufacturing and Inventory Control: Therese Connell
Composition: DSCS/Absolute Service, Inc.
Cover Design: Scott Moden
Cover Image: © Jeffrey Van Daele/ShutterStock, Inc.
Printing and Binding: Malloy, Inc.
Cover Printing: Malloy, Inc.

Library of Congress Cataloging-in-Publication Data
Falvo, Donna R.
    Effective patient education : a guide to increased adherence / Donna R. Falvo. —4th ed.
        p. ; cm.
    Includes bibliographical references and index.
    ISBN-13: 978-0-7637-6625-2 (alk. paper)
    ISBN-10: 0-7637-6625-9 (alk. paper)
1. Patient education. 2. Patient compliance. I. Title.
    [DNLM: 1. Patient Education as Topic—methods. 2. Patient Compliance. 3. Patient-Centered Care.
    W 85 F197e 2011]
    R727.4.F35 2011
    615.5071—dc22   2009038850

6048

Printed in the United States of America
14 13 12 11 10   10 9 8 7 6 5 4 3 2 1

This book is dedicated to my husband, Richard: without his love, patience, and support, this book, as well as the 30 years of my career, would not have been possible.

Contents

About the Author

Dr. Donna R. Falvo is a registered nurse, licensed psychologist, and certified rehabilitation counselor. During the span of her career, she has been a staff nurse, nursing instructor, counselor, and professor of family and community medicine and rehabilitation counseling. She is a former Mary Switzer Scholar and was elected to Sigma Xi National Scientific Research Society in 1995. She served as Chair of the Society of Teachers of Family Medicine's Group on Patient Education and served on the Steering Committee for the National Patient Education Conference sponsored by the American Academy of Family Practice and the Society of Teachers of Family Medicine. She was elected President of the American Rehabilitation Counseling Association in 1998. Most recently, she has served as a Dimension Expert in Information, Education, and Communication for the National Research Corporation (NRC)–Picker Institute and was a speaker at the NRC Picker Symposium. She has conducted a number of invitational workshops on patient education, sponsored by organizations such as the American Hospital Association, American Physical Therapy Association, Society of Teachers of Family Medicine, as well as a number of universities and private corporations. She is also author of the book *Medical and Psychosocial Aspects of Chronic Illness and Disability*. She is currently a professor of Rehabilitation Counseling and Psychology in the Department of Allied Health, University of North Carolina School of Medicine in Chapel Hill, North Carolina.

Preface

It is generally recognized that patients have a right to be fully informed about and be active participants in matters related to their health and health care. The general assumption is that patients who are fully informed will be better able to make informed choices that will in turn increase their health status. Currently, patients have access to more information than ever before; however, a large number of patients continue to ignore or neglect recommendations that are designed to help them maintain or improve their health or to manage their condition. Despite efforts to inform patients, many still are not willing or able to follow the advice or recommendations they are given.

Although patient education involves providing patients with information, mere provision of information does not appear to be enough. In order to be effective, patient education must also involve *patient teaching*. Patient teaching is an active process of communication built on mutual trust and respect, which in turn fosters a partnership between patient and health professional. It facilitates open sharing of information so that mutually agreed on goals can be established and barriers to following recommendations can be identified and overcome.

Patients enter the healthcare system with preexisting beliefs, attitudes, fears, anxieties, previous experiences, and individual life and family circumstances, all of which impact their receptivity to information and their ability and willingness to incorporate information into their daily lives. Only by identifying and incorporating individual patient variables into patient teaching can the health professional tailor teaching so it is relevant and comprehensible to the individual patient. Patient teaching involves helping patients gain knowledge, learn skills, and change attitudes so they are able to manage manifestations of their condition; cope with the emotional impact of illness or changing roles; prevent illness, complications, or disability from occurring; make different lifestyle adjustments; and manage complex treatment regimens. Centering patient teaching on individual needs helps the health professional identify issues, supports, and barriers that may impact on the patient's willingness and/or ability to incorporate information into his or her daily life. Patient education is an organized, structured program that serves as a vehicle utilized by health professionals to provide patients with information and to facilitate learning. Patient teaching, however, is centered on the patient and is the process by which learning is made possible.

This new edition of the book emphasizes a patient-centered approach to patient teaching and provides exploration of issues confronting health professionals conducting patient teaching and issues confronting patients when attempting to follow recommendations. It provides specific teaching and communication strategies that will help health professionals conduct patient teaching more efficiently and effectively. Although based on established theories, the book takes a clinical approach, using case examples to illustrate points rather than focusing on theory. The book emphasizes partnership between patient and health professional in order to reach mutually agreed on outcomes defined as increased adherence to recommendations.

The goal of effective patient teaching in patient education is to help patients make informed choices and to provide guidance and support that provides them with the best opportunity to achieve their optimal health potential.

—Donna R. Falvo

CHAPTER 1

Patient Adherence as an Outcome of Effective Patient Teaching

ADHERENCE VERSUS COMPLIANCE

Previously, health care was provided in the context of a "disease-centered model" in which most decisions about a patient's treatment were made by health professionals with little consultation with the patient (Stanton, 2002). The focus of the disease model was on the particular illness rather than the patient as a whole (Steckel, 1982). In this model, it was expected that all patients seeking health care would follow or *comply* with recommendations they received. It was assumed that patients seeking health advice believed that the health professional knew best and, consequently, that they would logically follow recommendations. The possibility that there could be disagreement with the health professional's recommendations, that recommendations may not be presented clearly or accurately by the health professional, or that the patient did not have the resources to follow recommendations was rarely considered.

The term *compliance* denotes a power differential between patient and health professional. It suggests that the patient is passively following recommendations and implies yielding to authority, rather than following a treatment plan based on a collaborative effort between the patient and health professional (Osterberg & Blaschke, 2005; Steiner & Earnest, 2000). Not only has the effectiveness of an authoritarian approach been questioned over the last few decades, increasing evidence has shown that this approach most often does not lead to the best health outcomes (Trostle, 1997). Although semantics may seem inconsequential, words used to describe a phenomenon significantly influence how the phenomenon is understood. Words chosen convey an underlying philosophical context. Consequently, because the word "compliance" has an authoritarian connotation, an attempt to diminish the paternalistic nature of the term has resulted in use of substitute words such as *adherence, alliance, collaboration,* or *concordance* to describe the extent to which patients follow advice and recommendations provided by the health professional. Although all of these words have been used to describe this phenomenon, the term compliance has largely been replaced by the term adherence. The substitution of the word adherence for compliance has coincided with a change of approach to patient care, an approach that is more *patient-centered,* focusing on the needs of patients rather than on the goals of the health professional.

A patient-centered approach to health care has shown increased patient satisfaction and better health outcomes (Aday et al., 2004; Balkrishnan, 2005; Balkrishnan et al., 2003; DiMatteo et al., 2002; Meryn, 1998; Sokol et al., 2005; Wagner, Austin, et al., 2001). In this approach, patients are treated as partners, are fully informed about health-related matters, are more involved in treatment planning and decision making, and are encouraged to accept more responsibility for their health care.

Given the positive impact that the patient-centered approach has apparently had on health care, it would seem that nonadherence would be a rare occurrence rather than a continuing healthcare issue. Adherence is, however, a complex and multidimensional issue that includes a multitude of dynamic behaviors and circumstances (Haynes et al., 2002b; Malouff & Schutte, 2004,).

Health professionals, even when attempting to use a patient-centered approach, may not have the awareness or understanding of the complexity of adherence and thus may be unable to fully incorporate strategies into patient interactions that would help patients achieve their optimal health outcomes (Vivian & Wilcox, 2000). Assuming the patient's condition has been accurately diagnosed and the appropriate treatment prescribed, the only way recommended preventative or therapeutic measures can be effective is if the patient is able to correctly follow recommendations and advice given by the health professional. Consequently, adherence, or more specifically nonadherence, must be identified, studied, and understood (Koltun & Stone, 1986). Adherence is a reflection of good communication and a relationship that is built on respect, active participation, and partnership between patient and health professional, not coercion or manipulation.

EXTENT OF NONADHERENCE

Today, when patients have access to more information than ever before, and advances in knowledge and sophistication of technology for prevention, diagnosis, treatment, or cure of disease have soared, patients continue to experience morbidity and mortality from conditions that could have been prevented or effectively treated. In some instances, treatment failure or iatrogenic causes account for some patient morbidity and even mortality; however, research has shown that in a large number of instances, the cause of treatment failure is that patients simply do not adhere to health recommendations.

In a 1996 study, 58% of emergency room visits were found to be directly related to nonadherence (Dennehy, Kishi, & Louie, 1996). In another study of reasons for emergency room visits, the high number of visits was found often to be a result of overuse or underuse of medication (Schneitman-McIntire et al., 1996). Since the acknowledgment of the high level of nonadherence more than 50 years ago (Davis, 1968b), the extent to which patients follow recommendations given to them by health professionals has been studied from a variety of perspectives, with a variety of types of recommendations, and a number of acute and chronic disease conditions. As a result of different conditions and associated recommendations, as well as different measures used, adherence rates vary along a continuum from never following recommendations to following recommendations 100% of the time. Regardless of the research approach used, the condition studied, or the measures used, the general consensus is that nonadherence with prescribed therapeutic regimens is, and continues to be, high (Blackwell, 1973; Haynes, 1999; Martin et al., 2005; Sackett & Haynes, 1976). Rates of nonadherence reported range from 15% to 93%, depending on the condition studied and the research methods used (Balkrishnan, 2005). Despite differences in reported adherence rates, nonadherence appears to be widespread with an approximate average of 25% across conditions (DiMatteo, 2004). Generally, adherence rates that are reported as part of a clinical trial demonstrate higher rates than other patients but, even then, adherence rates can run as low as 43% (Claxton, Cramer, & Pierce, 2001). Such findings suggest that a substantial proportion of individuals seeking medical treatment fail to receive maximum therapeutic benefits because of nonadherence to recommendations. The consequences of nonadherence are far-reaching.

CONSEQUENCES OF NONADHERENCE

Nonadherence has far-ranging individual, societal, and economic consequences. As a result of nonadherence, acute conditions that could have been cured may develop into chronic conditions; chronic conditions, which could have been controlled, may develop into debilitating illness; or disease may develop when it could have been prevented. Although considerable time and expense has been used to develop highly effective and relatively safe treatment regimens for multiple diseases, patients continue to be incapacitated or debilitated, or to even die from conditions for which effective treatments are available (Milgrom, Bender, & Wamboldt, 2001; Morrison, Wertheimer, & Berger,

2000). Likewise, although health risks for a number of serious diseases are known, millions of people continue to engage in unhealthy behaviors that predispose them to various diseases.

Consequences of nonadherence can be severe. Osteoporosis, although not always considered a serious condition, can be debilitating and life-threatening. Even though osteoporosis is treatable, nonadherence rates are high and resulting hip fractures take up one out of every five orthopedic beds (O'Connell & Sutcliffe, 2007). Poor adherence to antihypertensive medications has been found to lead to unnecessary complications, stroke, and early death (Chin & Goldman, 1997). Psychiatric patients with schizophrenia who are nonadherent with medications have been found to have an increased risk of rehospitalization, homelessness, and symptom exacerbation (Olfson et al., 2000). Nonadherence with medication for treatment of asthma has been found to be linked to asthma deaths (Birkhead, et al., 1989). Nonadherence in individuals with human immunodeficiency virus (HIV) may result in viral replication and disease progression (Hinkin et al., 2002). Individuals at risk for coronary heart disease who are nonadherent with recommendations may increase their risk of a debilitating and potentially fatal cardiac event (McDermott, Schmitt, & Wallner, 1997).

A variety of factors can contribute to nonadherence; however, a major factor is that patients often simply fail to follow the recommendations they have been given by their health professional. Hence, because of nonadherence, there is significant cost to the individual, to society as a whole, and to the health system in general.

The health benefit of properly treated and controlled disease is obvious. Many disease conditions, complications developing from disease, disability, and/or death resulting from disease can be forestalled or prevented through modifying health behaviors, adopting healthy lifestyles, and adhering to therapeutic regimens (Christensen et al., 2002; Hernandez, 1995; Johnson & Bootman, 1995; Kane et al., 2003; Liberman & Rotarius, 1999; Nicolucci et al., 1996). Adherence with treatment recommendations can also have an impact on general public health, especially in the treatment or eradication of infectious disease, such as tuberculosis or HIV (Freeman, Rodriguez, & French, 1996; Roberts & Mann, 2000). Failure to follow health recommendations has other impacts on society as well. Nonadherence, which results in increased morbidity, mortality, disability, or increased use of healthcare services, causes decreased productivity through lost work days, and drives up insurance and other healthcare costs (Feldman, 1982; Gerbino, 1993;).

Although there are instances in which nonadherence can have positive implications, such as when the treatment does more harm than good (Shine, 2002), in most instances, following recommendations for the treatment or prevention of disease has more positive consequences (Vermeire et al., 2001). The role of adherence with treatment recommendations in the control of chronic disease such as diabetes, heart disease, and hypertension has been shown to decrease morbidity rates and permanent disability, enabling patients to continue to live active and productive lives (Evangelista & Dracup, 2000; UK Prospective Diabetes Study [UKPDS] Group, 1998a).

Individual Consequences

The role of adherence for the individual, consequences of nonadherence can include progression of disease, which could have been forestalled, or development of disease, which could have been prevented. Individual consequences may be experienced with acute conditions, such as an infection, which could have been cured with a short course of medication, but progresses to a more serious condition because treatment recommendations were not followed, or with development of complications from a chronic condition because of nonadherence. In addition, nonadherence may interfere with curing a patient, causing serious complications from a disease that has not been adequately controlled (UKPDSUK Prospective D, 1998a).

Nonadherence has individual consequences in disease prevention as well. Engaging in healthy lifestyle behaviors can significantly decrease the risk of developing a number of diseases such as cancer, heart disease, stroke, or other serious illnesses (Burke & Dunbar-Jacob, 1995; Evangelista & Dracup, 2000). Development of chronic illnesses as a result of the contributions of tobacco use, excessive consumption of alcohol, sedentary lifestyle, or poor dietary practices are well known; however, many individuals fail to heed recommendations to change their behavior and live a more healthy lifestyle.

Societal Consequences

Although there can be exceptions, for the most part positive health outcomes from treatment rely largely on the degree to which patients follow health advice (Haynes et al., 2000; Horowitz & Horowitz, 1993; Haynes, Montague, & Oliver, 2001). When failure to follow recommendations results in the development of chronic disease, ramifications exist not only for the individual, but also for society as a whole. This also has implications for the effective use of healthcare resources. Nonadherence, which results in increased morbidity, mortality, or disability, causes decreased productivity through lost work days, drives up insurance rates, and places a burden on other social or healthcare programs that may be unable to keep pace with growing demand (Gerbino, 1993; Feldman, 1982).

Patients who seek medical attention but do not follow medical advice overutilize health services by receiving additional care that they may not have needed had they followed original treatment recommendations. The role and importance of patient adherence in treatment of acute conditions is one such example. Acute conditions, such as infections, can often be cured with short courses of medication or treatment. Patient failure to adhere to recommended treatment can result in progression of the condition or development of complications that require increased medical care and treatment with consequences of increased morbidity and, in some instances, mortality (Birkhead et al., 1989). Overutilization of services because of nonadherence taxes limited resources and is not only costly for society as a whole, but can also jeopardize availability of health services for others who may be seeking care. Nonadherence can also have an impact on general public health, especially in prevention, treatment, or eradication of infectious disease. Failure to obtain recommended vaccinations or follow precautions needed to contain disease can result in significant spread of disease. Negligence in adhering to medication regimens important in the cure or containment of conditions such as tuberculosis or HIV can result in producing organisms that become more resistant to treatment (Freeman, Rodriquez, & French, 1996).

Adherence with outpatient therapy is important to reduce patient risk of developing additional complications as well as to reduce costs. Patients who miss appointments misuse the time of the health professional and perhaps have wasted a time slot that could have been used by another patient.

Nonadherence can also interfere with the ability to determine treatment efficacy for various diseases. Measurement of effectiveness of a new treatment is based on the assumption that patients have accurately complied with treatment protocol. If patients have not accurately followed treatment recommendations, it is difficult to determine the extent to which treatment is effective.

Economic Consequences

Nonadherence not only affects patients' and society's well-being, but has economic consequences as well. The financial costs of nonadherence can be high (Aday et al., 2004; Balkrishnan, 2005; Balkrishnan et al., 2003). Expenditures associated with patient nonadherence resulting in increased hospitalizations or additional visits to healthcare providers can cause a large economic burden that has been estimated as amounting to billions of dollars per year (Breen & Thornhill, 1998; DiMatteo, 2004; Martin et al., 2005; McDonnell & Jacobs, 2002; Sullivan, Krelling, & Hazlet, 1990). Ensuring the success of treatment becomes increasingly important as healthcare costs rise. As healthcare costs rise, there is increased tendency to decrease costs by decreasing hospitalization days. Consequently, patients are expected to assume more responsibility for their own care in the home setting. Patients' failure to follow recommendations in the outpatient setting can result in complications that require increased medical attention or readmission to the inpatient facility. Diagnostic procedures or additional treatments may be needed, which increase not only costs but perhaps risks to patients continued health as well.

Nonadherence produces substantial adverse effects on quality and cost of care directly by disrupting or negating potential benefits of therapies or preventive measures prescribed, and indirectly by exposing patients to unnecessary diagnostic procedures and additional treatment that may otherwise not have been needed.

Ensuring the success of treatment becomes increasingly important as healthcare costs rise. Nonadherence not only jeopardizes patients' health but also has economic consequences for the healthcare system. In an era when efficacious therapies exist, or are rapidly being developed, the health and economic consequences of such high instances of nonadherence are alarming. The consequences of nonadherence seem apparent, but the effects may not be fully appreciated. High rates of nonadherence can have a profound impact on both the health of the individual and the healthcare system. Chronic conditions that could have been prevented increase general health costs for society. Engaging in healthy lifestyle behaviors can significantly decrease risk of developing a number of diseases such as cancer, heart disease, stroke, or other serious illnesses, all of which are not only costly to the individual, but also to society (Burke & Dunbar-Jacob, 1995; Evangelista & Dracup, 2000).

As medical care becomes more sophisticated and effective in its ability to treat and prevent disease, patient adherence becomes more crucial. Nonadherence is costly; it wastes medical expertise and healthcare resources as well as being harmful to patients. Highly advanced medical procedures and treatments are of limited use in improving health status if patients neglect to follow recommendations.

TYPES OF NONADHERENCE

Patient nonadherence can take many forms, including failure to keep appointments, take medication as directed, follow recommended dietary, exercise, or other lifestyle changes or restrictions, follow other aspects of treatment, and follow recommended preventative health practices. Nonadherence in any of these areas can have varying effects, depending on the seriousness of the condition and the degree of nonadherence. Specific examples of types of patient nonadherence and their potential effects will help illustrate the scope of the problem.

Appointment Keeping

A patient's failure to keep an appointment can have serious consequences for the individual, but is also an inefficient use of time by the health professional who has set aside a specified period to work with that patient. The missed appointment may be for a regular checkup, follow-up of a previously treated medical problem, evaluation, diagnostic procedure, or referral to a specialist for evaluation of care.

Patients who fail to keep an appointment for a regular checkup run the risk of allowing early stages of disease to go undetected; a medical problem that could have been solved rather simply could become a major problem because of the lack of early intervention. Such was the case of Mrs. Lappas, a 50-year-old postmenopausal woman who failed to keep her appointment for a routine Pap smear. She had decided that during a time of economic strain such an examination was not worth the money. Some time later, when she began having abnormal vaginal bleeding, she consulted her physician. At that time, she was diagnosed as having cervical cancer that had become far advanced, requiring extensive surgery and yielding a rather poor prognosis for her longevity. Earlier detection of the disease could have had an impact not only on how the disease was treated but on the patient's prognosis as well.

Appointments for follow-up of a previously treated condition can also be a source of nonadherence. A study of psychiatric patients demonstrated consequences of nonadherence with follow-up appointments (Nelson, Maruish, & Axler, 2000). The study examined whether patients discharged from an inpatient psychiatric facility would have lower rehospitalization rates if they kept their follow-up appointments after discharge. Results showed that patients who failed to keep their outpatient follow-up appointments after discharge from the inpatient facility were two times more likely to be rehospitalized in the same year as those patients who had kept at least one follow-up appointment. When annual rates for readmission were examined, it was discovered that patients who kept follow-up appointments after discharge from the psychiatric facility had a 1 in 10 chance of being rehospitalized when compared to those patients who had been discharged but who were not compliant with follow-up appointments. The readmission rate for these patients was one in four.

Other potential consequences of a missed follow-up appointment can be illustrated in the case of Mr. Jones who was found to have hypertension. His physician prescribed an antihypertensive medication and told him his blood pressure should be closely monitored. The physician asked Mr. Jones to come for a follow-up appointment every month to assess the effectiveness of the medication. Mr. Jones experienced no symptoms, and consequently saw no reason to return for follow-up visits. Six months after the initial visit, having gone to no follow-up visits, Mr. Jones experienced a stroke.

Referral appointments with specialists may also be missed; such failure can postpone diagnosis and treatment of specific disease entities. Such was the case of Mr. Ling. During a routine examination by his dentist, a growth was found in Mr. Ling's mouth. The dentist, concerned about the growth, immediately referred him for evaluation by an ear, nose, and throat specialist. The dentist informed Mr. Ling of the importance of having the growth evaluated. Being a busy man, however, Mr. Ling continued to postpone consultation. A year later, when Mr. Ling began to have difficulty breathing and swallowing, he consulted his regular physician who found the growth had grown considerably. On further evaluation, the growth was found to be cancerous.

Not all missed appointments have the consequences described in the preceding examples; however, patients' failure to keep appointments can affect healthcare delivery, not only in terms of time and money, but also in delays of treatment.

Nonadherence with Medication

Nonadherence with prescribed medication regimens can also take several forms and can result in a number of serious consequences. Numerous examples of consequences of medication nonadherence can be found in literature; a study by Marinker and Shaw (2003) found that half of the medicine prescribed for patients with chronic illness is not taken as prescribed. Adherence rates for medication are often higher among individuals with acute conditions; however, adherence rates for medication are significantly lower for individuals with chronic conditions, especially after the first 6 months (Cramer et al., 2003; Dew et al., 1996; Haynes, McDonald, & Garg, 2002; Jackevicius, Mamdani, & Tu, 2002; Cramer, Rosenheck, Kirk, Krol, & Krystal, 2003). In a study of individuals who were being treated for osteoporosis, up to two thirds stopped taking their medication within 1 year (O'Connell & Sutcliffe, 2007).

Adherence rates are usually calculated as the percentage of the prescribed doses of medication the patient actually takes over a specific period of time, including taking the medication in the right amount at the right time (Johnson, Williams, & Marshall, 1999; Osterberg & Blaschke, 2005). There is no common standard of what constitutes adequate medication adherence. Depending on the condition, and the medication, adherence rates as low as 80% of the time may also produce satisfactory results (Osterberg & Blaschke, 2005). In other instances, the seriousness of the condition and the nature of the medication may necessitate near 100% adherence.

Nonadherence with medication may consist of never having the prescriptions filled, altering the prescribed dose (taking either too much or too little of the medication), or varying the time interval at which the medication is taken (Matsui et al., 2000). Other patients may neglect to follow the full course of treatment, stopping the medication as soon as their symptoms subside. Nonadherence with medication can have deleterious effects. The following examples illustrate these points.

Mrs. Cellini was pregnant with her third child. During her prenatal checkup, it was discovered that she had a urinary tract infection. She was given a prescription for treatment. The family had a limited income, and because her daughter had also needed medication, Mrs. Cellini reasoned that her first priority was her daughter's medication. Consequently, Mrs. Cellini's urinary tract infection progressed to pyelonephritis, necessitating hospitalization.

Underutilization of a drug may deprive patients of anticipated therapeutic benefits, possibly resulting in worsening of the condition being treated. Patients who discontinue use of a medication after symptoms subside but before the condition is fully cured may run the risk of recurrence of the condition because the shorter course of therapy was not enough to eradicate it. This may necessitate additional visits to the health professional and may have deleterious effects on the patient. In addition, the health professional who is unaware of the patient's nonadherence and who sees the condition as neither improved nor controlled may prescribe higher doses of the drug or additional drugs, exposing the patient to an increased possibility of adverse side effects if he or she decides to take all the prescribed drugs at different intervals. In other circumstances, if drugs are not used up, patients may store them, potentiating inappropriate use of the medications by themselves or others at a later time.

The seriousness of lack of adherence with a prescribed medication regimen can vary from one situation to another. In those cases in which medication is a continual, ongoing part of controlling the disease itself, such as in hypertension or diabetes, failure to follow recommendations can have life-threatening consequences. Virginia, an 18-year-old individual with insulin-dependent diabetes, was repeatedly treated at the local hospital emergency room for hyperglycemia. Her physician, attributing the problem to inadequate amounts of insulin, continued to alter the dosage accordingly. Eventually, she was brought into the emergency room in a diabetic coma. Upon more careful questioning of family members, the nurse discovered that Virginia had frequently neglected to take her insulin in the prescribed amounts. The problem had not been the amount of insulin prescribed, but Virginia's failure to take it accurately.

In other cases when medication is intended to prevent a medical problem from becoming a more serious threat to health, nonadherence can also have serious consequences. Julie, a 4-year-old girl, was brought to the neighborhood health clinic by her mother because of a cold, fever, and sore throat. She was diagnosed as having strep throat and was placed on a regimen of penicillin.

The nurse explained to Julie's mother that the medication was not only to help Julie's sore throat but also to prevent the infection from involving other parts of the body. Before the course of treatment was complete, the family went to visit Julie's grandparents for the weekend and forgot to take along the medication. Upon returning from the visit, the parents never resumed Julie's medication regimen; she seemed so much better, and she had missed several days of the medication anyway. Julie later developed rheumatic fever.

Less serious medication nonadherence may still have an impact on the healthcare system itself by causing patients with recurring symptoms to be readmitted to the hospital or to return to outpatient clinics for treatment conditions that could have been cured had recommendations been followed initially. The healthcare provider is thus diverted from caring for other individuals who may have a more serious need for health care.

Nonadherence does not always refer neglecting to take medications. Taking more medications than recommended can also have consequences. Medications are not without side effects. Patients who err on the side of excess run the risk of drug interactions, drug toxicity, and a variety of other impairments related to side effects from misuse or overuse of prescribed therapeutic medications.

Adherence to Dietary Recommendations

Dietary recommendations are frequently required in the management of various conditions, control of health problems, or prevention of potential future disease states. In obesity, diet consists of restricting behaviors and is usually a lifelong process. Motivation for weight loss may vary for individuals. In some individuals, weight loss may be recommended because of current health problems, such as after myocardial infarction. In some instances, dietary restrictions may be recommended to prevent future health problems, such as diabetes, and in other instances, individuals may attempt to lose weight just to look better. In each instance, the motivation for weight loss is different depending on the individual, what weight loss means to them, and the consequences of weight loss. Persons in a weight loss clinic may lose weight initially only to gain it back. Controlling obesity is marked by remissions and exacerbations.

In other instances, dietary recommendations may be additive, such as in an eating disorder like anorexia or bulimia. Restrictions may be needed in conditions such as celiac disease. Dietary changes may constitute a major portion of disease treatment, such as patients on hemodialysis for end-stage kidney diseases who are asked to adhere to a strict regimen of fluid and diet restrictions or individuals who are taught to regulate and monitor food intake. Dietary and other lifestyle changes require significant discipline and motivation on the part of the patient. Recommendations associated with lifestyle changes can be some of the most difficult recommendations for patients to follow, but can also have some of the most severe consequences if the patient fails to follow them (Brown, 1990; Morgan, 2000). Take the example of Ms. Burnett. Ms. Burnett, a 20-year-old single woman, was pregnant with her first child. During one of her prenatal visits, the nurse noted that Ms. Burnett's blood pressure was elevated, there was protein in her urine, and she had had a substantial weight gain since her last visit. Upon questioning Ms. Burnett, the nurse found that she had been eating large quantities of junk food, including potato chips and other foods high in calories and salt. Ms. Burnett was referred to the dietitian for consultation. In addition, her physician restricted her activity, asking her to elevate her feet as much as possible to reduce swelling when out of bed and to remain in bed as much as possible. Ms. Burnett, however, was a student working her way through school and continued working part-time at a fast food restaurant where one of the perks was free food. She continued to stand for long periods during work and continued to eat the free food she was provided as part of her job. Eventually, she began having blurred vision and headaches. She consulted her physician and was promptly admitted to the hospital for treatment for preeclampsia.

Adherence with Lifestyle Recommendations

Lifestyle changes, such as smoking cessation or cardiovascular exercise for prevention of heart and lung disease, may be recommended in order to maintain health and prevent disease from occurring. In other instances, lifestyle changes constitute a major portion of disease treatment, such as patients with diabetes who are taught exercise and other self-care behaviors, such as foot care, or individuals with rheumatoid arthritis who are asked to exercise, or obtain rest. Other lifestyle changes may include avoiding drug abuse, cutting down on alcohol consumption, or work recommendations.

Adherence with Other Aspects of Treatment

Treatment modalities other than keeping appointments, taking medications, and following dietary and other lifestyle restrictions may also be prescribed. Examples include treatments such as postural drainage for individuals with cystic fibrosis, applying heat or cold to areas of the body, wrapping extremities with elastic bandages for sprains or strains, applying warm soaks, changing bandages, and so forth. Nonadherence even to these rather mild, noninvasive forms of treatment can have serious consequences, as is illustrated by the case of Mr. Schmidt. He had circulatory problems in his lower extremities for some time as a result of arteriosclerosis. Although he had been warned about the dangers of attempting his own foot care, he tried to remove a callous from his right foot. As a result, he sustained an injury that subsequently became infected. Upon consulting his physician, he was instructed to soak his foot several times a day, and to keep it under a heat lamp for 30 minutes three times a day. Mr. Schmidt, a farmer, discounted the importance of the instructions and continued to do farm chores, stating that he did not have time to sit around three times a day and pamper his foot. Although he used the heat lamp sporadically, he stopped soaking his foot altogether. The wound did not heal; the infection became worse, his foot became gangrenous, and he was eventually admitted to the hospital for amputation.

Adherence with Preventive Health Practices

Preventive practices may be primary in that they prevent disease or injury from occurring. Failure to follow primary prevention practices include not fastening a seatbelt, not wearing a helmet when riding a bicycle, or not adhering to recommendations during the prenatal period that could lead to complicated birth or low birth weight. Secondary prevention refers to delay in diagnosis, such as a failure to find cancer that could have been eradicated but needs more extensive surgery or ignoring mammography when location of a tumor could have resulted in lumpectomy rather than mastectomy. Tertiary prevention is retarding progress of disease and avoiding complications.

The role of prevention in maintaining health has been known for more than 40 years. As early as 1964, the Surgeon General of the United States Public Health Service issued a warning based on an accumulation of evidence that smoking is hazardous to health (Luther, 1964). It is now widely accepted that tobacco use is related to heart disease, stroke, emphysema, and cancer (Aubry, Wright, & Myers, 2000; Bartecchi, Mackenzie, & Schrier, 1994; He et al., 2001; MacKenzie, Bartecchi, & Schrier, 1994 He, Ogden, Bazzano, Vupputuri, Loria, & Whelton, 2001). The influence of diet and exercise on people's health and well-being has also been well-publicized. The importance of weight control in reducing risk from heart disease (Rao et al., 2001), hypertension (Hooker-Whitman, 2002), osteoarthritis (Hart & Spector, 1993), diabetes (Roth, 2002), and recently, cancer (Calle et al., 2003) is widely accepted. The importance of good dental hygiene in preventing tooth loss and gingivitis, which has been linked to other inflammatory processes in the body, is also recognized (Gustafsson, Hakansson, & Klinge, 2002).

A variety of health professionals try to teach patients how to prevent disease from occurring and promote good health. Physicians, nurses, dietitians, dentists, and a variety of other health professionals and professional organizations give countless recommendations to patients about how to stay healthy and prevent disease. Programs designed to help people follow preventive health practices have been established with varying degrees of effectiveness.

Nonetheless, countless numbers of patients fail to heed the advice of health professionals and other sources of information on disease prevention. Thousands of people still smoke, eat foods they know are bad for them, overeat, fail to exercise, or neglect dental care.

Obviously, patients who ignore preventive health advice also run a considerable risk of developing diseases and conditions that can result in disability or death. They may also require other therapeutic treatment, another potential area of nonadherence.

Lack of adherence to preventive measures can be illustrated by the case of Mr. Martinez. Approaching middle age, Mr. Martinez had an extensive family history of heart disease. Soon after moving to a new city with his family, he established health care for himself and his family at a nearby family practice clinic. During his first visit to the clinic for treatment of a cold, the nurse noted that he smoked nearly three packs of cigarettes and consumed nearly 20 cups of coffee daily, slept a maximum of 5 hours a night, and generally consumed large amounts of alcohol on a regular basis. The nurse talked with Mr. Martinez about aspects of prevention, giving him a variety of brochures on the subject to take home. The physician outlined an exercise program for Mr. Martinez, referred him to a smoking cessation clinic, and talked with him about ways to cut down on his coffee and alcohol consumption. Throughout the next year, each time Mr. Martinez came to the clinic, the family practice staff continued to reinforce the importance of prevention to avoid heart disease as well as a number of other ailments; however, he continued to ignore the advice given, stating that given his family history, his days were numbered anyway and he might as well make the most of life while he could. Almost 2 years to the day after moving to the city, Mr. Martinez was hospitalized with his first heart attack.

The nurse and the physician, as well as other members of the clinic staff, felt very frustrated. Not only had Mr. Martinez's nonadherence endangered his health, but also considerable time and effort had been spent helping Mr. Martinez learn ways to modify his behavior to adhere more closely to prescribed preventive health measures. Now he was being treated for a condition that was partly caused by his own failure to put the recommendations into practice, behavior that could possibly have prevented his heart attack from occurring.

RESEARCH ON ADHERENCE

The importance of health recommendations to the health and well-being of patients, the healthcare system, and society as a whole has caused adherence to be the focus of research for decades (Oldridge, 2001). Over the past 50 years, research on patient adherence has grown rapidly (DiMatteo, 2004). In that time period, more than 32,550 citations related to adherence have been added to PubMed, not to mention the 10,087 adherence citations found in PsycINFO (Martin et al., 2005). The increased interest in the study of patient adherence has been brought about by many factors, including recognition of the extent of nonadherence, the potential health cost of nonadherence, increased prevalence of chronic disease, increased use of prescription drugs, and the patient's need for self-management of his or her condition (Haynes, 2001).

The health benefit of properly treated and controlled disease is obvious. Many conditions and complications, as well as disability and/or death resulting from disease, can be forestalled or prevented by modifying health behaviors, adopting healthy lifestyles, and adhering to therapeutic regimes (Christensen et al., 2002; Hernandez, 1995; Johnson & Bootman, 1995; Kane et al., 2003; Liberman & Rotarius, 1999; Nicolucci et al., 1996). To increase adherence, it is logical that the health professional should have some understanding of its causes. A number of factors that have been thought to contribute to nonadherence with health recommendations have been studied extensively. These factors include those specific to the patient, those related to the disease or treatment, and those specific to the health professional (Amundson, 1985; Chambers et al., 1999; Daneri, 1999; Davis, 1968b; DiMatteo & DiNicola, 1982).

Health professionals hold a variety of misconceptions about patient nonadherence and its causes as well as its cures. In many instances, health professionals' lack of understanding of the adherence issues can be a factor in nonadherence. For example, health professionals frequently have misconceptions about the extent of patient nonadherence (Roth & Caron, 1978). At first glance, it seems irrational that a patient seeking and paying for health advice would choose not to follow it. However, studies indicate that a large number of patients fail to follow the recommendations they receive from their health professionals. Various studies have demonstrated that the ability of healthcare professionals to recognize nonadherence is poor and that they grossly underestimate the extent of nonadherence in patients with whom they have been working (Burnier, 2000; Charney, 1972; Haynes et al., 2000; Murri et al., 2004; Roth & Berger, 1960). If health professionals are unaware of patients' nonadherence, causes for it cannot be identified and thus corrected. This, in turn, can result in patients' unnecessary exposure to additional treatments and tests, as well as the possibility of worsening of the condition itself.

A frequently held misconception is that nonadherence is common only in outpatient practices, when, in fact, patient nonadherence can occur in any setting in which recommendations are given. Even hospitalization does not guarantee adherence (Blackwell, 1997). In an early study by Roth and Berger (1960), 75 hospitalized patients in a gastrointestinal ward were prescribed liquid antacid. Although nurses in the ward did general supervision, the actual taking of the medication was left up to individual patients. Despite the inpatient setting and general supervision by health professionals, patient adherence with taking the medication as prescribed was shown to be less than 50%.

Health professionals may also have misconceptions about patients who are at risk of nonadherence. It is often assumed that patients who are uneducated or from lower socioeconomic groups are less likely to follow recommendations; however, research has not shown this to be the case. Variables such as age, gender, race or ethnic background, education level, marital status, socioeconomic level, and religion have been studied as determinants of patient adherence. Few demographic variables have consistently been shown to be related to patient nonadherence (Lutfey & Wishner, 1999; Turk & Meichenbaum, 1991). Although such inconsistent findings may be attributed in part to differences in research design, study population, and technique used for measuring adherence, the fact that many other researchers have not been able to accurately identify patients who do not adhere to recommendations suggests that patient variables are not a reliable explanation for nonadherence. Although demographic variables may be factors in nonadherence for individual patients, they certainly do not appear to be influential for the patient population as a whole.

Other possible reasons for nonadherence have also been studied; these include features of the disease itself, its diagnosis and severity, its symptomatology, and its chronicity. Again, it seems logical that where failure to follow medical advice would be the most harmful, patient adherence would be greatest. Although findings in this area are inconclusive, in many instances this also has not seemed to be the case (Dew et al., 1996). Classic early studies found that patients with less severe medical problems were actually more likely to follow through with medical advice than those with more severe illness (Davis, 1968a).

Some early studies found patients' increased perception of disease severity to be significantly related to the likelihood of adherence (Becker, Drachman, & Kirscht, 1972). Leventhal's classic work (1971), however, suggested that for asymptomatic individuals, low levels of perceived severity were not sufficiently motivating to produce increased adherence, while very high levels of perceived seriousness raised fear and anxiety and were inhibiting, thus decreasing the chances that patients would adhere to treatment recommendations. Other studies have shown little consistent correlation between any disease features and how closely patients follow medical advice (Haynes, 1979). Findings from classic studies suggest that adherence, as related to a disease condition, are based on individual differences rather than factors generalizable to patients as a group.

Adherence was originally viewed as a patient-related phenomenon. Early classic studies looked toward patient-related variables as a way of understanding and predicting patient nonadherence. However, given results from many of the early studies, which indicated that sociodemographic and disease features had little consistent correlation with patient adherence, researchers turned to other variables that might be found to explain the phenomenon. When studying features of the therapeutic regimen itself, several features were found to be correlated with patient adherence. Early studies found that the greater the extent to which patients must alter personal habits, behavior, or other aspects of lifestyle as part of their treatment, the less likely they were to follow recommendations (Davis, 1967; Donabedian & Rosenfeld, 1964). In addition, researchers found that the less complicated the treatment regime, the higher the rate of compliance (Cohen, 1979; Lane, 1983). Over the last 2 decades, many researchers have replicated studies utilizing these variables, and these findings have been confirmed (Coutts, Gibson, & Paton, 1992; Kolton & Piccolo, 1998; Spector, 1985).

Measurement of Nonadherence

Adherence has been measured in a variety of ways in research settings as well as in clinical practice. Methods used include direct observation, patient self-report or patient journals, report from family members, pill counts, electronic measures such as metered dose inhalers or electronic recording devices, blood or urine assays, prescription records from pharmacists, and patient outcome (Farmer, 1999). Each method has advantages and disadvantages, and some methods are more useful for some types of recommendations than others. However, no method has been found to be a panacea (Alcoba et al., 2003; Wagner, Justice, et al., 2001). Measurements of adherence that may be useful for recommendations that include medication or appointments may not be useful for other recommendations that involve lifestyle changes or treatment recommendations the patient carries out at home. As a result of the different levels of sophistication and objectivity each of these measures offer, findings from research studies as well as health professionals' estimate of the degree to which patients follow recommendations vary considerably.

In clinical practice, one widely used method for measuring adherence is simply asking the patient (Osterberg & Blaschke, 2005). This method, although simple and inexpensive does not, however, always produce the most accurate results. Patients overestimate or distort the degree to which they follow recommendations because they have not kept accurate track of how often they adhere, because they want to please the health professional, or because they fear reprimand. Studies have shown, however, that asking about adherence in an open and nonjudgmental way can increase accuracy of self-report of adherence (Schoenthaler et al., 2009).

A number of measures have been utilized for assessing medication adherence. One common measure of adherence is pill count (counting medications left in the patient's medication bottle). Although this method may seem more reliable than self-report, it also has its flaws. Even though medication may be missing from the bottle, there is no assurance that the patient actually took the medication, or if they did take the medication, that they took it accurately. In addition, this method addresses only one type of adherence—that of taking medication—and does not take into account the variety of other recommendations that may have been made in conjunction to taking medication. Pharmacy measurement of prescription filling or of having prescriptions refilled at the right time provides information regarding patient adherence with regard to obtaining medication, but again, provides no measurement of whether the patient actually takes the medication or does so accurately, and does not address other types of adherence that may be part of the total therapeutic regimen.

Directly observing therapy, such as patients taking medication, may seem to be a more accurate way of measuring adherence, but extensive use of direct observation is not usually feasible for most patients. Direct observation with regard to medication is also not a fail-safe method. Patients may hide medication in their mouth and then discard it when they are not being observed. Direct observation is most useful in measurement of adherence to recommendation that involves an appointment. It is relatively easy and inexpensive to determine whether or not a patient made and kept an appointment.

More accurate direct measures of adherence are those that involve medication levels or metabolite in the blood, or measurements of biological markers. These measures can, however, be costly, and may not take into account that patients may adhere prior to measurement being taken, but then be nonadherent the remainder of the time.

Electronic devices for measuring adherence can also be expensive and require some degree of patient cooperation. In addition, although useful for some conditions and types of recommendations, electronic devices are not suitable for measuring adherence for all recommendations.

The ultimate measure of adherence would seem to be positive health outcome; however, this is also not always the case. In some instances, positive health outcomes defined by the original treatment goal, may or not be directly related to adherence. For instance, an individual placed on a nutritionally sound diet and exercise regime in order to lose 25 pounds may, rather than follow the diet and exercise as prescribed, resort to other drug supplements and starvation instead. Direct measure of weight loss of 25 pounds, in this instance, would be an inaccurate and misleading measure of the degree to which patient actually followed the recommendations.

INTERVENTIONS TO INCREASE ADHERENCE

Many different interventions alone, or in combination, have been developed and tested for effectiveness in increasing adherence. With growing interest in factors of the therapeutic regime itself as potential determinants of adherence, a number of studies related to strategies and interventions specifically designed to enhance the likelihood of increased adherence have been conducted (Haynes et al., 2000; Peterson, Takiya, & Finley, 2003; Petrilla et al., 2000).

Technological Devices

Technology used to develop devices to assist individuals to remember to take their medications has been used for more than 40 years (Azrin & Powell, 1969; Eshelman & Fitzloff, 1976). Electronic reminder devices have the potential to assist patient ability to adhere with medical recommendations. Electronic reminders may consist of beepers, pillbox alarms, wristwatch alarms, or other forms that prompt the patient to take medication at a certain time (Wise & Operario, 2008).

Although many additional devices such as computer-generated reminder charts, computer-assisted patient monitoring, and other electronic devices have been developed over the years to improve adherence, and some studies have shown an increase in patient adherence as a result of using such devices, technology alone has been found to be insufficient to solve the problem. One flaw in the strategy of using many devices is the assumption that forgetfulness is the major factor that causes nonadherence. Even when forgetfulness is a factor, device use still requires patients to remember to fill it and to be motivated to use it. It might seem reasonable to assume that if patients cannot remember their medications, they may also be unable to remember to use the device designed to increase adherence. Although a device may be helpful to some patients, the method has not been shown to be the panacea for all problems with adherence. Because of the variability of adherence in different patients with different conditions, technological means to increase patient adherence are best suited as one strategy that may be used according to specific patient need and in the context of collaborative relationship between patient and health professional (Wise & Operario, 2008).

Behavioral Techniques

Other strategies include specific behavioral techniques involving differential reinforcement, extinction, shaping, modeling, and desensitization (Azrin & Powell, 1969; Eshelman & Fitzloff, 1976). These methods have been found to have varying degrees of success for some regimens, although still not a panacea. To succeed, behavioral approaches require motivation and cooperation by patients themselves. Patients must be willing to follow through with these techniques on their own in the home environment, or to see the health professional responsible for instituting the techniques on a regular basis. The more frequent the interaction between patient and health professional, the more likely the technique will be successful in increasing adherence. Use of behavioral techniques, which over time has shown success in many instances, can be costly in terms of the health professional's time. If the patient is motivated enough to carry out the techniques independently, then much of the adherence battle has already been won. Behavioral techniques are less useful when patients who are nonadherent have little motivation to carry out the regimen, let alone the behavioral techniques designed to improve adherence with the regime itself. Before behavioral techniques can be implemented, the patient must also clearly understand what he or she must do. Even if the health professional has explained the procedure, the explanation may have been given in terms the patient did not understand, or the patient may view the procedure as an impossible task.

Another problem with the strict use of behavioral techniques to increase adherence is the accurate identification of the target behavior to be changed. The behavior the health professional considers in need of change may, in fact, not be the behavior that needs to be changed, or that the patient wants to change. The case of Ms. Grossman, an obese college student, is an example of such an occurrence. Ms. Grossman had been going to the obesity clinic for several months without success. A variety of behavioral techniques had been implemented to help her control her eating behavior. She seemed motivated, visiting the clinic regularly and appearing genuinely sincere about carrying out the plans she had been given. After several months, when she still had not lost weight, the nurse at the clinic questioned her more closely about her behavior away from the clinic. Although Ms. Grossman had adhered with the recommendations to control her eating at home, her downfall appeared to be her eating behavior in public. She ate a meal at noon daily at the student center, and other food intake occurred at social events on weekends. Painfully shy, Ms. Grossman tended to overeat when in a group. While she was eating, she did not have to engage in conversation. In addition, at social events she hovered at the food table so she did not have to mingle in a group or be forced to sit alone, waiting for someone to approach her to talk. The target behavior originally identified as contributing to her obesity was daily eating behavior. It became more obvious that the behavior that actually contributed more to her obesity was her social behavior. Once the target behavior was correctly identified and work began on helping her improve her social skills, her weight reduction program became successful.

Although behavioral techniques were used with varying degrees of success in increasing adherence, most studies concluded that adherence dropped when the specific interventions or programs designed to increase adherence were discontinued (McKenney et al., 1973).

Patient Contracting

Patient contracting is another type of intervention intended to increase patient adherence. Patient contracting is a process in which measurable and observable elements of expected behavior are explicitly outlined in a contract that is acceptable to all parties (Steckel, 1982). Stark and colleagues (1987) introduced behavioral contracting as a method to increase adherence of an 11-year-old girl with cystic fibrosis to her chest physiotherapy treatment. The technique produced positive changes in adherence, in her physiological measures, and in family functioning during the contracting period and at 9-week follow-up.

Although this application of behavioral contracting can show success for short-term therapies, over time and without additional interventions, adherence tends to decrease (Roby, Kominski, & Pourat, 2008). Likewise, although behavioral contracting has been found to be helpful in increasing adherence for some individuals, not all patients are receptive to the contracting approach and individual circumstances may change the effectiveness.

Reminder Postcards

Other strategies have also been developed in an attempt to increase adherence. Wolosin (1990) studied the effect of appointment scheduling and reminder postcards on women's likelihood of adhering with recommendations for mammography screening. One group of women was examined, told about mammography, and instructed to make an appointment for themselves, whereas another group had appointments scheduled for them at the visit, which were followed up with reminder postcards. The women who had appointments scheduled for them had higher rates of adherence with recommendations for mammography screening than did those who had to make their own appointments. Although this intervention apparently increased adherence with recommendations, variability of patient populations and socioeconomic differences in different locations and other extraneous variables make generalization of results questionable. In addition, even though adherence was apparently increased, the question of whether such an intervention merely maintains dependence as opposed to helping patients accept responsibility for their own health must be asked.

Patient Teaching as an Intervention to Increase Adherence

Information giving would appear to be an important intervention in increasing adherence. Patients cannot be expected to adhere to a treatment plan they do not understand. It would seem reasonable to speculate that the better informed a patient is about his or her condition and treatment, the more adherent the patient would be. Studies, however, have not consistently shown this to be the case (Bartlett, 1983; Blessing-Moore, 1996; Sands & Holman, 1985). In a study of diabetic patients, knowledge about diabetes and its control was increased with an educational program, but adherence with the medical regimen was not (Watts, 1980).

Patients may be able to repeat facts without having a true understanding of the material presented. Although some information, such as knowledge of what the therapeutic regimen requires and how and when to do it, is especially relevant to patient adherence, acquisition of knowledge is not necessarily followed by appropriate action (Blessing-Moore, 1996).

Although presenting a patient with information about their condition and treatment, it would appear from the research that information giving alone is insufficient to produce significant increases in adherence.

ROLE OF THE HEALTH PROFESSIONAL IN ADHERENCE

One variable that has been studied with increasing interest is the role the health professional might play in influencing patient behavior and increasing adherence. As researchers began to study the health professional-patient relationship in the context of patient adherence, interesting findings began to emerge. Poor communication has been found to be one of the most important factors in determining the extent to which patients adhere to treatment recommendations (McLane, Zyzanski, & Flocke, 1995; Kirchner, 2000). A positive influence on patient adherence appeared to be strongly related to skills of health providers involving communication and explanation (Schmidt, 1977). Communication in this context appears to go beyond verbal exchange of information, extending to the very relationship between patient and health professional.

Communication style and patient satisfaction with care have been associated with higher levels of adherence with recommendations (Bultman & Svarstad, 2000; DiMatteo, Reiter, & Gambone, 1994). Communication has been found to be a key component to increase adherence, especially when it engenders collaboration between the patient and the health professional and enables the patient to make informed choices (DiMatteo, 2004; Roter, 1995). The ability of health professionals to demonstrate warmth and concern for patients (Falvo, Woehlke, & Deichmann, 1980), to demonstrate empathy (Luborsky et al., 1985), and to generate a trusting, cooperative environment that provides patients with freedom of choice appear to be important components in the relationship between patient and health professional in the facilitation of adherence

(Langer, 1999). Helping patients feel comfortable discussing concerns or perceived difficulties with the recommended treatment by demonstrating empathy is built on a relationship of trust (Waeber, Burnier, & Brunner, 2000). This type of relationship helps patients feel that the health professional is listening and understands their feelings, concerns, and limitations without judging them. Health professionals who take time to explain elements of treatment in an informative and nonthreatening manner encourage patient participation and enhance the likelihood of adherence with recommendations (Miller, 1997). Having an open relationship between patient and health professional so that patients' concerns are accepted and in which the patient and health professional work together to develop a mutually agreeable plan appears to be a major factor in promoting patient adherence (Milgrom, Bender, & Wamboldt, 2001).

PATIENT EDUCATION, PATIENT TEACHING, AND ADHERENCE

Providing patients with information about their condition, treatment, risks, and benefits are essential parts of patient care, and as previously described, providing patients with information has been an intervention used to increase adherence. It stands to reason that providing patients with this type of information is an important factor in patient adherence because patients are unable to follow recommendations unless they have knowledge and understanding of what they are to do. Having knowledge and understanding of the condition and treatment alone, however, has not been found to be a strong predictor of adherence (Bernard-Bonnin et al., 1995; Dolde et al., 2003).

Perhaps one of the difficulties is equating *patient education* with *patient teaching*. Merely providing patients with information is not patient teaching, and information acquisition by patients is not necessarily education. Education is a concept describing an organized, structured process or program with the goal of imparting information to facilitate learning. Teaching, on the other hand, is an active process of facilitating and enhancing the individual's ability to apply what he or she has learned.

Education in any setting is complex, and consists of organized programs of which teaching is a part. In a highly mechanized age when so many materials to enhance learning are available, and when so many sources of information are produced, it is not surprising that many people think of patient education simply as the transfer of information to patients without considering that the real goal is patient teaching, in which patients are not only provided with information, but helped to incorporate it into their daily lives. Although the transfer of information is a part of the educational process, teaching in any setting usually consists of goals that include more than providing information, which individuals then regurgitate. Goals of teaching generally consist of techniques and strategies that help individuals gain knowledge, skills, or attitudes that they will be able to incorporate into their lives. Patient teaching then involves more than merely providing the patient with information. The goals of patient teaching are more than simply repeating directions to patients or handing out printed materials. Rather, the goal of patient teaching is to enable the patient and his or her family to manage and cope with his or her condition and treatment, or prevent disease, disability, or complications from occurring (Porché, 2007).

Effective patient teaching, which is part of structured patient education, is an integrated process that encompasses precise clinical skills, including data gathering, individualization of instructions, support, evaluation, and follow-up of patient success, in implementing the recommendations. Patient teaching may take place in minutes or in hours. It may take place in one 1-hour session, or it may last over weeks, months, or years. How patient teaching is conducted is dependent on the situation and the needs of the patient.

PATIENT-CENTERED TEACHING TO INCREASE ADHERENCE

Adherence is complex and multidimensional, and nonadherence is costly. There may be a variety of reasons for patients' failure to follow medical recommendations, including cost of treatment, complexity of regime, and length of treatment. On the other hand, nonadherence may also represent patients' rational choice to not follow recommendations if they feel to do so would jeopardize their quality of life, interfere with their personal goals, or if they view nonadherence as a way to maintain control and autonomy.

The foundation of patient teaching is not only assessing the learning needs of the patient and the best way to present information, but it also involves tailoring the teaching and the recommendations to the patient's specific needs and circumstances at home. Previously, there had been a tendency to oversimplify both patient teaching and patient adherence. There appears to be no cookie-cutter approach to either patient teaching or interventions to increase adherence that works for all patients with all conditions. Factors in both patient teaching and patient adherence are much more complex. There is no single strategy for promoting adherence that has been found to be effective for all patients and all conditions (Levensky & O'Donohue, 2006). Effective communication and collaboration between health professional and patient, guided by factual information and experience of the health professional, allows patients to make informed choices about an agreed upon recommendation (Quill & Brody, 1996; Salzman, 1995). Patient teaching is a process by which patients gain knowledge, skills, or attitudes that enable them to attain or maintain positive health outcomes (American Academy of Family Physicians, 2000). Patients have a right to receive appropriate information that enables them to participate in decision making as well as participate in their own care (The Joint Commission, 2001). By providing patients with clear, factual, and unbiased information, identifying and acknowledging their concerns and limitations, altering treatment plans as appropriate, and conducting evaluation and follow-up, increased adherence is more likely to result (Bender & Milgrom, 1996; Butler, Rollnick, & Stott, 1996; Graziani, Rosenthal, & Diamond, 1999; Roter et al., 1998). In addition, involving the patient in decision making and problem solving has been reported to contribute to improved treatment adherence, and ultimately, to positive patient outcomes (Bosch, Capblanch, & Garner, 2003; Hook, 2006). The remainder of this book is devoted to helping health professionals achieve these skills.

REFERENCES

Aday, L. A., Begley, C. E., Lairson, D. R., & Balkrishman, R. (2004). *Evaluating the healthcare system: Effectiveness, efficiency, and equity* (pp. 93–120). Chicago: Health Administration Press.

Alcoba, M., Cuevas M. J., Perez-Simon, M. R., Mostaza, J. L., Ortega L., Ortiz de Urbina J., Carro, J. A., Raya C., Abad M., Martin, V, & HAART Adherence Working Group for the Province of Leon, Spain. (2003). Assessment of adherence to triple antiretroviral treatment including indinavir: Role of determination of plasma levels of indinavir. *Journal of Acquired Immunity Deficiency Syndrome, 33*(2), 253–258.

American Academy of Family Physicians. (2000). Patient education: Recommended core educational guidelines for family practice residents. *American Family Physician, 62*(7), 1712–1714.

Amundson, L. H. (1985). Review of patient compliance: I. Magnitude and determinants. *Continuing Education*, September, 621–630.

Aubry, M. C., Wright, J. L., & Myers, J. L., (2000). Smoking and pulmonary and cardiovascular diseases: The pathology of smoking-related lung diseases. *Clinics in Chest Medicine, 21*, 11–35.

Azrin, N. H., & Powell, J. (1969). Behavioral Engineering: The use of response priming to improve prescribed self-medication. *Journal of Applied Behavior Analysis, 2*, 39–42.

Balkrishnan, R. (2005). The importance of medication adherence in improving chronic-disease related outcomes: What we know and what we need to further know. *Medical Care, 43*(6), 517–520.

Balkrishnan, R., Rajagopalan, R., Camacho, F. T., Huston, S. A., Murray, F. T., & Anderson, R. T. (2003). Predictors of medication adherence and associated health care costs in an older population with type 2 diabetes mellitus: A longitudinal cohort study. *Clinical Therapeutics, 25*, 2958–2971.

Bartecchi, C. E., Mackenzie, T. D., & Schrier, R. W. (1994). The human costs of tobacco use. (First of Two Parts). *The New England Journal of Medicine, 330*, 907–912.

Bartlett, E. E. (1983). Restoring credibility to the field of patient education. *Patient Education Newsletter, 6*(6), 11.

Becker, M. H., Drachman, R. H., & Kirscht, J. P. (1972). Predicting mothers compliance with pediatric medical regimens. *Journal of Pediatrics, 81*, 843–854.

Bender, B., & Milgrom, H. (1996). Compliance with asthma therapy: A case for shared responsibility. *Journal of Asthma, 33*, 99–202.

Bernard-Bonnin A. C., Stachenko, S., Bonin, D., Charette, C. & Rousseau, E. (1995). Self-management teaching programs and morbidity of pediatric asthma: A meta-analysis. *Journal of Allergy and Clinical Immunology, 95*(Part 1), 34–41.

Birkhead, G., Attaway, N. J., Strunk, R. C., Townsend, M. C, & Teutsch, S. (1989). Investigation of a cluster of deaths of adolescents from asthma: Evidence implicating inadequate treatment and poor patient adherence with medications. *Journal of Allergy and Clinical Immunology, 84*(Part 1), 484–491.

Blackwell, B. (Ed.). (1997). *Treatment compliance and the therapeutic alliance.* Newark, NJ: Hardwood Academic Publishers.

Blackwell, B. (1973). Drug therapy: Patient compliance. *New England Journal of Medicine, 289*, 249–252.

Blessing-Moore, J. (1996). Does asthma education change behavior? To know is not to do. *Chest, 109*, 9–19.

Bosch-Capblanch, X., Abba, K., Prictor M., & Garner, P. (2007). Contracts between patients and healthcare practitioners for improving patients' adherence to treatment, prevention and health promotion activities. *Cochrane Database of Systematic Reviews* (Protocol) 4, CD004808.

Breen, R., & Thornhill, J. T. (1998). Noncompliance with medications for psychiatric disorders. *CNS Drugs, 9*, 457–471.

Brown, S. (1990). Studies of educational interventions and outcomes in diabetic adults: A meta-analysis revisited. *Patient Education and Counseling, 16*, 189–215.

Burke, L. E., & Dunbar-Jacob, J. (1995). Adherence to medication, diet, and activity recommendations: From assessment to maintenance. *Journal of Cardiovascular Nursing, 9*, 62–79.

Butler, C., Rollnick, S., & Stott, N. (1996). The practitioner, the patient and resistance to change: Recent ideas on compliance. *Canadian Medical Association Journal, 154*, 1357–1362.

Bultman, D. C., & Svarstad, B. L. (2000). Effects of physician communication style on client medication beliefs and adherence with antidepressant treatment. *Social Science and Medicine, 40*, 173–185.

Burnier, M. (2000). Long-term compliance with antihypertensive therapy: Another facet of chronotherapeutics in hypertension. *Blood Pressure Monitor, 5*(Suppl. 1), S31–S34.

Calle, E. E., Rodriguez, C., Walker-Thurmond, K., & Thun, M. J. (2003). Overweight, obesity, and mortality from cancer in a prospectively studied cohort of US adults. *New England Journal of Medicine, 348*, 1625–1638.

Chambers, C. V., Markson, L., Diamond, J. J., Lasch, L., & Berger, M. (1999). Health beliefs and compliance with inhaled corticosteroids by asthmatic patients in primary care practices. *Respiratory Medicine, 93*, 88–94.

Charney, E. (1972). Patient-doctor communication: Implications for the clinician. *Pediatric Clinics of North America, 19*, 263–279.

Chin, J. H., & Goldman, L. (1997). Correlates of early hospital admission or death in patients with congestive heart failure. *American Journal of Cardiology, 79*, 1640–1644.

Christensen A. J., Moran, P. J., Wiebe, J. S., Ehlers, S. L., & Lawton, W. J. (2002). Effect of as behavioral self-regulation intervention on patient adherence in hemodialysis. *Health Psychology, 21*(4), 393–397.

Claxton, A. J., Cramer, J., & Pierce, C. (2001). A systematic review of the associations between dose regimens and mediation compliance. *Clinical Therapy, 23*, 1296–1310.

Cohen, S. J. (1979). *New directions in patient compliance.* Lexington, MA: Lexington Books.

Coutts, J. A., Gibson, N. A., & Paton, J. Y. (1992). Measuring compliance with inhaled medication in asthma. *Archives of Diseases of Childhood, 67*, 332–333.

Cramer, J., Rosenheck, R., Kirk, G., Krol, W., & Krystal, J. (2003). Medication compliance feedback and monitoring in a clinical trial: Predictors and outcomes. *Value Health, 6*, 566–573.

Daneri, G. (1999). Medication adherence failure in schizophrenia: A forensic review of rates, reasons, treatments, and prospects. *Journal of the American Academy of Psychiatric Law, 27*, 426–444.

Davis, M. S. (1968a). Physiologic, psychological and demographic factors in patient compliance with doctors orders. *Medical Care, 6*, 115–122.

Davis, M. S. (1968b).Variations in patient compliance with doctors advice: An empirical analysis of patterns of communication. *American Journal of Public Health, 58*, 274–288.

Davis, M. S. (1967). Predicting non-compliant behavior. *Journal of Health and Social Behavior, 8*, 265–271.

Dennehy, C. E., Kishi, D. T., & Louie, C. (1996). Drug related illness in emergency department patients. *American Journal of Health System Pharmacy, 53*(12), 1422–1426.

Dew, M. A., Roth, L. H., Thompson, M. E., Kormos, R. L., & Griffith, B. P. (1996). Medical compliance and its predictors in the first year after heart transplantation. *Journal of Heart and Lung Transplantation, 15*, 631–645.

DiMatteo, M. R. (2004). Variations in patients; adherence to medical recommendations: A quantitative review of 50 years of research. *Medical Care, 42*(3), 200–209.

DiMatteo, M. R., & DiNicola, D. D. (1982). *Achieving patient compliance: The psychology of the medical practitioner's role.* New York: Pergamon Press.

DiMatteo, M. R., Giordani, P. J., Lepper, H. S., & Croghan, T. W. (2002). Patient adherence and medical treatment outcomes: A meta-analysis. *Medical Care, 40*, 794–811.

DiMatteo, M. R., Reiter, R. C., & Gambone, J. C. (1994). Enhancing medication adherence through communication and informed collaborative choice. *Health Communication, 5*, 253–266.

Dolder, C. R., Lacro, J. P., Leckband, S., & Jeste, D. V. (2003). Interventions to improve antipsychotic medication adherence: Review of recent literature. *Journal of Clinical Psychopharmacology, 23*(4), 389–399.

Donabedian, A., & Rosenfeld, L. S. (1964). Follow-up study of chronically ill patients discharged from the hospital. *Journal of Chronic Diseases, 17*, 847–862.

Eshelman, F. N., & Fitzloff, J. (1976). Effect of packaging on patient compliance with an antihypertensive medication. *Current Therapeutic Research, 20*, 215–219.

Evangelista, L. S., & Dracup, K. A. (2000). A closer look at compliance research in heart failure patients in the last decade. *Progress in Cardiovascular Nursing, 15*, 97–103.

Falvo, D., Woehlke, P., & Deichmann, J. (1980). Relationship of physician behavior to patient compliance. *Patient Counseling and Health Education, 2*, 185–188.

Farmer, K. C. (1999). Methods for measuring and monitoring medication regimen adherence in clinical trials and clinical practice. *Clinical Therapeutics, 21*, 1074–1090.

Feldman, R. H. L. (1982). A guide for enhancing health care compliance in ambulatory care settings. *Journal of Ambulatory Care Management, 5*, 1–15.

Freeman, R. C., Rodriquez, G., & French, J. F. (1996). Compliance with AZT treatment regimen of HIV seropositive injection drug users: A neglected issue. *AIDS Education and Prevention, 8*, 58–71.

Gerbino P. (1993). Forward. *Annals of Pharmacotherapy, 27*(Suppl.), S3–S4.

Graziani, C., Rosenthal, M. P., & Diamond, J. J. (1999). Diabetic education program use and patients perceived barriers to adherence. *Family Medicine, 31*, 358–363.

Gustafsson, B. K., Hakansson, J., & Klinge, B. (2002) Oral health and cardiovascular disease in Sweden. *Journal of Clinical Periodontology, 29*, 254–259.

Hart, D. J., & Spector, T. D. (1993). The relationship of obesity, fat distribution and osteoarthritis in women in the general population: The Chingford study. *Journal of Rheumatology, 20*, 331–335.

Haynes, R. B. (1979). Determinants of compliance: The disease and the mechanics of treatment. In R.B. Haynes (Ed.), *Compliance in health care* (pp. 49–62). Baltimore: Johns Hopkins University Press.

Haynes, R. B. (1999, April). Compliance: The state of the science. *Conference PRM Proceedings.* Waltham: MA.

Haynes, R. B. (2001). Improving patient adherence: State of the art, with a special focus on medication taking for cardiovascular disorders. In L. E. Burke & I. S. Ockene (Eds.), *Compliance in Healthcare and Research* (pp. 3–21). Armonk, NY: Futura.

Haynes, R. B., McDonald, H. P., & Garg, A. X. (2002a). Helping patients follow prescribed treatment: Clinical applications. *Journal of the American Medical Assocation, 288*, 2880–2883.

Haynes, R. B., McDonald, H. P., Garg, A. X., & Montague, P. (2002b). Interventions for helping patients to follow prescriptions for medications. *Cochrane Database System Review,* (2), CD000011.

Haynes, R. B., Montague, P., Oliver, T., McKibbon, K. A., Brouwers, M. C., & Kanani, R. (2000). Interventions for helping patients to follow prescriptions for medications. *Cochrane Database System Review,* (2), CD000011.

He, J., Ogden, L., Bazzano, L., Vupputuri, S., Loria, C., & Whelton, P. (2001). Risk factors for congestive heart failure in US men and women. *Archives of Internal Medicine, 161*, 996–1002.

Hernandez, C. A. (1995). The experience of living with insulin dependent diabetes: Lessons for the diabetic educator. *The Diabetic Educator, 21*, 33–37.

Hinkin, C. H., Castellon, S. A., Durvsula, R., Hardy, D. J., Lam M. N., Mason K. I., Thrasher, D., Goetz, M. B., & Stefaniak, M. (2002). Medication adherence among HIV+ adults: Effects of cognitive dysfunction and regimen complexity. *Neurology, 59*(12), 1944–1950.

Hook, M. L. (2006). Partnering with patients—a concept ready for action. *Journal of Advanced Nursing, 56*(2), 133–143.

Hooker-Whitman, J. (2002). Medical complications of obesity. *Clinics in Family Practice, 4*, 2.

Horowitz, R. I., & Horowitz, S. (1993). Adherence to treatment and health outcomes. *Archives in Internal Medicine, 153*, 1863–1868.

Jackevicius, C. A., Mamdani, M., & Tu, J. V. (2002). Adherence with statin therapy in elderly patients with and without acute coronary syndromes. *Journal of the American Medical Association, 288*, 462–467.

Johnson, J. A., & Bootman, J. L. (1995). Drug-related morbidity and mortality: A cost of illness model. *Archives of Internal Medicine, 155*, 1949–1956.

Johnson, M. J., Williams, M., & Marshall, E. S. (1999). Adherent and nonadherent medication taking in elderly hypertensive patients. *Clinical Nursing Research, 8*, 318–335.

Kane, S., Huo D., Aikens, J., & Hanaauer, S. (2003). Medication nonadherence and the outcomes of patients with quiescent ulcerative colitis. *American Journal of Medicine, 114*, 39–43.

Kirchner, J. T. (2000). Patient compliance in filling new prescriptions. *American Family Physician, 62*, 201–206.

Koltun, A., & Stone G. C. (1986), Current trends in patient noncompliance research: Focus on diseases, regimes, programs and other provider disciplines. *The Journal of Compliance in Health Care, 2*, 21–32.

Kolton, K. A., & Piccolo, P. (1998). Patient compliance: A challenge in practice. *Nurse Practitioner, 13*, 37–50.

Lane, S. D. (1983). Compliance, satisfaction and physician-patient communication. In R. N. Bostrom (Ed.), *Communication Year Book 7* (pp. 772–799). Beverly Hills, CA: Sage.

Langer, N. (1999). Culturally competent professionals in therapeutic alliances enhances patient compliance. *Journal of Health Care for the Poor and Undeserved in Nashville, 1*, 19–26.

Levensky, E. R., & O'Donohue, W. T. (2006). Patient adherence and nonadherence to treatments: An overview for health care providers. In W. T. O'Donohue & E. R. Levensky (Eds.), *Promoting treatment adherence: A practical handbook for health care providers* (pp. 3–14). Thousand Oaks, CA: Sage.

Leventhal, H. (1971). Fear appeals and persuasion: The differentiation of a motivational construct. *American Journal of Public Health, 61*, 1208–1224.

Liberman, A., & Rotarius, T. (1999). Behavioral contract management: A prescription for employee and patient compliance. *The Health Care Manager, 18*, 1–10.

Luborsky, L., McLellan, A. T., Woody, G. E., O'Brien, C. P., & Auerbach, A. (1985). Therapist success and its determinants. *Archives of General Psychiatry, 42*, 602–611.

Lutfey, K. E., & Wishnet, W. (1999). Beyond compliance: Is adherence improving the prospect of diabetes care. *Diabetes Care, 22*, 635–639.

Luther, T. (1964). *Smoking and health: Report of the advisory committee to the surgeon general of the public health service.* PHS Publication No. 1103.

MacKenzie, T. D., Bartecchi, C. E., & Schrier, R. W. (1994). The human costs of tobacco use (second of two parts). *The New England Journal of Medicine, 330*, 975–980.

Malouff, J. M., & Schutte, N. S. (2004). Strategies for increasing client completion of treatment assignments. *The Behavior Therapist, 27*(6), 118–121.

Marinker, M., & Shaw, J. (2003). Not to be taken as directed: Putting concordance for taking medicines into practice. *British Medical Journal, 326*, 348–349.

Martin, L. R., Williams, S. L., Haskard, K. B., & DiMatteo, M. R. (2005). The challenge of patient adherence. *Therapeutics and Clinical Risk Management, 1*(3), 189–199.

Matsui, D., Joubert, B. I., Dykxhoorn, S., & Rieder, M. J. (2000). Compliance with prescription filling in a pediatric emergency department. *Archives of Pediatric and Adolescent Medicine, 154*, 195–198.

McDermott, M. M., Schmitt, B., & Wallner, E. (1997). Impact of medication nonadherence on coronary heart disease outcomes. A critical review. *Archives of Internal Medicine, 157*, 1921–1929.

McDonnell, P. J., & Jacobs, M. R. (2002). Hospital admissions resulting from preventable adverse drug reactions. *Annals of Pharmacotherapy, 36*, 1331–1336.

McLane, C. G., Zyzanski, S. J., & Flocke, S. A. (1995). Factors associated with medication noncompliance in rural elderly hypertensive patients. *American Journal of Hypertension, 8*, 206–209.

McKenney, J. M., Slining, J. M., Henderson, H. R., Devins, D. & Barr, M. (1973). The effect of clinical pharmacy services on patients with essential hypertension. *Circulation, 48,* 1104–1111.

Meryn, S. (1998). Improving communication skills: To carry coals to Newcastle. *Medical Teacher, 20*(4), 331–337.

Milgrom, H., Bender, B., & Wamboldt, F. (2001). Psychological factors and patient adherence. *Immunology and Allergy Clinics of North America, 21*(3). 589–604

Miller, N. H. (1997). Compliance with treatment in chronic asymptomatic disease. *American Journal of Medicine, 102,* 43–49.

Morgan, L. (2000). A decade review: Methods to improve adherence to the treatment regime among hemodialysis patients. *Nephrology Nursing Journal, 27,* 299–304.

Morrison, A., Wertheimer, A. I., & Berger, M. L. (2000). Interventions to improve antihypertensive drug adherence: A quantitative review of trials. *Formulary, 35,* 234–255.

Murri, R., Ammassari, A., Trotta, M. P., DeLuca, A., Meizi, S., Minardi, C., et al. (2004). Patient-reported and physician-estimated adherence to HAART: Social and clinic center-related factors are associated with discordance. *Journal of General Internal Medicine, 19*(1), 1104–1110.

Nelson, E. A., Maruish, M. E., & Axler, J. L. (2000). Effects of discharge planning and compliance with outpatient appointments on readmission rates. *Psychiatric Services, 51,* 885–889.

Nicolucci, A, Cavaliere, D., Scorpiglione, N., Carinci, F., Capani, F., Tognoni, G., et al. (1996). A comprehensive assessment of the avoidability of long-term complications of diabetes. A case-control study. SID-AMD Italian Study Group for the Implementation of the St. Vincent Declaration. *Diabetes Care, 19,* 927–933.

O'Connell, N., & Sutcliffe, A. (2007). Improving adherence in osteoporosis. *Practice Nurse, 33*(4), 49–50.

Oldridge, N. B. (2001). Future directions: What paths do researchers need to take? What needs to be done to improve multi-level compliance? In L. E. Burke & I. S. Ockene (Eds,), *Compliance in Healthcare and Research* (pp. 331–347). Armonk, NY: Futura.

Olfson, M., Mechanic, D., Hansell, S., Boyer, C. A., Walkup, J., & Weiden, P. J. (2000). Predicting medical noncompliance after hospital discharge among patients with schizophrenia. *Psychiatric Service, 51,* 216–222.

Osterberg, L., & Blaschke, T. (2005). Adherence to Medication. *New England Journal of Medicine, 353*(5), 487–497.

Peterson, A. M., Takiya, L., & Finnley, R. (2003). Meta-analysis of trials of interventions to improve medication adherence. *American Journal of Health-System Pharmacy, 60,* 657–665.

Petrilla, A. A., Benner, J. S., Battlemman, D. S., Tierce, J. C., & Hazard, E. H. (2005). Evidence-based interventions to improve patient compliance with antihypertensive and lipid-lowering medications. *Journal of Clinical Practice, 59*(12), 1441–1451.

Porche, R. A. (2007). *The Joint Commission Guide to Patient and Family Education* (2nd ed.). Oakbrook Terrace, IL: Joint Commission on Accreditation of Health Care Organizations.

Quill, T. E., & Brody, H. (1996). Physician recommendations and patient autonomy: Finding a balance between physician power and patient choice. *Annals of Internal Medicine, 125,* 763–769.

Rao, S. V., Donahue, M., Pi-Sunyer, F. X., & Fuster, V. (2001). Obesity as a risk factor in coronary artery disease. *American Heart Journal, 142,* 1102–1107.

Roberts, K. J., & Mann, T. (2000). Barriers to antiretroviral adherence in HIV infected women. *AIDS Care, 12,* 377–386.

Roby, D. H., Kominski, G. F., & Pourat, N. (2008). Assessing the barriers to engaging challenging populations in disease management programs. *Disease Manage Health Outcomes, 16*(6), 421–428.

Roter, D. (1995). Advancing the physician's contribution to enhancing compliance. *J Pharmacoepidemiology and Drug Safety, 3*(2), 37–48.

Roter, D. L., Hall, J. A., Merisca, R., Nordstrom, B., Cretin, D., & Svarstad, B. (1998). Effectiveness of interventions to improve patient compliance: A meta-analysis. *Medical Care, 36*, 1138–1161.

Roth, H. P., & Caron, H. S. (1978). Accuracy of doctors' estimates and patients' statements on adherence to a drug regimen. *Clinical Pharmacological Therapy, 23*, 361–370.

Roth, A. (2002). Diabetes mellitus and obesity. *Primary Care, 29*, 279–295.

Roth, H., & Berger, D. (1960). Studies on patient cooperation in ulcer treatment: Observation of actual as compared to prescribed antacid intake on a hospital ward. *Gastroenterology, 38*, 630–633.

Sackett. D. L., & Haynes, R. B. (1976). *Compliance with therapeutic regimens.* Baltimore: Johns Hopkins University Press.

Salzman, C. (1995). Medication compliance in the elderly. *Journal of Clinical Psychiatry, 56*(Suppl. 1), 18–22.

Sands, D., & Holman, E. (1985). Does knowledge enhance patient compliance? *Journal of Gerontological Nursing, 11*, 23–29.

Schmidt, D. D. (1977). Patient compliance: The effect of the doctor as a therapeutic agent. *Journal of Family Practice, 4*, 853–856.

Schneitman-McIntire, O., Farnen, T. A., Gordon, N., Chan, J., & Toy, W. A. (1996). Medication misadventures resulting in emergency department visits at an HMO medical center. *American Journal of Health-System Pharmacy, 53*(June 15), 1416–1422.

Schoenthaler, A., Chaplin, W. F., Allegrante, J. P., Fernandez, S., Diaz-Gloster M., Tobin, J. N., et al. (2009). Provider communication effects medication adherence in hypertensive African Americans. *Patient Education & Counseling, 75*(2), 185–191.

Shine, K. I. (2002). Health care quality and how to achieve it. *Academic Medicine, 77*, 91–99.

Sokol, M. C., McGuigan, K. A., Verbrugge, R. R., & Epstein, R. S. (2005). Impact of medication adherence on hospitalization risk and healthcare cost. *Medical Care, 43*(6), 521–530.

Spector, S. L. (1985). Is your asthmatic patient really complying? *Annals of Allergy, 55*, 552–556.

Stanton, M. W. (2002). Expanding patient-centered care to empower patients and assist providers. (Publication No. 02-0024). Retrieved May 14, 2009, from http://www.ahrq.gov/qual/ptcareia.htm.

Stark, L. J., Miller, S. T., Plienes, A. J., & Drabman, R. S. (1987). Behavioral contracting to increase chest physiotherapy. A study of a young cystic fibrosis patient. *Behavioral Modification, 11*, 75–86.

Steckett, S. B. (1982). *Patient contracting.* Norwalk, CT: Appleton-Century-Crofts.

Steiner, J. F., & Earnest, M. A. (2000). The language of medication-taking. *Annals of Internal Medicine, 132*, 926–930.

Sullivan, S., Kreling, D. H., & Hazlet, T. K. (1990). Noncompliance with medication regimens and subsequent hospitalizations: A literature analysis and cost of hospitalization estimate. *Journal of Research in Pharmaceutical Economics, 2*, 19–23.

The Joint Commission. (2001). *2001 Hospital accreditation Standards.* Oakbrook Terrace, IL: Joint Commission on Accreditation of Healthcare Organizations.

Trostle, J. A. (1997). The history and meaning of patient compliance as an ideolog. In D. S. Gochman (Ed.), *Handbook of health behavior research III: Provider determinants* (pp. 109–124). New York: Plenum Press.

Turk, D. C., & Meichenbaum, D. (1991). Adherence to self-care regimens: The patient's perspective. In J. Sweet, R. Rozensky, & S. Tovian (Eds.), *Handbook of clinical psychology in medical settings* (pp. 249–268), New York: Plenum Press.

UK Prospective Diabetes Study Group. (1998a). Intensive blood glucose control with sulphonylureas or insulin compared with conventional treatment and risk of complications in patients with type 2 diabetes: UKPDS 33. *Lancet, 352* (9131), 837–853.

UK Prospective Diabetes Study Group. (1998b).Tight blood pressure control and risk of macrovascular and microvascular complications in type 2 diabetes: UKPDS 38. *British Medical Journal, 317,* 703–713.

Vermeire, E., Hearnshaw, H., Van Royen, P., & Denekens, J. (2001). Patient adherence to treatment: Three decades of research. A comprehensive review. *Journal of Pharmacy and Therapeutics, 26,* 331–342.

Vivian, B. G., & Wilcox, J. P. (2000). Compliance communication in home health care: A mutually reciprocal process. *Qualitative Health Research, 10,* 103–116.

Waeber, B., Burnier, M., & Brunner, H. R. (2000). How to improve adherence with prescribed treatment in hypertensive patients? *Journal of Cardiovascular Pharmacology, 35* (Suppl.), S23–S26.

Wagner, E. H., Austin, B. T., Davis, C., Hindmarsh, M., Schaefer, J., & Bonomi, A. (2001). Improving chronic illness care: Translating evidence into action. *Health Affairs, 20*(6), 64–78.

Wagner, J. H., Justice, A. C., Chesney, M., Sinclair, G., Weissman, S., Rodriguez-Barradas, M, & VACS 3 Project Team. (2001). Patient and provider reported adherence: Toward a clinically useful approach to measuring antiretroviral adherence. *Journal of Clinical Epidemiology, 54*(Suppl. 1), S91–98.

Watts, F. N. (1980). Behavioral aspects of the management of diabetes mellitus: Education, self-care and metabolic control. *Behavior, Research and Therapy, 18,* 171–180.

Wise, J. & Operario, D. (2008). Use of electronic reminder devices to improve adherence to antiretroviral therapy: A systematic review. *AIDS Patient Care and STDs, 22*(6), 495–502.

Wolosin, R. J. (1990). Effect of appointment scheduling and reminder postcards on adherence to mammography recommendations. *Journal of Family Practice, 30,* 542–547.

CHAPTER 2

Toward a Model of
Patient-Centered Teaching

Health professionals have always given patients information about their condition and treatment, as well as information about disease prevention or how to avoid complications from illness and/or injury from occurring; however, in the past, the type and amount of information given to patients was determined mainly by the health professional and was based on the signs, symptoms, and standard treatment for a particular medical diagnosis rather than on specific psychosocial and cultural issues that may affect the patient's daily life (Lubkin & Larsen, 2002). The main focus of patient teaching usually was not information the individual patients wanted or needed to know based on their individual circumstances, but rather on information the health professional predetermined to be important.

Previously, many health professionals believed patients neither had the background to fully understand nor the interest in receiving detailed information about their medical condition or treatment. There was also the belief that full disclosure of information to patients could be detrimental, and might open the door for patient's misinterpretation of information, causing the patient needless anxiety. Consequently, it was the health professional who determined what information patients were given (Goldstein et al., 1998). As a result, the amount and type of information given to patients was often limited. In some instances, patient teaching amounted to limited information or instructions such as, "Just take the two pink pills everyday to help your blood pressure."

Likewise, patients also frequently held beliefs that they had limited medical knowledge or experience, and that they would be unable to understand detailed medical information about their condition and treatment. Therefore, they often remained passive, asking few questions, and placing full faith in the healthcare professionals to give them complete and appropriate information. Information

33

was often given to patients as an afterthought, and presented in a disorganized way, with little attention given to whether patients actually understood the information, or if they would actually be able to carry out recommendations. In part, this was because of the health professional's assumption that patients would automatically follow all the recommendations. If a health professional discovered that a patient did not follow recommendations, rather than exploring reasons recommendations were not followed or problem solving with the patient to increase their ability or willingness to follow recommendations, the health professional frequently labeled the patient as "uncooperative" or "difficult."

The aforementioned culture and atmosphere of health care was centered on the health professional and steeped in paternalism; patients had limited access to information and limited participation in decision making about their care. The general approach to giving patients information has, of course, changed. Although many social and political factors have contributed to this change, one significant factor serving as a catalyst was the publication of the "Patient's Bill of Rights" by the American Hospital Association in 1975. This document addressed not only patients' rights to considerate and respectful care, but also their right to current information on diagnosis, treatment, and prognosis, their right to receive information in understandable terms, and their right to receive information that would enable them to make informed decisions about any recommended treatment or procedure (American Hospital Association, 1975). Another factor contributing to change was advances in medical treatment and technology, which enabled more people to manage and live with chronic conditions they may have succumbed to in the past. As a result, patients required more information and skill training than had been previously required. At the same time, as a result of managed care, patients were being discharged from hospitals earlier and given greater responsibility for managing their own care and treatment at home. As sources of information became more readily available (e.g., the Internet), patients gained greater access to a wide array of resources that provided information about medical conditions, treatments, and ramifications of treatment choices—information that previously would not have been readily available to them. Today, many patients no longer accept a passive role, but rather become involved in their own health and health care and actively seek information about their condition, care, and treatment.

Changes in the philosophical basis of patient teaching changed the general attitude about giving patients information; however, the actual process of giving patients information was slower to change. Although health professionals were willing to provide complete and abundant information to patients, the type of information given was still often determined by the health professional and provided in a disease-centered rather than patient-centered way. Patients with the same medical condition were frequently presented with standard information about that condition, regardless of their individual needs. As a result, despite patient teaching efforts, the degree to which patients adhered to medical recommendations was not significantly improved. As different patient teaching interventions were evaluated, it became increasingly evident that information alone was insufficient to bring about positive health outcomes and that one formula for patient teaching does not suit all.

Part of "considerate and respectful care" outlined in the 1975 Patient's Bill of Rights meant respecting patients' individuality and autonomy. Relating to patient education, this would imply that the focus of patient teaching should be patient-centered and tailored to the individual rather than on the health professional's predetermined idea of what the patient should be told. In order to be effective, the patients' perspective must be considered; their values, culture, preferences, and key concerns must be solicited and addressed (Teutsch, 2003). Not all patients need or want the same type of information, just like not all medical conditions are experienced by patients in the same way. Even though they may be experiencing the same medical condition, life circumstances are not the same for every patient. Patients' values, beliefs, preferences, goals, and view of quality of life differ. Preferences for treatment and care also differ, as does the level of support patients receive from family and friends. The psychological and social impact and the meaning of disease and illness are different for each patient when taken in the context of their life and experiences. Therefore, in order to be effective, it would appear that patient teaching must be patient-centered. This means eliciting and respecting the patient's specific needs, and incorporating these into the teaching plan and recommendations, as well as taking into account the patient's particular circumstances, and the context of their values and goals as applied to their daily life (Hartog, 2009).

MAKING PATIENT TEACHING PATIENT-CENTERED

Patients can be given information in a variety of settings, for a variety of reasons, and under a variety of circumstances. Information can be given inpatient or outpatient settings. Information giving can be directed toward helping patients and families understand a medical condition or toward helping them learn ways to prevent disease or complications from occurring. It can be directed toward helping patients and families understand how to carry out treatment recommendations or toward helping patients understand a procedure they are about to undergo.

Regardless of the purpose of giving patients information, in order to provide patient-centered teaching, health professionals need a framework for understanding the patient so that information can be delivered in a way that will be the most meaningful and useful to the patient. Such a framework enables patients to apply information and carry out recommendations in the context of their daily life.

Gathering all patient information that is necessary to provide individualized patient-centered teaching may seem like a complex, time-consuming, and impossible task in an already harried schedule. However, information gathering and patient-centered teaching does not have to be a conducted in a formal teaching session or during a certain time frame. Every patient encounter offers opportunities to learn more about the patient and to provide information tailored to the individual's needs. Broadening the view of patient teaching from a single intervention to being an intrinsic part of each patient encounter also broadens the opportunities for health professionals to collect information about patients, provide patients with information, answer questions, reinforce information, check the patients' understanding of information, and monitor the effectiveness of past patient teaching efforts. Each interaction also provides an opportunity for health professionals to build trust and rapport, factors that are critical to effective patient teaching.

Routine procedures, physical exams, or times when patients pick up a prescription all provide opportunities to not only gather information about patients, but to give information to patients as well. Health professionals need only be aware of the opportunity and seize it, using a conscious and organized effort to gather and relay information that will make patient teaching patient-centered and more effective. Learning how to conduct efficient and effective patient teaching and incorporating it into daily interactions as an organized and structured part of each patient encounter can save health professionals time in terms of increased patient adherence.

Increased patient adherence can decrease the possibility of unnecessary return visits and phone calls and can potentially decrease development of complications or progression of a condition as a result of decreased adherence. In those instances when patients require additional patient teaching, the benefits of patients who are better able and willing to follow treatment plans can make up for any extra time spent in patient teaching. When patients feel that health professionals understand their concerns, have explained their condition and treatment in terms they understand, have individualized the treatment plan to their specific needs, and have conducted patient teaching in personalized, warm, and understanding manner, a positive effect on patient adherence can result (Green, 1987). Patient teaching, when conducted effectively, promotes the greatest benefit for the patient and health professional alike.

PATIENT-CENTERED TEACHING AND PATIENT ADHERENCE

Patients have access to an abundance of information from a variety of sources, yet nonadherence to medical recommendations continues to be a major health problem. The individual with diabetes who fails to follow dietary guidelines despite extensive patient teaching, the individual with bipolar disorder who discontinues their medications despite numerous explanations about how medications can help them manage their condition, or the patient who stops their antibiotic treatment prematurely even though they have been repeatedly advised of the importance of completing the full course of medication are all examples of individuals who had sufficient information, but still did not follow recommendations. Studies indicate that information alone is insufficient to motivate patients to follow recommendations or to improve clinical outcomes (Chaplin & Kent, 1998; Macpherson, Jerrom, & Hughes, 1996).

Given these examples, some health professionals may decide that providing patients with information about their condition and treatment, although legally and ethically mandated, is an exercise in futility with regard to patient adherence. Information alone does not guarantee that patients will follow medical advice, and they will be less likely to follow recommendations they do not understand. Equally important, patients will be more likely to follow recommendations when they feel their needs have been considered and that they will benefit from following treatment recommendations. Furthermore, when patients are able to apply information to their own situation and life circumstances, they will be more likely to follow recommendations.

Take for an example the case of Mr. Karnes. During a routine physical exam, Mr. Karnes, a 68-year-old male, learned he had an elevated prostate-specific antigen (PSA). His physician explained that PSA could be an indicator of prostate cancer and suggested a biopsy. He provided Mr. Karnes with a number of patient education materials that described conditions of the prostate and the implications of PSA testing, as well as procedure, risks, and benefits of the biopsy. The physician informed Mr. Karnes that although the biopsy was a routine minor procedure, there were some potential complications that could occur. The physician arranged a follow-up visit with Mr. Karnes a week later to discuss setting up an appointment for the biopsy. When Mr. Karnes returned, he told the physician he had decided not to have the biopsy performed. He stated that given his age, and the data showing that prostate cancer's tendency to be slow growing, he felt that avoiding the potential for associated complications of biopsy outweighed any benefits he would receive. His physician expressed concern about the decision and continued to strongly encourage him to have the biopsy, emphasizing the safety of the procedure. Mr. Karnes felt that his physician neither understood his position, nor respected his concerns; he continued to refuse the biopsy and ultimately decided to change physicians.

Although the benefits of biopsy of the prostate in diagnosing prostate cancer when there is elevated PSA may be debated, the major issue demonstrated by this case is one in which patient teaching was not focused on the patient, but rather, on the views of the health provider. A patient-centered way of approaching this interaction may have been to explore Mr. Karnes' concerns, assess his level of understanding of the potential consequences of having versus not having the biopsy, and then acknowledging and accepting his choice. Because risks and benefits of the biopsy had been provided, and the patient's understanding of the information, including those risks and benefits, had been assessed and found to be adequate, Mr. Karnes' choice could have been acknowledged. In this way, trust and rapport in the relationship with his physician could have been maintained, and opportunity for continued dialogue left open while preserving Mr. Karnes' autonomy.

Patient-centered teaching describes an approach to patient teaching that consciously takes the patient's perspective into consideration. Patients want to be treated with dignity and respect; when they experience a medical condition, or when treatment is recommended, they become concerned about how such events will affect their lives. They want to know the implications of the condition and the treatment, as well as the impact on their ability to function in their own environment. They want to be involved in decision making and to know what to expect if they do or do not follow recommendations and what, if any, alternatives may be available.

PATIENT TEACHING VERSUS PATIENT LEARNING

Patient-centered teaching is not simply a matter of providing patients with information about a particular condition, explaining risks and benefits of procedures, repeating directions to be followed, or distributing printed materials. Instead, it is a process involving the health professional's precise clinical skills in terms of information gathering, individualization of information giving, and treatment planning. Although patient teaching can be a formally scheduled intervention where a specific time is set aside for teaching, it more frequently takes place as an exchange between patients and health professionals in a healthcare setting during a regular clinical encounter.

By definition, one cannot be a teacher unless there is a learner. Therefore, merely giving information to patients does not mean that learning has occurred. To be effective, information must be presented in a way that makes it relevant and comprehensible. It must be delivered when patients are ready and motivated to learn, and it must be presented in an environment conducive to learning. In order to be an effective teacher, the health professional must be able to identify the information the patient needs to know and the information the patient wants to know. The health professional must also consider the patient's beliefs, feelings, perceptions, motivation, and his or her readiness to learn.

The relationship between teaching and learning is an interdependent one, and part of an interactive process consisting of a systematic set of actions directed toward a goal. Just as the goal of teaching in any educational setting is more than the mere transfer of information so the learner is able to regurgitate facts, the goal of patient teaching is to help the patient learn so he or she is able to incorporate the information into his or her daily life and apply it in a useful way that will help improve the potential for positive health outcomes. To reach this goal, patient teaching cannot happen by chance; it must be based on an organized and structured sequence of events between patients and health professionals.

Patient-centered teaching is an individualized process. The task of the health professional as teacher is to identify the specific needs of the individual patient, to present information according to those needs, and to work with the patient to set realistic and appropriate goals in accordance with the patient's life circumstances and priorities.

Viewed in this way, patient teaching requires the same problem-solving skills that other clinical interventions demand. Just as the same antibiotic is not ordered for all infections or the same diet therapy given to every person with a particular illness, neither should all patients receive the same type of patient teaching. A treatment is not prescribed without collecting data to arrive at a diagnosis, and the treatment prescribed is not based solely on a standard diagnosis, but rather on the patient's individual profile and symptoms. To be effective, patient teaching requires a similar process. There must be assessment of the patient and his or her individual needs, as well as assessment of his or her ability to carry out the recommendations given.

Although it may seem that patient teaching under these criteria could be a time-consuming process, conducting patient teaching in a haphazard way without using a structured and organized approach can also be time-consuming and ineffective. Conducting patient-centered teaching does not require the health professional to change roles from health professional to teacher. Patient-centered teaching can be conducted at many points during clinical interactions with patients. Health professionals must, however, be aware of teachable moments, be able to identify patient needs, and be able to make a conscious and organized effort to conduct patient teaching in a way that will be most meaningful to the patient.

IDENTIFYING THE NEED TO KNOW

The goal of patient teaching is to assist patients in obtaining knowledge, skills, or attitudes that will maximize their potential for positive health outcomes. The question becomes, however, who defines these "positive health outcomes"? Patients and health professionals may have different views, and unless the health professional is aware of patient views and perceptions, conducting effective patient-centered teaching will be hampered.

Health professionals should refrain from being so anxious to provide patients with information that the patient's perceptions and needs are ignored. Before giving information, the health professional should gather information from the patient that may enhance patient teaching and the ability to formulate strategies that would enable patients to achieve mutually acceptable goals. Such a process involves identifying factors that have an influence on the patient's behavior and motivation. This helps the health professional work with the patient to determine strategies within the patient's frame of reference that will optimize the patient's ability to carry out recommendations to improve health status.

A patient's individual needs may refer to the immediate teaching situation, or to needs that will support or deter the patient from following recommendations. For instance, in the immediate teaching situation when the patient is in pain, anxious, or generally distracted from receiving information at that time, teaching efforts are likely to be ineffective. Under these circumstances, no matter how crucial patient teaching may be, conducting patient teaching despite the patient's needs will result in less than satisfactory results. Individual needs can also refer to supports that can enhance a patient's ability to carry out recommendations or to barriers that may interfere with following recommendations. Physical, psychological, social, or cultural barriers can interfere with a patient's receptiveness and ability to learn or carry out recommendations. It does little good to give patients recommendations they are unwilling or unable to follow.

The patient's current level of knowledge must also be considered. Does the patient have insufficient knowledge to carry out the recommendations? Does he or she lack understanding of why the recommendations are important, thus decreasing the chance that the recommendations will be followed? Does the patient have an accurate perception of consequences of following or not following recommendations? Should information be presented in a different way or in a different format that would increase the patient's understanding? Should the information be broken into smaller parts so the patient can absorb information in a more gradual style?

Patients' attitudes and beliefs about their condition and treatment, and in some instances about health care in general, can also contribute to their willingness and ability to carry out recommendations. Is the patient motivated to carry out the treatment plan? Is he or she fearful about the diagnosis, treatment, or prognosis? Has the patient accepted the condition as well as the need for treatment? What are the patient's beliefs about their condition or treatment? How does he or she perceive the severity of the condition? What meaning does the condition have for the patient's family or for the individual personally?

Although knowledge and attitude are important contributors to the patient's ability and willingness to follow medical recommendations, some recommendations also include the patient's physical ability to perform a task. Take Mr. Marshall, a 72-year-old man with failing eyesight and severe rheumatoid arthritis deforming his hands. Mr. Marshall also has type II diabetes and is told he needs to add insulin injections to his treatment repertoire. The diabetic educator may find that Mr. Marshall is enthusiastic about learning how to give himself insulin injections and expresses excellent understanding of the need to monitor his glucose levels closely, balancing them with insulin; however, if the diabetic educator does not consider the difficulty Mr. Marshall may have in drawing up the accurate amount of insulin, his knowledge and enthusiasm will not be enough to help him effectively manage his condition. Only when his special needs are considered, and Mr. Marshall is made aware of assistive devices available and how to use them to draw up and inject insulin, will his ability to follow recommendations be enhanced. In addition to assessing patients' knowledge and motivation, health professionals must also assess individual patients' level of skill and physical ability to carry out the treatment plan.

Social factors and their impact on patients' ability or willingness to follow recommendations must also be assessed if patient teaching is to be effective. Social influences may either impede or facilitate both learning and the patient's ability to follow the recommendations given. For instance, Andrea, a 16-year-old, is a cheerleader at her high school and has moderate asthma, which exercise seems to exacerbate. She has been shown how to use an inhaler and has been able to demonstrate that she is able to use it appropriately. Andrea is concerned, however, that if others see her use the inhaler, it may hurt her chances to remain on the cheerleading squad. Despite her understanding of her condition and treatment, and her ability to carry it out, social factors may interfere with her willingness to follow treatment recommendations. By considering her concerns, the health professional can work with her in partnership to arrive at a plan to help her control her symptoms in the context of her needs.

Other social factors to be considered in patient teaching are the amount and type of social support the patient receives. What type of social support does the patient have? How well does the patient's system of social support function? Will family, friends, employers, or others with whom the patient has contact support him or her in achieving treatment goals, or will their influence interfere with the way the patient follows the recommendations? Take the case of Mr. Casey. Mr. Casey recently had cardiac bypass surgery and during cardiac rehabilitation met with the dietitian to discuss the need to reduce fat intake and to eat more fruits, vegetables, and whole grains. He appeared to have a good understanding of the information, and was able to accurately choose more healthy food choices when escorted by the dietitian to the cafeteria. Other members of the cardiac rehabilitation team noted, however, that Mr. Casey's wife frequently bragged about how much Mr. Casey enjoyed her homemade biscuits and sausage gravy, and how much she looked forward to making them for him again when he returned home. Without considering the influence Mr. Casey's wife may have on his ability or willingness to carry out the dietitian's recommendations, the effectiveness of patient teaching is limited.

Other issues involve patient's ethnic, cultural, or religious values that may conflict with recommendations, or with the patient's willingness to carry them out. Only when these issues are identified can the health professional problem solve with the patient in order to develop an alternative plan that is acceptable to the patient, and will assist them achieve appropriate health outcomes.

Environmental factors may also help or hinder a patient's ability to learn or to carry out recommended procedures. Does the patient have adequate physical supports to carry out recommendations or do factors such as inadequate housing, inadequate transportation, or a scarcity of other resources make carrying out the recommendations more difficult, or even impossible? Does the individual's daily schedule, responsibilities, or work schedule make it impossible to follow recommendations? For instance, it may be futile to ask a young single mother of three to rest in bed for the next 2 weeks if consideration has not been given to whether any type of child care may be available during that time.

At times, medical recommendations alone may be too complex for the patient to carry out. Rather than taking numerous medications at different times during the day, is it possible for the patient to receive a long-acting injection that serves the same purpose? Are other medications available that would serve the same purpose, but require fewer doses? Can some of the recommendations be added after the patient has mastered more immediate recommendations?

Of course, it is also important to assess the basic teaching environment itself. Is the environment conducive to learning? Is it comfortable and free from interruptions or distractions? Is sufficient privacy available? Are lighting and acoustics adequate?

Identifying individual, social, environmental, and medical factors about each patient provides information that can be used to determine the most appropriate approach to patient teaching and to develop a plan that would enhance the patient's ability to carry out recommendations. It is important to consider both supports and barriers. Factors that are viewed as supports can be reinforced to increase the patient's continuing ability and willingness to follow through with recommendations. Identifying potential barriers can help the health professional to open dialogue that will facilitate problem solving with the patient. Through open discussion and problem solving, potential alternative solutions may be identified that could enhance the patient's ability to reach optimal outcomes.

Assessing the patient's strengths and limitations influences the health professional's choice of words, the depth of information given, its sequence according to the patient's priorities, and the type of teaching intervention used. For example, if Mr. Smith, a patient with Parkinson's disease, is discouraged about his condition, its progressive nature, and about his inability to control it, patient teaching about the neurology of Parkinson's disease will probably be of little benefit. At this point, teaching might be directed to encouraging Mr. Smith to talk about his feelings or informing him about Parkinson's disease support groups that may be available where he can meet and talk with others who might be sharing similar experiences. In other instances, if the health professional discovers that the patient's main problem is not lack of understanding of the condition or the treatment involved, but merely difficulty remembering to implement the recommendations, teaching may be directed toward developing methods to help the patient remember the prescribed treatment.

Effective patient-centered teaching encompasses a deliberate problem-solving approach. The process of patient teaching involves a series of steps in which information about the patient is gathered, assessed, and incorporated into a plan for patient teaching. This plan includes helping the patient apply the information to their daily life, as well as evaluating short- and long-term effectiveness.

There are many levels of patient teaching and many circumstances in which it can take place. Although the exact approach may differ according to the setting and the type of patient teaching needed, many general principles remain the same. To be effective, health professionals must have an organized, structured approach to patient interactions so that information about the patient can be gathered and incorporated into the teaching plan. In so doing, health professionals are best able to meet patients' information needs and reach optimal outcomes.

GATHERING PATIENT INFORMATION

Gathering information about the patient is necessary in order to conduct patient-centered teaching, but it may seem like a nearly impossible task. If information gathering is incorporated into total patient care, however, it should take very little time. Information gathering requires awareness of the patient as an individual, astute observation, and active listening by health professionals. Systematic assessment enables health professionals to individualize patient teaching, thus maximizing the probability that it will be effective. Information gathering and assessment provides a basis for developing a teaching plan that is best suited to the individual patient's needs and goals. The plan can then be evaluated to see how effective it was in actually meeting those needs.

Much information is available from everyday interactions with patients, especially if the health professional has an ongoing relationship with the patient. Considerable information has probably been gathered over time through numerous patient interactions. Although obtaining some information from the patient may involve formal interaction, much information—both objective and subjective—can be gained in routine patient interactions. Every patient contact is an opportunity for information gathering. Information about patients can be collected from many sources and in many ways; simple observation can provide valuable information if the health professional makes a conscious effort to observe cues from patients.

For example, in an outpatient setting, simply glancing into the waiting room can offer a wealth of information. Who brought the patient to the clinic? What types of interactions does the patient appear to have with them? This information can provide the health professional potential information about social support and family interaction. Does the young mother of three have difficulty controlling her children in the waiting room? Is the older patient always accompanied by an aide rather than his or her adult son who lives with them and is out of work? Observation of patients' general appearance, manner of dress, hairstyle, and general affect can also provide important information. Does general appearance seem to indicate a pride in appearance? Is the patient disheveled? Has the patient's appearance or grooming changed?

Health professionals may also observe a variety of nonverbal cues, such as the patients' facial expressions, posture, or general body movements, which may be indicative of their general mood or general sense of well-being. Some health professionals routinely escort the patient from the waiting room themselves in order to increase opportunity for gathering this type of information. When preparing the patient for an exam, does the patient's expression indicate fear, anxiety, sadness, or anger, or does the patient appear calm and relaxed? While waiting for the health professional, does the patient engage in foot tapping, squirming, or other signs of restlessness? Does the patient seem distraught, or are they peaceful?

Observations provide the health professional with cues for follow-up. For instance, if the health professional observes the patient foot tapping or squirming, the health professional may say something like, "You seem a little restless today." This statement opens the possibility of dialogue that can offer additional insight into the patient's state of mind, which can have implications for patient teaching.

Informal information is also available to the health professional in the hospital setting. Glancing into a patient's room at visiting hours helps the health professional gain information regarding who visits the patient regularly and what type of interaction takes place. While distributing medications or performing treatments, other general observations can be made about the patient's general affect. Does the patient appear apprehensive or assured? Do they appear to be physically comfortable or are there signs indicating they may be in pain or experiencing some other type of physical discomfort that might interfere with patient teaching?

Skilled observation can be an extremely valuable assessment tool when combined with other sources of information such as the patient's chart. A brief review of the chart can provide demographic information, as well as information about a patient's health history. This may also be a clue to past experiences and may influence a patient's reaction to their condition, their treatment, or the health care he or she is currently receiving. Notes on the chart by other health professionals may help supply information about the patient's reactions, strengths, or other specific characteristics that can be helpful when individualizing a patient teaching plan.

Perhaps the most valuable source of information can be obtained from the patients themselves. Information can be gained from patients informally—through casual conversation—and formally—through structured interview. In casual conversation, astute health professionals may begin to note clues about a patient's lifestyle, who they feel close to, their general attitude and feelings about their condition and treatment, and their openness to receiving more information.

Through simple verbal interchange, health professionals can also determine anger, anxiety, and sadness from a patient's tone of voice as well as from words spoken. Information about learning capabilities can be gained by noting the patient's language structure and level of communication. Such information can be obtained any time there is contact, such as while preparing the patient for an exam, while carrying out a treatment, or while conducting a physical examination. Gathering information in the normal context of patient care requires no extra time, but rather, provides for a more efficient use of time already spent.

A more formal approach involving information gathering from the patient directly is in the form of an informational interview. This enables the health professional to gather additional information not available from other sources and to validate or re-evaluate perceptions formulated about the patient from other information sources. This formal approach has the specific purpose of gaining additional information as well as establishing a relationship of trust that can facilitate patient teaching. Information gathering should be a prelude to direct patient teaching that builds rapport and provides the opportunity to assess the patient's knowledge, beliefs, and attitudes more completely. Beginning with an open-ended question provides the health professional with information that can be used as a starting point for patient teaching as illustrated in the following example:

> Mrs. Ellis, I wanted to talk with you about your hypertension, or high blood pressure, today and to answer any specific questions you may have about it. It would help me to know something about the information you already have about your condition. Could you tell me a little bit about what you know about high blood pressure or hypertension, and what it means to you?

Such open-ended questions provide healthcare professionals with valuable information by allowing patients to respond in their own words. Through this approach, the health professional gains information about the patient's understanding of his or her condition and about his or her feelings concerning that condition, as well as any questions and priorities. This type of information may be obtained not only by listening to patients' words, but also by observing their willingness to talk about their condition, and by observing other nonverbal cues made by patients while talking about their condition.

The time needed for this type of formal information gathering depends on the patient's needs and the complexity of information about the condition or recommendations. Some patient teaching can be incorporated into this initial information gathering session. If questions are raised in the explanation of the patient's condition, the health professional need not wait for a formal teaching session to answer them. Questions that at first may seem irrelevant can indicate a patient's greatest area of interest. By answering questions promptly and honestly, health professionals not only acquire patient's attention, but further enhance patient trust in the health professional as someone who is genuinely interested. This trust and rapport may be one of the most important factors in effective patient-centered teaching. One approach to this part of the process is illustrated in the following case.

Mr. Oliver had been hospitalized because of ulcerative colitis that resulted in surgical resection of the colon with resulting ileostomy. The nurse on the surgical ward noted from reviewing Mr. Oliver's chart that he was Caucasian, 42 years of age, and divorced. From observation, the nurse also noted that Mr. Oliver, a certified public accountant, appeared concerned about his business while in the hospital, and he had numerous phone conversations with his business associates. He had few visitors other than his 18-year-old daughter, who visited him daily. During his daily care, the nurse discovered that Mr. Oliver engaged in few recreational activities other than bicycling on weekends with his daughter, who would be going away to college in the fall. Although pleasant, Mr. Oliver appeared restless, tense, and very anxious to return to work.

After the initial postoperative period, when Mr. Oliver was experiencing relatively little pain, the nurse began more formal information gathering as a prelude to teaching him about how to manage his ileostomy at home. The nurse chose a time when Mr. Oliver's roommate in the next bed had been taken to the radiology department, thus allowing more privacy for the interaction and lessening the chance of distractions. The nurse found Mr. Oliver going over some bookwork that one of his colleagues had brought him.

> *Nurse*: Mr. Oliver, I hope I'm not interrupting. I wanted to talk with you about instructions you are to follow when you go home. Should I come back later?
> *Mr. Oliver*: No, now is fine—anything to get me out of here sooner so I can get back to work.
> *Nurse*: It sounds as if getting back to work is pretty important to you.
> *Mr. Oliver*: Well, aside from my daughter, that's about the only social outlet I have. I don't know how my surgery is going to affect my relationship with my coworkers. . .everything will be much different now.
> *Nurse*: How do you feel things will be different?
> *Mr. Oliver*: Well, first I'm not sure what to say to people. They'll all want to know why I've been gone. I'm embarrassed to tell them all the details.
> *Nurse*: Well first of all, who you tell is up to you. For those people you don't feel comfortable relaying detailed information to, you might just say that you had abdominal surgery.
> *Mr. Oliver*: That's good advice. I hadn't thought of that. Of course, I'll also really miss going bicycling with my daughter.
> *Nurse*: There's no reason why you can't still go bicycling with your daughter. You may need to wait several weeks until your ileostomy is fully healed, but you can continue most of the activities you were doing before you had your surgery.
> *Mr. Oliver*: Wow, that makes me feel a lot better.
> *Nurse*: Great! Why don't we begin with talking about the specific management issues of your ileostomy that are going to maximize your ability to do the things you like to do.

The nurse was sensitive to Mr. Oliver's needs for information at the moment. Rather than pursuing her predetermined patient teaching plan, she was flexible enough to address Mr. Oliver's immediate concerns rather than pursuing her own preset agenda. In addition to helping lower Mr. Oliver's anxiety so that he was more ready to learn, the interaction also served to facilitate rapport and trust between the patient and the health professional.

Looking at specific points in the interaction, several principles can be identified. The nurse's first statement, offering to come back at a later time, not only demonstrated that the nurse was sensitive and respectful of the Mr. Oliver's time but also revealed something about his motivation and readiness to learn as well. His motivation seemed high, and he seemed receptive to receiving information at that time. The nurse explored Mr. Oliver's statement about work, which helped her determine one source of his anxiety. She was also able to offer reassurance and support about his ability to still engage in activity with his daughter. In the interaction, the nurse conveyed sensitivity to Mr. Oliver's concerns and identified specific sources of anxiety. Information the nurse gained from her interaction with Mr. Oliver provided useful insight that could be used in formulating an effective patient-centered plan for patient teaching.

The case of Mr. Oliver illustrates assessment of patient needs in an inpatient facility. Because health professionals have the opportunity to interact with patients for extended periods of time, information may be collected throughout the hospital stay. Although interactions with patients in outpatient facilities are shorter, the same process of information collection, assessment, and formulation of a patient teaching plan can be used. If patients are regular patients at the outpatient facility, health professionals may have opportunities over extended periods of time to develop an extensive information base about patients and their families that can be used in formulating an effective plan for patient teaching.

Information collection, assessment, and formulation of a patient teaching plan are key components of effective patient-centered teaching. Because the probability that patients will follow recommendations is greater when the plan is developed around their individual needs, the significance of this process cannot be overstated.

DEVELOPING A TEACHING PLAN

Information gathering requires a systematic, conscious effort, and the information gathered must be incorporated into a systematic plan to meet patients' individual needs. Once information about the patient has been gathered and assessed, the next step is to develop an individualized plan that will enable the client to incorporate recommendations into their everyday life.

The plan should incorporate patient goals as well as the goals of the health professional. The approach of the plan should reflect patients' individual needs as well as their strengths. Part of effective patient-centered patient teaching is to set goals in collaboration with the patients that they feel are realistic and achievable. For instance, take the case of Mr. Wright, an attorney who has been smoking two packages of cigarettes a day for the last 20 years. He states he is under considerable stress in his job and that smoking helps him keep his stress under control. He has developed chronic bronchitis, and has received instruction about antibiotics prescribed, as well as information about humidification and expectorants. The physician has also used this as an opportunity to discuss the importance of smoking cessation, a recommendation to which Mr. Wright seems highly resistant. Although Mr. Wright acknowledges the role smoking cessation has in decreasing morbidity, he feels unsure he can follow through with this recommendation because of his long history of smoking. The physician works with Mr. Wright to establish a plan whereby he will gradually decrease the number of cigarettes he smokes per day, with an initial goal of cutting down to one pack a day rather than two. Although total and immediate smoking cessation is ideal, it is not a goal that Mr. Wright feels is attainable at this time. In working with Mr. Wright to establish intermediate goals, however, the physician establishes a plan that is realistic for Mr. Wright, and a goal that once attained may be modified to include further reduction in smoking.

Because patient teaching takes place under a wide range of circumstances, there is no standard format that applies to all situations. In the case of Mr. Wright, his goals may be different from the goals of his physician. Although Mr. Wright may be willing to consider cutting down on cigarette consumption, he may be unwilling to accept the goal of his physician, which may be total smoking cessation. Individual goals of patient teaching may include helping Mr. Wright understand the importance of taking his antibiotics on a regular schedule and completing the antibiotic regimen, how to use humidification, and the use of expectorant. In addition, part of the teaching plan is also to discuss the role cigarette smoking plays in the development and recurrence of chronic bronchitis. It is important that the physician address Mr. Wright's perception of the role cigarette smoking plays in development and recurrence of chronic bronchitis, rather than focusing only on Mr. Wright's ability to regurgitate facts. The physician notes that Mr. Wright discusses considerable stress in his job, and appears to rely partially on cigarettes to reduce the stress. The physician may discuss other ways of reducing stress or provide referral for Mr. Wright to a stress reduction clinic. With increased sensitivity and understanding of how dependent Mr. Wright appears to be on cigarettes, the physician is able to approach the issue in a nonjudgmental way, arrive at an alternative plan for smoking reduction, and provide the support needed for Mr. Wright to begin to reduce his daily cigarette intake. Mr. Wright appeared receptive to attempting to reduce his cigarette intake; therefore, the physician may not need to spend additional time preparing him to receive information.

In another situation with a different patient, someone not as receptive or perhaps someone having more difficulty accepting the need to decrease smoking, the situation may be different. A major portion of the teaching plan might be devoted to building trust with the patient, working to help the patient express feelings about his or her condition and treatment, and helping the patient toward gradual acceptance of his or her condition and treatment.

In the case of Mr. Wright, patient teaching focused on knowledge, with some teaching of skills related to specific relaxation techniques. Attitudes were also assessed, because Mr. Wright appeared to have significant emotional ties to using cigarettes as a way of reducing stress. Because Mr. Wright was being seen in an outpatient setting, teaching interactions took place during an office visit, but the interactions may also extend over several visits, to provide support and assess his success with following recommendations.

Depending on the receptiveness of the patient, the complexity of the regimen, and the degree of patient understanding, patient teaching may be extended over several office visits. The process of assessment and collection of information, as well as development of a teaching plan, remains the same regardless of the circumstances surrounding patient teaching, although the scope and focus of assessment and information gathering might be narrowed in various circumstances.

The purpose of the patient teaching plan is to help health professionals develop and structure clear, concise descriptions of planned teaching actions based on patient need. Different patients need different amounts and different types of information. Effective patient-centered teaching addresses the specific needs, goals, and motivation of the patient, rather than only providing the information that the health professional considers to be important. In beginning to formulate a plan, the health professional should ask:

- What type of information, skills, and support does the patient need to effectively manage their condition?
- What type of information does the patient want?
- What issues are the most important to the patient?
- What are patient's supports and strengths?
- What factors could serve as potential barriers that would prohibit the patient from learning or following recommendations?
- What potential alternatives may be appropriate?

Although an important part of patient teaching is giving patients information that will enable them to follow recommendations in their own environment, another important part is identifying supports and barriers that may help or hinder their ability to follow through with the plan. Some conditions involve complex information and may require several teaching sessions and several teaching approaches. Complex teaching situations may require the use of several team members teaching patients about different aspects of their condition or recommendations they are to follow. For instance, in the case of Mr. Wright, a respiratory therapist may talk with him about using humidification devices and a physical therapist may discuss chest physiotherapy with him. Less complex regimens may require a shorter interaction with only one health professional.

The importance of setting realistic goals cannot be overemphasized. The most comprehensive patient teaching cannot be effective if patient needs and goals are not considered, and if the goals established are not realistic within the patient's frame of reference. Analysis and synthesis of information must be done by the health professional throughout the teaching interaction. Further processing of information is done in formulating the problem base and subsequently, the teaching plan. A patient-centered approach to patient teaching takes into account the patient's learning needs, potential barriers to learning or carrying out the recommendations, and the patient's strengths.

IMPLEMENTATION OF THE TEACHING PLAN

Implementation involves carrying out the teaching plan that has been developed based on information gathered. Obviously, the most carefully designed plan is of no value if it is not implemented. When more than one health professional is involved in patient teaching, the approach for implementing the teaching plan should be consistent among all health professionals involved in patient teaching. Although having one health professional responsible for patient teaching may be ideal, this is not always possible, especially when there are a number of health professionals involved in care or responsible for providing the patient with information. In these instances, consistency of information and consistency of approach to patient teaching can be accomplished through regular communication between health professionals. If more than one professional is involved in patient teaching, each member of the team must be aware of what the patient has been told, the level of patient understanding, patient response, and any additional learning needs that have been identified. Such communication prevents redundancy and promotes consistency, thus increasing the probability that patient teaching will be effective.

Whether implementation of the patient teaching plan involves a one-to-one interaction or whether several health professionals are involved, it provides another opportunity for additional information collection and assessment that can determine the need for alteration of the plan or approach to patient teaching. If additional barriers to patient teaching or the patient's ability to carry out the recommendations are identified during the implementation phase, the teaching plan and implementation phase may need to be altered. If the patient appears distraught over the recent awareness of the implications of their medical condition, the approach to patient teaching may need to be changed. To be effective, patient teaching must be flexible. Information given during a teaching session may need to be altered according to new patient needs identified during the teaching interaction. In some instances, there may be a need for alteration of the original treatment plan itself. In such cases, patient teaching must be altered to fit the alternative treatment plan.

The case of Ms. Hernandez can be used to illustrate this point. Ms. Hernandez was a new patient seen by a physician in an outpatient clinic for the first time for a urinary tract infection. The physician, through observation and talking with the patient, assessed Ms. Hernandez as being pleasant, relatively well spoken, well dressed, and apparently receptive to learning more about her condition than simply how to take the medication. From the original interaction, the physician learned that Ms. Hernandez had not had a urinary tract infection before. The physician therefore proceeded with a teaching plan that included a brief description of urinary tract infection, measures that might prevent reoccurrence, and a description of the recommendations to be followed and its importance. Implementation of the teaching plan was as follows:

Physician: Ms. Hernandez, in examining a sample of your urine under the microscope, I've confirmed my diagnosis of urinary tract infection. Urine normally contains no bacteria or germs, but since there were some found in your urine, this indicates that an infection is present. Because you have no other symptoms of fever or back pain, I believe it is confined to the bladder, which is the storage place for urine.

Ms. Hernandez: Is this the same thing as a kidney infection?

Physician: No, the kidney is located higher up in your lower back. This infection is only in your bladder, which is located in your lower abdomen. It's important to treat the infection in your bladder early, however, so the infection doesn't become chronic and doesn't eventually infect the kidney. There are several different factors that can predispose to urinary tract infection and several ways in which urinary tract infections can consequently be prevented. A common source of infection, especially for women, is the rectum. One way you can prevent contamination of the urinary tract, which can predispose to infection, is to wipe from front to back after going to the bathroom. Another factor that predisposes to bladder infections is allowing long periods of time to elapse without emptying the bladder. Some people go all day without urinating. This causes organisms that may have entered the bladder, but would normally have been washed out, to begin to grow and an infection can become full blown. In addition, the bladder stays flushed out if you drink enough fluids.

Ms Hernandez: I already wipe from front to back. I'm not much of a water drinker, but maybe I could drink juice or orange drink or something to increase my fluid intake.

Physician: Good. Even four to six glasses of liquid a day are a good start. Now I'd like to explain how to take the medications I'll be giving you to treat the infection. The medicine is a double-strength antibacterial agent that will kill the germs causing the infection. You'll need to take one pill every 12 hours for 10 days. It's important that the medication is taken at 12-hour intervals so that the level of the medicine in your body remains high enough to kill the germs or bacteria, so try not to miss any doses. After taking the medication for a few days, you may find that your symptoms disappear. It's important that you continue taking the mediation every 12 hours for the full 10 days, otherwise the bacteria may not be killed, and the symptoms may reoccur in a few days. I would like to have you return for an appointment at the end of the 10 days so we can test your urine again and make sure the organism is gone. If it isn't, we will begin further treatment. Is there anything about any of the recommendations that you feel you may have difficulty doing?

Ms. Hernandez: How expensive do you think the medicine is? I've just quit my job and become a full-time student. My money is really tight now. I don't think I can afford both the medication and the return appointment.

Physician: Let me see if we have some free samples of the medication. If not, I can give you samples of a comparable medication that I know we have in stock, and it's just as effective. Both the medication and return appointment are very important. Because you're a student though, didn't you pay a health fee to cover visits to the student health service?

Ms. Hernandez: Yes, I did.

Physician: Then at the end of 10 days why don't you go there and have your urine retested. The visit will be free there. I'll call Dr. Marin at the health service and make the arrangements.

The physician organized patient teaching based on the preliminary assessment of Ms. Hernandez's needs. Ms. Hernandez was made aware of the importance of taking the medication as directed and was taught measures of prevention. During the teaching interaction, however, barriers to carrying out the recommendations were identified. By maintaining flexibility, the physician was able not only to include alternative recommendations for treatment but also to teach Ms. Hernandez how she could follow the recommendations despite the barriers. The physician consequently helped increase the probability that time spent in patient teaching would have a positive outcome.

DOCUMENTATION OF PATIENT TEACHING

A coordinated, consistent approach to patient teaching requires good communication among members of the healthcare team. Although some communication can take place through word of mouth, another method occurs through documentation in the patient records. Documentation prevents redundancy by communicating what has been taught and is also a way of communicating what still needs to be taught, the patient's level of understanding, and what needs to be reinforced.

Documentation of the teaching interaction may specify strengths or barriers that were identified, alternative approaches that were discussed, or strategies implemented to overcome barriers that were identified. Because information about the patient's needs identified in initial teaching are immediately apparent, teaching by other health professionals can be more efficient and additional time does not have to be spent rediscovering information that was already identified.

Documentation is especially important when several health professionals are involved in patient teaching or when patient teaching takes place over several sessions. Documentation helps remind health professionals of information that has been given in previous teaching sessions and what additional information still needs to be provided. This is especially useful when patient teaching takes place over an extended period of time as, for example, for a prenatal patient for whom patient teaching extends throughout the course of the pregnancy. Although some patient information is determined by the trimester of pregnancy, each patient has different information needs and priorities. Consequently, not all prenatal teaching follows the same pattern. By documenting information that has been provided at every visit, the health professional is able to organize teaching according to a patient's needs and priorities, and avoid the risk of neglecting pertinent information that may not have been provided earlier.

To be useful, documentation need not be elaborate, nor need it take an inordinate amount of time. In some instances, when information is complex or is given to many patients with similar conditions, such as with prenatal patients, documentation may consist of a simple check sheet that can be placed on the chart with space for comments about individual patients. In other instances, documentation may consist of a simple note on the patient's chart as part of the regular records. In either instance, documentation is an important component of patient teaching. It also helps make patient teaching effective by providing a means of communication among health professionals, so that all involved are aware of patient information that has been given as well as the patient's response to it.

EVALUATION OF PATIENT TEACHING

Patient teaching is only effective when it achieves its intended goal. As part of the process, goals or desired outcomes must be established before they can be evaluated. In the absence of evaluation, there is no way of knowing whether or not patient teaching was effective. Giving information to patients without determining teaching effectiveness is an inefficient exercise. Evaluation is essential to effective patient-centered patient teaching.

Evaluation consists of measuring the effectiveness of patient teaching on both a short-term and long-term basis. Evaluation of the effectiveness of patient teaching on a short-term basis measures only the effectiveness of the immediate interaction in reaching the goals established for that particular interaction. For example, if a session is devoted to teaching a patient who has been newly diagnosed with type I diabetes how to accurately draw up and inject insulin, the objective for the teaching session may be to have the patient perform the activity. If the patient is able to perform the activity accurately, the teaching session may be considered a success. This does not mean, of course, that the patient will continue to draw up the insulin and inject it accurately at home, or be able to determine when additional insulin may be needed. Effective patient-centered teaching cannot focus only on short-term goals. Likewise, if a teaching interaction in an outpatient setting is directed to having a patient understand the purpose of each medication and when to take each medication, their ability to accurately repeat the purpose and schedule for medication may be evaluated as a short-term goal of teaching, but does not guarantee that the patient will be able to follow the recommendations at home.

The ultimate goal of patient teaching is not merely to enable patients to perform a skill or repeat information in the presence of a health professional. The ultimate goal of patient teaching is to enable patients to carry out recommendations in their home environment when they are not under direct supervision. Long-term evaluation of the effectiveness of patient teaching then is the extent to which the patient is actually able to follow the recommendations given in accordance with the plan jointly established by the patient and the health professional.

Evaluation of Short-Term Goals

If the patient does not have a clear understanding of what is to be done and why it is important, or if the patient cannot perform the desired behavior in the presence of the health professional, it is unlikely that the patient will be to able to carry out the recommendations at home. By evaluating a patient's understanding of the information at the end of the teaching session, the health professional can determine whether additional teaching is necessary or additional problem solving is needed to enable to the patent to reach long-term goals.

Short-term evaluation of patient teaching interaction can be accomplished in a variety of ways. If the patient is to perform a behavior, return demonstration is the most logical way to evaluate how well the patient understood the information and how well he or she can perform the task. If patient teaching is directed toward increasing the patient's understanding about his or her condition or treatment, asking the patient to describe the condition or recommendations can assess success. A simple phrase such as, "Just so I can be sure I've given a clear explanation of how you are to take your medicine, could you tell me how you're going to take the medicine when you go home?" provides the health professional with the opportunity to assess the patient's understanding and adjust information as necessary. In each of these instances, the purpose of evaluation is to help the health professional identify lack of knowledge or areas of misunderstanding that need to be remediated before long-term goals can be reached.

Evaluation of Long-Term Goals

Informal means of short-term evaluation may involve conversations with patients in which misunderstanding or misinformation is identified, such as the following example:

> *Nurse*: Hi Ms. Anderson. Nice to see you. I'm here to take your blood pressure before you see Dr. Mason. How are you doing?
> *Ms. Anderson*: Oh, I'm doing great. After Dr. Mason put me on the blood pressure medication, I took it for a whole week, but I feel so much better now. Because I'm not feeling like I'm under a lot of pressure, I just discontinued the medicine . . . but if I start feeling stressed again, I'll start taking the medication again.

Although Ms. Anderson may have appeared to understand the information in the initial teaching session, her statement above is an indication that more information is needed. Reassessment of the extent to which immediate goals were reached may supplement, validate, or invalidate the original evaluation of teaching effectiveness. Such information enables health professionals to identify problems and provide additional information, assistance, support, or resources to enable the patient to carry out recommendations accurately.

Not all health professionals have the opportunity to evaluate formally whether or not patients have followed recommendations. In a hospital, a nurse who has conducted patient teaching may not see the patient again after discharge to determine whether or not teaching was effective. If there has been adequate documentation and adequate communication between health professionals, however, evaluation may still be conducted. For example, the patient's physician, if aware of what teaching the patient received in the hospital, should be able to evaluate the extent to which the patient followed recommendations when seeing the individual for a regular clinic visit. Although the nurse may not have a direct means for evaluating teaching effectiveness, consequent re-admissions of the patient for the same condition may be an indirect means of evaluation. Other means of evaluation available to health professionals in a hospital setting may be telephoning the patient after discharge, or contacting the patient's physician or clinic nurse for follow-up to assess success in follow-ing recommendations.

Teaching conducted in an outpatient setting may be more easily evaluated if the patient is seen regularly. When patient teaching is documented, the degree to which patients were able to follow the recommendations can be assessed at subsequent visits. Methods of evaluation are varied. In some instances, objec-tive methods of measuring effectiveness may be used, whereas in others, evalua-tions may be more subjective. If the dietitian has taught a patient about a weight reduction diet and at a subsequent clinic visit the patient's weight continues to reduce at the anticipated rate, the dietitian may evaluate the teaching as being effective. If the physician conducting prenatal teaching stressed the importance of prenatal care, and notes that the patient regularly returns for prenatal visits, teaching may be said to be effective. In instances when measures are not as readily observable, other techniques may need to be used. If the person with dia-betes continues to have elevated blood glucose levels despite alterations of insu-lin dose, the health professional may suspect that the patient has not followed the recommendations and thus the patient teaching has not been effective. Fur-ther assessment of patient knowledge, skill, or attitude may help the health pro-fessional determine where the problem lies and what type of remediation may be necessary. Health professionals must be aware, however, that other factors may also influence the patient's failure to reach treatment goals. Are there compli-cations for the condition or treatment that were unforeseeable? Did the patient receive the correct diagnosis? Was the treatment the correct treatment?

Evaluating teaching effectiveness by assessing the degree to which patients followed recommendations is productive only if accurate information is gained. Frequently, when patients are simply asked whether or not they actually fol-lowed recommendations, an affirmative answer may be obtained. Such evalu-ative techniques not only provide little useful information but also preclude gaining further information that could be helpful in assessing barriers that pre-vented the patient from following the plan. Unless barriers are actually identi-fied, alternatives cannot be provided. Less direct questioning of patients can yield useful information and can continue to build the trust and rapport needed between patent and health professional if teaching is to be effective. In addi-tion, if done in a nonjudgmental way, such evaluative techniques communicate that the health professional is interested in helping the patient carry out recommendations and that those recommendations are truly important.

Remarks such as, "Tell me how you've been taking your medication," "How many pills do you have left?" or in the case of diet instruction, "Tell me what you had for breakfast this morning and for dinner last night," yields more information than questions such as "Are you taking your medications?" or "Are you following your diet?"

Evaluation of patient teaching is conducted to identify problems that may prevent patients from following recommendations. The health professional must remember that the purpose of patient teaching is to help patients gain the knowledge, skills, or attitudes that will enable them to carry out recommendations in their own environment and in accordance with their goals. Patient teaching is not conducted to coerce patients into following advice. Positive health outcomes are more likely if health professionals understand the patient's perspective and if patients and health professionals work together as a team and maintain a relationship of mutual respect. Evaluation is a means of reassessing the effectiveness of patient teaching. If the original teaching plan was not effective, then new strategies must be incorporated to assist being better able to follow recommendations in accordance with their goals.

REFERENCES

American Hospital Association. (1975). *Statement of Patient Education.* Chicago: American Hospital Association.

Chaplin, R., & Kent, A. (1998). Informing patients about tardive dyskinesia: Controlled trial of patient education. *British Journal of Psychiatry, 172,* 78–81.

Goldstein, M. G., DePue, J. D., Monroe, A. D., Lessne, C. W., Rakowski, W., Prokhorov, A., et al. (1998). A population-based survey of physician smoking cessation counseling practices. *Preventive Medicine, 27,* 720–729.

Green, L. W. (1987). How physicians can improve patient's participation and maintenance in self-care. *Western Journal of Medicine, 147,* 346–349.

Hartog, C. S. (2009). Elements of effective communication—Rediscoveries from homeopathy. *Patient Education and Counseling, 77*(2), 172–178.

Lubkin, I. M., & Larsen, P. D. (2002). *Chronic illness: Impact and interventions* (5th ed.). Sudbury, MA: Jones and Bartlett.

Macpherson, R., Jerrom, B., & Hughes, A. (1996). A controlled study of education about drug treatment in schizophrenia. *British Journal of Psychiatry, 168,* 709–717.

Teutsch, C. (2003, September). Patient-doctor communication. *Medical Clinics of North America, 87*(5), 1115–1145.

CHAPTER 3

Enhancing Patient Motivation: Increasing Adherence

MOTIVATION IN PATIENT TEACHING

Motivation determines the extent to which people engage in particular behaviors. Usually, motivation is related to a goal, and typically, that goal has positive meaning for the individual. Patient motivation is a significant factor in preventing, as well as managing, medical conditions (Elliot et al., 2000; Grahn, Ekdahl, & Borquist, 2000; Rose & Walker, 2000; Wagner & McMahon, 2004), and plays a significant role in the success of patient teaching, and especially in positive health outcomes. If patients are not motivated to learn strategies of prevention, are not motivated to learn about their condition and its management, or are not motivated to follow recommendations, health professionals may find that their own efforts of patient teaching are of little consequence.

When, despite extensive patient teaching efforts, patients do not seem receptive to learning, or neglect to follow recommendations, it is easy to attribute these failures to "lack of motivation" or to label the patient as "unmotivated." However, in evaluating the situation more closely, the "unmotivated" patient may simply be (1) a patient who is unaware of how information or recommendations contribute to his or her health status, (2) a patient whose goals do not match those of the health professional, or (3) a patient who may not attribute the same positive meaning to end results as does the health professional (Koumans, 1969).

Patients have the right to self-determination, in which they make their own decisions, develop their own goals, and decide how to achieve those goals. This does not mean, however, that the health professional has no role in helping the patient achieve their optimum health status. Health professionals have a significant role in providing needed information, fostering knowledge and skill development, fostering self-confidence, and facilitating problem solving.

Exploring the patient's view of recommendations, including his or her perception of positive and negative aspects of recommendations, can help the health professional identify the goals and values of the patient and identify supports or barriers that may enhance or impede his or her ability to follow recommendations. Identifying the patient's goals and perceptions provides the health professional with information that can serve as a springboard for discussion, collaboration, and problem solving.

Effective patient teaching is affected by patient motivation at each level. First, the patient must be motivated to gain or hear information. Second, they must be motivated to learn the new information or skill. Lastly, the patient must be motivated to incorporate the information or skill into their daily lives and circumstances. The patient may be receptive to learning information about their condition, treatment, or prevention, but they may be unwilling, unable, or unready to make the changes or implement the interventions that recommendations require. In order for patient teaching to be effective, patient motivation must be considered at all levels. This includes the motivation to hear and learn the information as well as to incorporate the given recommendations into everyday life.

INTRINSIC AND EXTRINSIC FACTORS IN MOTIVATION

Patient motivation to learn or follow recommendations may be related to both intrinsic and extrinsic factors (Lane & Barry, 1970). Whether intrinsic or extrinsic, these factors lead to a propensity to pursue goals with energy and to persevere even when there are setbacks and frustrations.

Intrinsic Factors

Intrinsic motivation may be related to either physical or psychological factors. An example of how physical factors can affect motivation is the case of Mr. Gorden. Mr. Gorden was a patient with severe gout who experienced several painful gout attacks in 1 month. The attacks were not only extremely painful, but also interfered with his ability to work. Mr. Gorden consulted a physician, who placed him on a prophylactic daily dose of colchicine to prevent future attacks. Mr. Gorden was intrinsically motivated to follow the recommendations and adhered to the recommendations precisely.

Other intrinsic factors that can affect motivation are psychological factors. For instance, patients may be more receptive to hearing information or following recommendations if they believe the information will be of benefit, or that the recommendations will help them reach a desired goal. An example is the case of Mrs. Rosen. Mrs. Rosen suffered from rheumatoid arthritis for several years. In the most recent year, she experienced increasing pain, stiffness, and fatigue. Her granddaughter's wedding was approaching, an event she looked forward to attending, but had concerns that the pain and fatigue may interfere with her ability to attend. She made an appointment with her physician to ask if there were additional treatments or approaches that she could use that would increase her stamina. The physician discussed the importance of physical exercise and joint protection, and also referred Mrs. Rosen to a rheumatoid arthritis psychoeducational group where she could receive peer support and discuss coping strategies used by others with rheumatoid arthritis. Because Mrs. Rosen had a specific goal, she sought information, participated in recommended activities, and was receptive to making any changes that were needed in order to help her reach her goal. Intrinsic factors can also negatively affect a patient's motivation for learning or following recommendations. If the patient does not perceive that they will benefit from following recommendations, or if they have anxiety about their diagnosis, apprehension regarding uncertainty of whether the recommendations will be effective, or lack of confidence in their ability to manage recommendations, they may not be motivated to learn or to follow recommendations. Mr. Roberts' case is an example of how intrinsic factors can have a negative influence on motivation and affect adherence. Mr. Roberts recently discovered he is living with human immunodeficiency virus. Since his diagnosis, he has experienced significant stress related to the uncertainty and unpredictability of his condition, and feels he is unable to plan for the future. In addition, he feels overwhelmed by the medication regimen and his ability to mange it. He finds that he consistently forgets some of his medications and at other times does not take them because of his concern for the possibility of toxic effects. Unless the health professional recognizes the impact Mr. Roberts' anxiety, apprehension, and lack of confidence has on his ability to manage his condition and applies appropriate interventions to help him deal with issues he is experiencing, his motivation for following recommendations will be limited.

Extrinsic Factors

Extrinsic factors that impact a patient's motivation to learn or to follow recommendations are related to relationships or factors outside of the individual and within their environment. Extrinsic factors may be related to the degree of social encouragement or reinforcement from family or friends, or to external rewards individuals receive for reaching their goal. Benefits to health status from social support have been well documented (Cohen et al., 1997). An example of the positive effects of social influence on health status can be illustrated by the case of Mr. Johnson, a man who sustained an injury to his left leg a few weeks before a planned camping trip with his son. Both had looked forward to the trip for months and were greatly saddened by the prospect that Mr. Johnson's leg injury may mean that they would not be able to carry out their plans. The physician recommended that Mr. Johnson go to physical therapy as well as do a series of strengthening exercises at home. The physical therapy sessions were inconvenient because they needed to be scheduled during Mr. Johnson's work day and interrupted his daily work schedule; however, his supervisor was supportive of his need for therapy and rearranged the work schedule so Mr. Johnson could attend the sessions. Likewise, the home exercises were time consuming, meaning that Mr. Johnson would be unable to carryout household chores for which he was usually responsible. However, his son and other family members encouraged him and assumed some of the tasks he would normally have done. The social support and encouragement Mr. Johnson received served as a motivator for him to follow the recommendations that would enable him to recover so that he would be able to take the camping trip with his son.

Extrinsic factors can also, however, have a negative influence on an individual's motivation to follow recommendations. An individual's social network or societal attitudes can create a sense of dependency or inadequacy that hinders his or her ability or willingness to follow treatment recommendations. Take, for example, Mrs. Thompson, who lives with her daughter and has chronic obstructive pulmonary disease. As her condition progressed and breathing became more difficult, her physician referred her to the pulmonary rehabilitation center where she participated in a structured program of education, smoking cessation, exercise conditioning, energy conservation, and physiotherapy, as well as psychosocial counseling. She progressed well in the program and appeared to be motivated to continue the techniques she had learned. At home she attempted to maintain a program of regular exercise in order to build stamina and to assist her daughter with daily household activities by using the energy-conserving techniques she had learned. Her daughter, however, discouraged Mrs. Thompson from exercising or helping with household tasks, insisting that she was "overdoing it." Mrs. Thompson's daughter criticized her mother's efforts stating, "You don't understand how ill you really are. You have difficulty breathing when you exercise; you should think about how difficult this will be for me if you make your condition worse by doing more than you should do." Mrs. Thompson's daughter refused to let her assist with household tasks or do anything for herself, continuing to insist that activity only made things worse. Mrs. Thompson began to be more dependent on her daughter, believing that she could not do many of the things she had done. Eventually, she decided to forgo most of the strategies and techniques she had learned at the pulmonary rehabilitation center.

Other external factors, such as economic or environmental issues, can also have a negative impact on motivation, and consequently, on adherence. Take, for example, Mrs. Parker, who was on an anticoagulant, and needed to have her blood tested regularly to check coagulation levels. In order to reach the clinic to have her blood drawn, however, she needed to take a bus from her apartment. The cost of the bus was $2 each way. Because Mrs. Parker was on a limited budget, spending $4 for a round-trip bus ticket meant that she would have less money for groceries for her two young grandchildren who lived with her. Consequently, Mrs. Parker chose not to have her blood drawn as frequently as recommended.

MOTIVATION TO GAIN INFORMATION

Motivation to seek or gain new information stems from recognition of the need to know. Patients cannot be motivated to learn unless they believe they need the information, or need to learn a skill. The need to know may be first identified by either the health professional, or the patient. When the patient identifies a need to know, they will be more likely to seek information. For example, an individual who is contemplating entering a sexual relationship, but who wishes to avoid pregnancy, may be much more motivated to seek information about contraception than an individual who is not engaging in sexual activity. When the patient identifies the need for information, they will obviously be more motivated to seek information and to learn information once it is presented. The patient who asks, "What type of precautions should I take to prevent getting malaria on my trip to Africa?" or, "Exactly how do I go about changing my dressings after I go home?" has clearly recognized the need for information. In these instances, the patient has identified a lack of knowledge or skill they perceive that they need. Obviously, the more the patient recognizes the need for the information or skill, and the more relevant and important they feel the information is, the more motivated they will be to seek information and incorporate it into their life by following recommendations given.

When the health professional has identified the patient's need to know, patient teaching consists not only of relaying information in a way the patient can understand, but also in a way that helps the patient appreciate why the information is important. The patient's need to know is not always easily recognizable. The health professional may not have the opportunity to observe the patient in situations that would make their need to know evident. Take, for example, Mr. Scott. Mr. Scott had a stroke that resulted in right-sided weakness and partial paralysis of his right leg. Throughout the stroke rehabilitation program, Mr. Scott was cooperative and appeared adept at problem solving when he was faced with an obstacle to reaching goals. He was released from the stroke rehabilitation unit to go home, and was mobile with a cane. At a follow-up visit, at the stroke rehabilitation unit, the physical therapist checked with Mr. Scott to identify any problems he may be having in performing activities at home. Mr. Scott denied any difficulty, stating that whatever problems he had experienced he had resolved. At this point, his son, who had accompanied him to the visit stated, "Yes, Dad has really been great about problem solving when he runs into a snag. . .like going to the bathroom. When he found he was unable to get up from the toilet stool, he just linked his cane over the towel rack in front of him and pulled himself up. Can't keep him down." Mr. Scott and his son were, of course, unaware of the potential danger of falling that his method produced, and the physical therapist, unaware of Mr. Scott's situation at home, would not have known that there was a need for additional patient teaching had it not been for the son's remark.

Patients may not always ask direct questions because they do not know what to ask or have not realized they have a need for information. Such is the case of Mrs. Landis, a 50-year-old Caucasian woman who has, for most of her life, had a sedentary lifestyle and poor diet. She has a history of heavy alcohol and tobacco use, as well as heavy use of caffeinated beverages. Her mother was severely disabled with osteoporosis. As she approached menopause, she was unaware of her risk for developing osteoporosis, and consequently did not seek medical advice regarding what might be done to reduce her risk. Mrs. Landis was unaware of her need to know.

Likewise, health professionals may assume or take for granted that patients have better understanding of the condition or recommendations than they really do. Ms. Dervy, a woman who had had type I diabetes for 5 years, is an apt example. She lived with her parents, but after she received a promotion at work, she was transferred to a new position at her company's branch office in another state and, for the first time, rented her own apartment. After moving, she became established as a patient at a local health clinic and made an appointment to see a physician for an initial visit. At the visit, the physician checked Ms. Dervy's medical record and conducted a brief physical exam. Assuming that because Ms. Dervy had had few incidences in which her blood sugar was out of control in the past, and because she had been diagnosed with diabetes for 10 years and had all the information she needed, he did not engage in any additional patient teaching, nor did he assess Ms. Dervy's knowledge about her condition. Three weeks later, Ms. Dervy came again for an office visit, this time with her blood sugar level out of control. Upon questioning Ms. Dervy, the physician found that since moving to her new location, Mr. Dervy frequently went out with fellow employees for dinner, and in addition to eating more in restaurants than she had done previously, was also often having wine with dinner. The physician found she actually had limited understanding of her diet, because her mother had assumed the responsibility for cooking her meals. In addition, Ms. Dervy was unaware that wine also needed to be calculated as calories in the diet plan. As illustrated by Ms. Dervy's case, in some instances, the health professional may be unaware of the patient's misunderstanding or misinterpretation of information, or the health professional may miss cues given by the patient that would indicate that he or she lacks knowledge in certain areas, or is deficient in a skill needed to carry out recommendations. Recognizing the patient's need to know opens an opportunity for the health professional to provide the patient with needed information and help them become aware of how the information is of benefit to them.

The health professional may identify the patient's need to know based on the patient's comments or on observation. For example, the nurse observed Mrs. Eaton, a new mother, diapering and dressing her baby awkwardly and failing to support the infant's head. Although it had not been a planned activity, the nurse began patient teaching, explaining principles about carrying and handling a new infant. In another example, the physician treating Mr. Ray, an older patient with failing eyesight, for a variety of chronic conditions, discovered that he was keeping most of his medications in one container, making it difficult for him to distinguish pills by color. The physician referred Mr. Ray to a nurse who then taught Mr. Ray how to separate pills and identify them so that the appropriate pill could be identified and taken at the right time.

Unless health professionals are aware of, or alerted to, cues that signal the need for information, patient teaching opportunities may be lost. An example of an indirect cue that may be an indication that patient teaching is needed is Mrs. Clark, a middle-aged woman who, at an annual check up, remarked, "I guess I'll be going through menopause soon. I hear so many stories about how it totally changes your life. It's sure not something I'm looking forward to. I guess there's nothing I can do; it's just part of being old. I just hope my husband understands that I'll be a different woman." Although perhaps not consciously aware that she needed information, Mrs. Clark nonetheless demonstrated a need for patient teaching, or at least a further exploration of her information base.

In other instances, there may be incongruence between the patient's and the health professional's views of the patient's need to know. The health professional may perceive the need for patient teaching when the patient does not. For example, consider the following response by Mr. Jenkins when he picked up his prescription at the pharmacy. After filling the prescription, because it was a new medicine, the pharmacist attempted to give Mr. Jenkins additional information about the medication, including possible side effects. Mr. Jenkins responded, "Oh, I trust the doctor. Whatever she ordered is fine. After all, she's the doctor; there's no reason why I should have to know all those details." In this instance, Mr. Jenkins obviously did not perceive a need to know. Blindly proceeding to give Mr. Jenkins information that he has obvious disinterest in receiving would be an inefficient use of the pharmacist's time and will likely result in little comprehension or retention of information. Although the pharmacist identified Mr. Jenkins' need to know, the pharmacist also realized that Mr. Jenkins was not motivated to receive the information. Coercing him into receiving information he is not ready to receive has little benefit. A better approach may be for the pharmacist to acknowledge Mr. Jenkins' trust in his physician, and at the same time provide him with written information regarding the medication and its side effects, encouraging him to discuss them with his physician at the next visit. A statement such as, "It sounds as if you have a really trusting relationship with your physician. Why don't I just give you this information about the medication and its potential side effects so you can discuss them with your physician at your next visit. I know this is information she will feel is important for you to have," would be appropriate in this situation.

GOALS AS MOTIVATORS

A patient's motivation to avail himself or herself to patient teaching, and to follow health recommendations, are related to his or her goals. Patients will be more motivated if they feel the information and recommendation will help them attain their goal. The patient's goals and priorities may differ significantly from those of the health professional, especially if goals were not determined collaboratively. For instance, patients may place more personal importance on factors that they perceive as having immediate value than on following recommendations that are directed toward achieving future benefits, especially if those benefits seem illusive.

For example, Mr. Conrad, in preparation for a cruise with friends, was interested in improving his appearance by losing 10 pounds before the cruise. When he consulted with his physician, his physician told him that he should lose much more than 10 pounds; he should lose at least 50 pounds as well as significantly lower his cholesterol or he could be at serious risk of developing heart disease and having a myocardial infarction. The physician referred Mr. Conrad to a dietitian who instructed him about caloric restriction, low-fat and low-cholesterol diets, and the importance of exercise. He was given reading material about the relationships between obesity, high cholesterol, and heart disease and demonstrated an understanding of principles of weight reduction and risk factors related to development of cardiac disease.

Mr. Conrad participated in the dietary consultation, read all the materials given to him by the dietitian, and from all indications was able to follow recommendations. He lost 10 pounds, went on the cruise, and then abandoned the dietitian's recommendations. Mr. Conrad's social life revolved around friends, and food was a large focus of his social interaction. He prided himself in the rich meals and desserts he prepared and enjoyed. He had gained popularity among friends because of his cooking and, from Mr. Conrad's standpoint, changing his eating and cooking habits would significantly interfere with his social interactions as well as his newfound popularity. His personal goal was an immediate one—to lose 10 pounds prior to a cruise. Although he restricted calories and exercised in order to lose the 10 pounds, he reestablished his former eating habits after returning from the cruise. He was less motivated to totally change his dietary habits in order to lose more weight or lower his cholesterol because to him, his current behavior seemed more rewarding than following the recommendations that in the dietitian's and physician's view would provide potential long-term benefits. To Mr. Conrad, avoiding the potential of possible future heart disease did not outweigh the immediate reward he felt from his current lifestyle.

In another example, Lynn, a long distance runner, successfully competed in a variety of running events, winning the majority of them. She had gained respect as a runner in sports circles and dreamed of being on the Olympic team. When she qualified for the Olympic trials, she was elated; however, prior to the trials, she sustained a knee injury that required surgery and subsequent rehabilitation. After surgery, it was recommended that in addition to extensive rehabilitation, she restrict her running activities for at least 8 months to prevent potential future injury. Although she participated in rehabilitation, concerned that lack of continuing her daily exercise routine would compromise her speed in the Olympic trials, she began her daily running routine early, rather than restricting running activities, a recommendation she felt would hamper her goal to be competitive in the Olympic tryout.

In both of the aforementioned examples, motivation to follow recommendations was based on the patient's short-term goals, not on the long-term goals of the health professional. Consequently, although in each example, the patient was motivated to follow recommendations to achieve their short-term goals, they were not motivated to follow the recommendations that were based on the health professional's goals.

MOTIVATION TO LEARN

How motivated a patient is to learn is determined by many factors, including levels of physical and psychological comfort. Although the patient's need to know may have been identified by either the patient or the health professional, the patient's motivation to learn at that time must also be assessed. Patients who may not be receptive learning at one time may be more receptive at another. Take, for example, Mrs. Lindsey, who was told by her physician that her mammogram was positive and that she would need a breast biopsy.

He proceeded to give her information regarding what the breast biopsy entailed, the procedure to be followed if the breast biopsy was positive, and the different treatment options depending on the tumor type. Mrs. Lindsey, still shocked at the news of a positive mammogram, heard little of the physician's explanation. Although she realized that she needed to learn what her treatment would entail, she was overwhelmed at the time and unable to absorb it. Consequently, the time spent providing in patient teaching was wasted. The time may have been better spent in acknowledging her feelings, and conveying empathetic support by offering a statement such as, "I know this was probably some unexpected news and a shock for you. I'm sure you would like some time to incorporate the news. Are there immediate questions you have right now, or would you like some time to think about it and come back at a later time?" The physician's response demonstrates concern and understanding, and gives Mrs. Lindsey the opportunity to ask questions at that time, but also provides her with the opportunity to return at a later time when she may be better able to concentrate on the information provided.

Patients who are experiencing pain or who are in some other way physically uncomfortable are also unsuitable candidates for learning about their present condition or treatment. Pain and physical discomfort are distractions from learning. The same patient may be quite motivated to learn about their condition and treatment at a later time when the pain has subsided or the discomfort has been alleviated. For instance, Mr. Atchley, who is being seen in the emergency room because of severe back strain, will probably not benefit from instruction about proper body mechanics to prevent future back strain until a later time when his back pain is relieved.

In addition to physical discomfort, patients may have other priorities that supersede learning, thus affecting their motivation to learn. Ms. Daly, a patient with allergies who has taken a lunch break from work in order to obtain a prescription from her physician for relief of acute allergy symptoms, may not be as attentive to learning detailed strategies regarding how to eliminate allergies in her home if she is concerned about being able to return to work on time. She may be far more motivated to learn the same information when there are fewer time constraints.

Patients' reactions to illness can also influence motivation to learn. Emotional upheavals are powerful distractions from learning. Such was the case of Mrs. Peterson, who had consulted her physician because of pain and lesions she had found around her perineal area. After examining her, the physician diagnosed Mrs. Peterson's condition as genital herpes and spent additional time explaining the condition to her. An outside observer might have rated the information given to Mrs. Peterson as very comprehensive and the physician's skill in conducting patient teaching extremely proficient. The physician explained the condition thoroughly and in terms that Mrs. Peterson could understand—had she been listening. Mrs. Peterson had become so upset by the diagnosis—believing it meant that her husband had been cheating on her—that she heard nothing more the physician had said. Even though the physician, from all indications, did an excellent job of patient teaching, Mrs. Peterson was not ready or motivated to learn. Consequently, little was gained from the time the physician spent doing patient teaching.

FEAR AS A MOTIVATOR

Fear was once thought to be a potent motivator the health professional could use to enhance patient adherence. Many health professionals held the belief that patients could be frightened into adherence with recommendations, so they presented vivid details emphasizing detrimental consequences of nonadherence. For instance, a person with a strong family history of heart disease who also smoked three packages of cigarettes a day may have been told in no uncertain terms of their potential early mortality if they did not change behavior. An individual with type II diabetes may have been told that unless they followed strict diet recommendations, they would most likely experience complications such as blindness or amputation.

It may seem as if individuals made aware of potential severe consequences of nonadherence would indeed be more likely to follow medical advice, but in most cases, the reverse has been found to be true. Studies indicate that scare tactics do little to motivate people to follow health advice, preventive or otherwise. Whereas some anxiety may be motivating, severe anxiety is incapacitating and can, in fact, can have the opposite effect. (Leventhal, 1971; Rudd, 1995). Severe anxiety may only lead to denial, so that patients reject information, ignore recommendations, or minimize ramifications of their condition. Information may be blocked out totally, or the patient may rationalize that although detrimental effects from the condition or from nonadherence may be experienced by some individuals, they will be immune to negative effects because they will "beat the odds." In other instances, the patient's anxiety may contribute to nonadherence out of a sense of hopelessness. For instance, the patient may believe that following recommendations is of no avail, taking on the attitude of "I might as well do what I want now, since I seem doomed anyway."

To persist in giving patients information, they are not ready or are too anxious to hear is ineffective and risks jeopardizing trust and rapport with the patient. Acknowledging a patient's anxiety and feelings and demonstrating acceptance of his or her anxiety builds a foundation for teaching at a later time when the patient may be more motivated to learn. Patients are not always aware of their level of anxiety. Helping patients recognize fear and anxiety creates an environment conductive to a discussion of fears, thus lowering anxiety and enhancing patient motivation to receive information and learn how to incorporate it into their life.

MOTIVATION TO FOLLOW RECOMMENDATIONS

The ultimate goal of patient teaching is not only to assist patients in obtaining necessary knowledge or skills; it is helping them identify strategies or interventions that will help them achieve their optimal health outcome, based on their goals and circumstances. In reaching the latter goal, health professionals must be able to collaborate with patients to determine goals that are appropriate for them, and identify factors specific to their individual circumstances that may either facilitate or impede their reaching the goal.

Some patients may be apprehensive about recommendations if they feel there is risk involved, or that the outcome may be uncertain. Some patients may lack confidence in their ability to carry out treatment recommendations, or have feelings of dependency, or lack self reliance, which contributes to poor adherence. Others may fear the change that recommendations imply and feel more comfortable with what is familiar rather than what is unknown. In other instances, if patients feel that the risks or costs of following recommendations outweigh the benefits, they may be less motivated to follow treatment advice.

The patient's social system may contribute to the patient's motivation to follow recommendations. A strong system of social support that offers reinforcement, support, and encouragement for following recommendations contributes to patient adherence. However, if the patient has little or no social support, poor adherence through lack of reinforcement or blatant discouragement for following recommendations will most likely have a negative impact on patient adherence.

Patient motivation to follow recommendations depends to a great extent on (1) their perception of the costs versus benefit of following recommendations, (2) perception of the probability of achieving the desirable health outcome if they follow the recommendations, (3) the degree of social support they receive, and (4) any environmental factors that serve as supports or barriers to their ability to adhere (Roessler, 1980).

ENHANCING PATIENT MOTIVATION TO CHANGE

Many factors impact a patient's ability and readiness to follow health recommendations. The impact of patient nonadherence varies with its magnitude of seriousness. Whereas some nonadherence may have minimal impact on the patient's immediate well-being, such as failing to brush his or her teeth after every meal, other instances of nonadherence, such as failing to restrict fluid between renal dialysis treatments, has significant impact on the patient's health, well-being, and overall quality of life. Many patients, however, have difficulty changing behaviors that may be detrimental to their health or that may interfere with treatment effectiveness. As health professionals continue to try to convince the patient that their behavior is not in their best interest, patients can become frustrated with the persistence of the health professional as well as with their own inability to change behavior. Both health professional and patient can become enmeshed in a cycle of failure, with ensuing guilt at having failed, and finally end the cycle by giving up.

Effective patient teaching helps patients gain understanding of the purpose and importance of recommendations so that they can make informed choices. However, another purpose of patient teaching is to collaborate with the patient to identify factors that might enhance or preclude their willingness or ability to follow recommendations, and then to jointly problem solve to enhance their motivation to change.

Enhancing motivation should not be confused with coercion or manipulation. Effective patient teaching that increases patient motivation uses a patient-centered approach, in which a partnership is formed between the patient and health professional so that motivation for change comes from the patient, rather than the health professional. This requires that the health professional strive to understand how the patient's ability to follow recommendations can be facilitated. By listening to patients and trying to understand their unique perspective and experience, health professionals establish an atmosphere of collaboration and partnership. In this sense, the health professional is placed in the role of consultant, never criticizing patients' efforts or failure to follow recommendations as expected. Patients may have their own reasons for not following recommendations. By providing empathy and support, as well as feedback and guidance, health professionals help patients consider implications of recommendations and enhance their ability to follow them.

STAGES OF CHANGE

Understanding patient resistance, lack of motivation, and nonadherence helps health professionals work more effectively to help patients achieve health-related goals. One model that has been used frequently over the last few decades to facilitate behavior change with addictive and health-related conditions is the Stages of Change model (Miller, Sovereign, & Drege, 1988; Prochaska, DiClemente, & Norcross, 1992; Rollnick, Kinnersley, & Stott, 1993). This model proposes that there are predictable stages of change. By understanding which stage of change an individual is in, interventions appropriate to that stage can be instituted to motivate individuals to change. Stages included in this model are precontemplation, contemplation, preparation, action, and maintenance (Prochaska, et al., 1992). The case of Mr. Johnson in the following paragraphs helps to illustrate these stages.

Precontemplation

In the first stage, that of precontemplation, patients may not be aware that a problem exists, may not fully understand the nature or extent of the issues regarding their condition or the ramifications of following or not following treatment recommendations, or may not be ready to change behavior as recommended. They may be resistant to information that could help them understand their condition or treatment, or could help them change. For instance, Mr. Johnson scoffed at the recommendation that he should give up smoking. Mr. Johnson stated he enjoyed smoking and that he knew many people who smoked for years with no untoward efforts. At this stage, barraging Mr. Johnson with additional information, no matter how factual, or emphasizing consequences of not following recommendations may only alienate him or increase his resistance to change. A more productive approach to patient teaching at this point may be to listen to Mr. Johnson and identify his perceptions about the effects of smoking and then, in a sensitive and empathetic manner, explore his understanding of consequences of following or not following health recommendations.

Contemplation

In the second stage, contemplation, the patient recognizes that there is a problem and that there needs to be change. At this stage, patients may begin to think about whether change is necessary and begin to weigh the pros and cons of maintaining or changing their current behavior. This stage of change is characterized by ambivalence about making a commitment to change. Change may be something the patient is considering for the future, but not necessarily now. At this stage, patients still feel the benefits of continuing their current behavior outweigh the cost of any behavior change that is proposed, and may overestimate benefits of current behavior and underestimate the cost. In the case of Mr. Johnson, at a later visit he mentioned that his best friend, also a smoker, had recently been diagnosed with lung cancer. Mr. Johnson stated he had begun to think that he should cut down at least on the number of cigarettes he smokes, but also is not sure he is ready to give up an activity that he enjoys so much. During the contemplation stage, health professionals should avoid pushing patients into change, but rather should encourage further dialogue about patients' questions, concerns, or thoughts related to the change that is being contemplated. At this stage, the health professional may assess how long the individual has been thinking of change, and whether they have attempted to make change previously.

Patients may be more receptive to receiving information regarding both positive and negative consequences of change during this stage. It is important that the health professional offer accurate, personally relevant information, and help the patient think through consequences while, at the same time, accenting the positive, engendering hope that it is possible to make the changes.

Preparation

When patients realize that change is necessary, they have reached the preparation stage. At this point, the patient plans to change in the near future, because they realize that the costs of their current behavior outweigh the benefits of changing. Although they may be considering different ways that the new behavior could be accomplished, they may not yet have set a specific goal. At a later visit, Mr. Johnson told the health professional that he had begun coughing daily and found that it was difficult for him to walk up one flight of stairs. He recognized that he needed to stop smoking and came to the health professional for assistance in doing so. At this point, effective patient teaching interventions are those that facilitate the patient's ability to move toward the goal they have identified and recognized as being important. The health professional should consider the patient's past experiences and assist the patient to develop a plan that takes into account his or her own life circumstances. Helping patients identify and establish an action plan with steps that are manageable and achievable should be the focus of patient teaching during this stage. Establishing short-term goals that lead to long-term change help patients achieve small measures of success that reinforce their overall efforts so they can see that they are making progress toward their long-term goals.

Action

The action stage of change occurs when patients are taking active steps to implement the plan to help them accomplish the change they perceive to be necessary. As a result of changes necessitated by the plan, the patient's familiar routine or environment may have changed, making them particularly vulnerable to returning to their former behavior. Depending on the nature of the change, the patient may miss behaviors they have given up and may find the new uncomfortable or unchallenging. At a follow-up visit, Mr. Johnson told the health professional that he had thrown out all cigarettes and ashtrays in his house, and purposefully avoided those situations that he found triggered his need for a cigarette. However, he also related that he thought of a cigarette every morning when he got up and when he was having his first cup of coffee and missed the "buzz" he always looked forward to in starting his day. At this stage, the health professional should never assume that because the patient has reached this stage that continued success is guaranteed. The health professional should reinforce success, provide support, evaluate effectiveness of the plan, and reevaluate any portions of the plan that seem to be less effective so that the plan can be revised.

Maintenance

Even when change has been accomplished and is integrated into the patient's daily life, change must be maintained. Sustaining change may be difficult and the patient may struggle to prevent relapse. Continued support, encouragement, and reinforcement helps patients maintain the changes they have made. In the case of Mr. Johnson, return appointments were scheduled at regular intervals to assess his continued success at smoking cessation and to identify any potential problems which could interfere with success. As Mr. Johnson continued to be successful in meeting his goal, appointments were made less frequently; however, at other visits for issues unrelated to smoking, his progress in continuing his new behavior was assessed. Continued feedback about patient progress in maintaining their behavior can be reinforcing in itself.

Relapse

Although not a stage of change, relapse can be expected. Despite success in achieving goals, relapses can occur in which patients revert to previous behavior. If relapse does occur, the patient should be helped to view the relapse as a learning experience rather than a failure. After maintaining abstinence from cigarettes for 6 months, Mr. Johnson reported to the health professional that during a particularly stressful time at work, he began smoking again. Relapses can occur at any time and require additional exploration and problem solving with the patient (Karalis & Wiesen, 2007). Mr. Johnson and the health professional discussed what had been learned from the event, and what could be done in the future to prevent future relapses from occurring. Patients can come to the health professional at any stage of the Stages of Change continuum. Recognizing the stage the patient is in, and tailoring interventions to the patient's readiness to change helps the health professional build rapport with the patient that facilitates change. Commending the patient on their previous success, reinforcing his or her efforts at achieving change, reevaluating his or her goals, identifying triggers and recognizing methods to prevent relapse, as well as reviewing the effectiveness of interventions and strategies used can help the patient achieve and maintain their goal.

MOTIVATIONAL INTERVIEWING AS AN INTERVENTION IN PATIENT TEACHING

The approach used in the Stages of Change model, motivational interviewing, was initially applied to individuals with addictive behaviors, and alcohol use in particular. In recent years, there has been more interest in applying this approach to patients in healthcare settings (Carels et al., 2007; Cook, Emiliozzi, & McCabe, 2007; Resnicow et al., 2002). It has been used with success in individuals with type I diabetes (Channon et al., 2007), schizophrenia, (Rüsch & Corrigan, 2002), and in patients with end-stage kidney disease (Karalis & Wiesen, 2007; Ossman & Szromba, 2004) to name a few. Although many of the principles of motivational interviewing have been found to be helpful in working with individuals with addictive behaviors, differences may exist when applying motivational interviewing to patients in healthcare settings, depending on the patient's medical condition and the type of behavior to be changed. Consequently, as is true for effective patient teaching interventions in general, one strategy or technique—in this case, motivational interviewing—does not suffice for all types of patient and in all situations. However, many of the underlying principles and concepts found in motivational interviewing are consistent with principles and concepts of patient-centered teaching. Effective patient teaching using the Stages of Change model, including motivational interviewing, demonstrates respect for patients, their views, and their values. As with most patient teaching efforts, effective patient teaching focuses on helping patients make informed decisions based on individual needs and circumstances.

Motivational interviewing has been described as a client-centered counseling approach to elicit behavior change by helping clients explore and resolve ambivalence about change (Rollnick, Mason, & Butler, 1999). It emphasizes personal choice and responsibility for decisions related to the future (Lang & Tigges, 2005) and is based on a partnership developed between patient and health professional (Ossman & Szromba, 2004). In motivational interviewing, the patient is viewed as the "expert," and the focus is on helping the patient develop realistic strategies to change the behavior in question (Kumm et al., 2002). Underlying principles that characterize this approach are (1) motivation for change comes from the patient, rather than the health professional, (2) patients often experience ambivalence when contemplating behavior change, (3) provider persuasion is not an effective means of helping patients resolve ambivalence, and (4) the role of the health professional is to elicit rather than direct ideas of change from the patient (Ossman & Szromba, 2004).

Specific elements of motivational interviewing include working with the patient to identify pros and cons of change, helping the patient gain confidence in his or her ability to change, promoting the patient's autonomy and involvement in decision making and choice, and accepting the patient's choice.

The focus of motivational interviewing is on the patient's values and goals, while also promoting the patient's responsibility for implementing change (Wagner & McMahon, 2004). It helps patients identify costs and benefits associated with different behaviors and helps them explore and resolve ambivalence they may have about behavior change (Rüsch & Corrigan, 2002). Patients often progress and then relapse through the stages of change. The role of the health professional is to assess where the patient is on the continuum, empower them to make change, and encourage and reward them even when the smallest change is made (Karalis & Wiesen, 2007).

SELF-EFFICACY

Self-efficacy is a term used to describe an individuals' belief that they have the ability to carry out a course of action to achieve certain goals (Bandura, 1977). No matter how motivated patients are to change, and no matter how willing or able they are to make changes, unless they believe they can control and exercise influence over what they do, or unless they believe in their ability to make change, they are most likely not to succeed in maintaining the changes they desired. If patients believe they have no power to produce the desired results, they will not be receptive to learning strategies to reach goals or to carrying out the strategies once they are implemented. Individuals can have either a strong or weak sense of self-efficacy. A patient's self-efficacy plays a major role in his or her ability to achieve treatment goals.

High Self-Efficacy

A patient with a strong sense of self-efficacy approached with particularly difficult treatment recommendations may generally see the recommendation as a challenging task to be mastered, demonstrate an active interest in learning information or skills related to the task and participate actively in learning, demonstrate a strong sense of commitment to carrying out the recommendations and reaching their goal, and take setbacks in stride.

Take, for example, Ms. Jones. Ms. Jones was a 28-year-old graduate student in English Literature. She had been having difficulty with intermittent symptoms consisting of double vision, increasing fatigue when she climbed stairs, and difficulty with balance. After seeing several specialists, she was diagnosed with multiple sclerosis. After her friends learned of her condition, they expressed concern about her ability to complete her graduate program given her diagnosis. When they attempted to provide sympathy, she reassured them saying, "This isn't the first time I've had an obstacle thrown in front of me. I'll make it through and do whatever it takes." She began to engage in extensive reading about multiple sclerosis, joined a multiple sclerosis support group, and volunteered at the local multiple sclerosis society. When she experienced an exacerbation of her condition, she merely viewed it as the nature of her condition, and made the needed adjustments.

Ms. Jones' case illustrates a patient with strong self-efficacy who became fully engaged in striving to manage her condition and achieve her goals.

Low Self-Efficacy

Patients who have low self-efficacy may react by avoiding recommendations that they find challenging or believing that challenging recommendations are beyond their capabilities. They may also focus on weaknesses and negative results and lose confidence in their ability to carry out recommendations.

Had Ms. Jones, in the previous example, had low self-efficacy, the outcome may have been quite different as illustrated in the following narrative. Upon learning she had multiple sclerosis, Ms. Jones became overwhelmed. She dropped out of graduate school, stating she would be unable to continue given her diagnosis. She found the management of her condition very difficult and became increasingly withdrawn. She declined to participate in the multiple sclerosis support group and spent most of her time watching television. When she had an exacerbation of her symptoms, she became increasingly pessimistic about her future.

The above scenario illustrates the importance of the patient's sense of self-efficacy in the management of their condition and in their ability to reach positive outcomes.

Development of Self-Efficacy

There are several ways that individuals develop self-efficacy (Bandura, 1994). The first is through mastery. When individuals successfully perform a task, their sense of self-efficacy is strengthened. For instance, Mr. Adams, at first overwhelmed with performing peritoneal dialysis at home, eventually became proficient at hooking up the machine and setting the dials appropriately. Through gaining competence after performing the task several times, his sense of self-efficacy was enhanced. When an individual does not perform the task adequately, however, the opposite is true. If Mr. Adams continually had difficulty hooking up the machine, or made countless errors when attempting to set the machine dials, his confidence in his ability to perform the task, and willingness to adhere to it, would soon be eroded.

Another way self-efficacy develops is by observing those who the individual sees as similar to him- or herself perform a task successfully. For example, Mr. Davis recently underwent surgery for partial removal of the colon as a result of cancer. Patient teaching regarding colostomy care included helping Mr. Davis learn how to do colostomy irrigation. One of the members of the ostomy club, who had had a colostomy for several years, routinely volunteered to meet with patients with a recent colostomy and to demonstrate colostomy irrigation. Although Mr. Davis, at first, doubted his ability to adequately care for his colostomy, and to perform the colostomy irrigation in particular, he gained confidence that he also would be able to perform the tasks successfully after talking with the ostomy club member about colostomy care and watching him perform colostomy irrigation.

Most people do not live in isolation. Consequently, the ability of the individual to change is also rooted within a broad network of social influence that can provide both constraints and resources. The third way self-efficacy can be developed is through encouragement from others. In the example of Mr. Davis, the nurses routinely praised him for how well he was taking care of his colostomy and offered him encouragement and support. In so doing, they helped Mr. Davis overcome any self-doubt he may have experienced, and helped him focus on continuing caring for his colostomy successfully. It is important, however, to avoid empty praise or condescending encouragement. To be most effective in helping individuals develop self-efficacy, praise should be wholehearted and consistent for recognition of real accomplishment.

Lastly, individual coping styles and responses also determine how the individual feels about their ability to handle a certain situation or perform a certain task. Take, for example, the contrasting cases of Ms. Styles and Mr. Morrison. Ms. Styles had been very sheltered as a child by her parents. She had developed little confidence in her ability to successfully achieve goals on her own. As an adult, she was involved in an automobile accident which resulted in the amputation of her lower leg. While still in the hospital, she was fitted with a prosthetic device and began ambulatory training. She became very nervous and upset every time a training session took place, and after attempting a few steps gave up, stating, "I'll never be able to use this to walk. I will be confined to a wheelchair for the rest of my life." Mr. Morrison, on the other hand, had a different experience. As he was growing up, his parents encouraged him to be self-sufficient and fostered his independence. When he experienced amputation of his leg after a motorcycle accident, he viewed learning to use the prosthetic device as a challenge. He completed the training in record time, and went on to participate in many extreme sports events, including surfing.

Self-Efficacy and Adherence

The extent to which patients follow health recommendations is dependent to a great extent on their perceived self-efficacy (Conner & Norman, 2005). The degree to which individuals will engage in treatment recommendations, how much energy they will expend, and how persistent they will be in following recommendations when they are faced with obstacles is influenced by how certain they feel that they will be able to carry out the task. When individuals believe they have no power to produce the desired results, they will be less likely to perform the behaviors associated with reaching a particular goal (Bandura, 1997).

REFERENCES

Bandura, A. (1994). Self-efficacy. In V.S. Ramachaudran (Ed.), *Encyclopedia of human behavior* (pp. 71–81). New York: Academic Press.

Bandura, A. (1977). Self-efficacy: Toward a unifying theory of behavioral change. *Psychological Review, 84*, 191–215.

Bandura, A. (1997). *Self-efficacy: The exercise of control.* New York: W.H. Freeman and Company.

Carels, R. A., Darby, L., Cacciapaglia, H. M., Konrad, K., Coit, C., Harper, J., et al. (2007). Using motivational interviewing as a supplement to obesity treatment: A stepped-care approach. *Health Psychology, 26*(3), 369–374.

Channon, S. J., Huws-Thomas, M. V., Rollnick, S., Hood, K., Cannings-John, R. L., Rogers, C., et al. (2007). A multicenter randomized controlled trial of motivational interviewing in teenagers with diabetes. *Diabetes Care, 30*(6), 1390–1395.

Cohen, S., Doyle, W., Skoner, D. P., Rabin, B. S., & Gwaltney, J.M. (1997). Social ties and suscepti-bility to the common cold. *Journal of the American Medical Association, 277*, 1940–1944.

Conner, M., & Norman, P. (Eds.). (2005). *Predicting health behaviour* (2nd rev. ed.). Buckingham, England: Open University Press.

Cook, P. F., Emiliozzi, S., & McCabe, M. M. (2007). Telephone counseling to improve osteoporosis treatment adherence: An effectiveness study in community practice settings. *American Journal of Medical Quality, 22*(6), 445–456.

Elliot, T. R., Uswatte, G., Lewis, L., & Palmatier, A. (2000). Goal instability and adjustment to physical disability. *Journal of Counseling Psychology, 47*, 251–265.

Grahn, B., Ekdahl, C., & Borquist, L. (2000). Motivation as a predictor of changes in quality of life and working ability in multidisciplinary rehabilitation: A two-year follow-up of a pro-spective controlled study in patients with prolonged musculoskeletal disorders. *Disability & Rehabilitation, 22*(15), 639–654.

Karalis, M. & Wiesen, K. (2007). Motivational Interviewing. *Nephrology Nursing Journal, 34*(3), 336–337.

Koumans, A. J. R. (1969). Reaching the unmotivated patient. *Mental Hygiene, 53*, 298–300.

Kumm, S., Hicks, V., Shupe, S., & Hagemaster, J. (2002). You can help your clients change. *Dimensions of Critical Care Nursing, 21*(2), 72–77.

Lane, J. M. Jr., & Barry, J. R. (1970). Client motivation. *Rehabilitation Research and Practice Review, 1*(4), 5–26.

Lang, N., & Tigges, B. B. (2005). Influence positive change with motivational interviewing. *The Nurse Practitioner, 30*(3), 44–53.

Leventhal, H. (1971) Fear appeals and persuasion: The differentiation of a motivational construct. *American Journal of Public Health, 61*(6), 1208–1224.

Miller, W. R., Sovereign, R. G., & Drege, B. (1988). Motivational interviewing with problem drinkers: II. The drinker's check-up as a preventive intervention. *Behavioral Psychotherapy, 16*, 251–268.

Ossman, S. S., & Szromba, C. (2004). Motivational interviewing: A process to encourage behavioral change. *Nephrology Nursing Journal, 31*(3), 346–347.

Prochaska, J. O., DiClemente, C. C., & Norcross, J. C. (1992). In search of how people change: Applications to addictive behaviors. *American Psychologist, 47*, 1102–1114.

Resnicow, K., DiIorio, C., Soet, J. E., Borrelli, B., Ernst, D., Hecht, J., et al. (2002). Motivational interviewing in medial and public health settings. In W.R. Miller & S. Rollnick (Eds.), *Motivational interviewing: Preparing people for change* (2nd ed., pp. 251–269). New York: The Guilford Press.

Rollnick, S., Kinnersley, P., & Stott, N. (1993). Methods of helping patients with behavior change. *British Medical Journal, 307,* 188–190.

Rollnick, S., Mason, P., & Butler, C. (1999). *Health behavior change: A guide for practitioners.* New York: Churchill Livingstone.

Roessler, R. T. (1980). Factors affecting client achievement of rehabilitation goals. *Journal of Applied Rehabilitation Counseling, 11,* 169–172.

Rose, J., & Walker, S. (2000). Working with a man who has Prader-Willi syndrome and his support staff using motivational principles. *Behavioural and Cognitive Psychotherapy, 28,* 293–302.

Rudd, P. (1995) Clinicians and Patients with hypertension: unsettled issues about compliance. *American Heart Journal, 130*(3 Pt 1), 572–579.

Rüsch, N., & Corrigan, P. W. (2002). Motivational interviewing to improve insight and treatment adherence in schizophrenia. *Psychiatric Rehabilitation, 26*(5), 25–32.

Wagner, C. C., & McMahon, B. T. (2004). Motivational Interviewing and Rehabilitation Counseling Practice. *Rehabilitation Counseling Bulletin, 47*(3), 152–161.

CHAPTER 4

Individual Factors in Patient Teaching and Patient Adherence

PSYCHOSOCIAL ISSUES IN PATIENT TEACHING

Patients with medical problems sometimes behave in ways that imperil their health. Some who have not yet developed symptoms of disease neglect measures that might prevent it. Others with chronic conditions fail to follow recommendations that would control their symptoms or that would prevent complications from occurring. The fact that patients would purposely behave in a manner that would make them vulnerable to disease or that would make their conditions worse seems totally irrational. It is widely recognized, however, that many patients neglect to take medications as prescribed, resist restriction of activities as recommended, and neglect to follow preventive measures.

If one of the goals of patient-centered teaching is to produce behavior change that helps patients to improve or maintain their health, then poor adherence with recommendations may be viewed as a failure in patient teaching. Such behavior can be frustrating and puzzling for the conscientious health professional devoted to increasing positive health outcomes through patient teaching. Why would patients deliberately act in ways deleterious to their health despite having received information indicating that they should behave otherwise? Why, for example, would patients with emphysema continue to smoke regardless of knowledge of the consequences of their behavior? Why do some patients neglect self-care even though they know they will be incapacitated by their condition if it is left untreated?

There is, of course, no single answer. All patients, as individuals, have different reactions, experiences, and motives that direct their behavior. Illness, or threat of illness, elicits many responses from individuals and their families. At times, responses are helpful; other times, responses deter patients from following the prescribed therapeutic regimen. In addition to patients' knowledge, many other factors have an impact on their ability and willingness to carry out recommendations. Psychosocial factors that can have a profound impact on patient teaching and its effectiveness both in terms of a patient's receptivity to information and his or her ability or willingness to carry out recommendations include the patients' psychological traits, past experiences, gender, age, culture or ethnic background, systems of support such as their family or other social group, financial circumstances, and physical environment.

Health professionals may be uneasy dealing with psychosocial factors, however. Some may be unaware of signs that could alert them to factors with an impact on the effectiveness of patient teaching. Others may be reluctant to act on psychosocial factors when they are identified. Some may believe that considering psychosocial factors is impractical because of time constraints.

If patient teaching is to be effective, psychosocial factors cannot be avoided. Giving patients information about their condition or treatment without considering factors that may facilitate or hinder their following recommendations is not only an inefficient use of time, but also leads to poor patient teaching outcomes. If, for example, the patient does not believe in taking medication, but medication is a necessary part of treatment, ignoring the problem while continuing to teach the patient about the medication is useless. Explaining the importance of treatment and how to take the medication does little good unless the health professional also considers the patient's beliefs and feelings and takes those factors into consideration.

In other instances, health professionals may avoid psychosocial factors because they seem overwhelming. Psychosocial factors may be avoided because of the health professional's own feelings of inadequacy in handling the problems presented. Again, merely relaying information and failing to address psychosocial issues is a futile effort. Without a firm understanding of the other factors that have an impact on the patient's receptiveness to information or his or her ability to follow recommendations, the health professional's efforts in patient teaching can end in frustration for both the patient and the health professional.

Gathering information about and assessing psychosocial factors should be part of every patient interaction. Health professionals need only be aware of available data sources, and identification of psychosocial issues need not involve extensive use of time. Likewise, if health professionals put psychosocial information into the right perspective, information need not be overwhelming, but rather can be helpful in working more effectively with the patient.

Patients frequently drop hints about factors that might influence their ability or willingness to follow recommendations. By listening to these hints and exploring them further, health professionals may be able to devise a plan with the patient that will help them be better able to follow recommendations.

Take, for example, Mrs. Delengato, a 32-year-old woman with a history of rheumatic fever. Mrs. Delengato was being treated for cardiac arrhythmias with several medications. The physician taught her about her heart condition and gave her clear and explicit instructions about her medication and behavioral restrictions. At a subsequent outpatient visit, however, it was noted that Mrs. Delengato frequently neglected to take her medication and continued to smoke one pack of cigarettes a day despite recommendations to stop smoking. During the clinic visit, Mrs. Delengato stated that she had recently experienced tachycardia, weakness, and pressure in her chest. In the course of describing her symptoms, she mentioned that her mother had had the same symptoms. Upon further exploration of her statement, Mrs. Delengato revealed that her mother had died at age 35 from a myocardial infarction, although she had had no previous history of cardiac problems. As the physician continued to talk with her, the patient revealed that she believed she was also destined to die at an early age. Mrs. Delengato felt that if her mother had had no previous history of heart disease and still died, that with her own history of rheumatic fever and subsequent health problems, there was little hope no matter what she did. Consequently, Mrs. Delengato had elected to do what she wanted, feeling the medications and restrictions were of little consequence. Because the physician had discovered this new information, he was able to alter his approach to Mrs. Delengato and alter patient teaching to address her fears and beliefs.

Patients have a set of norms and values—expressed or unexpressed—that are individually determined by their culture, socioeconomic status, ethnicity, gender, age, and life experiences. The meaning of illness and the consequences ascribed to following or not following recommendations are based on patients' values and norms. Patients' symptoms are also relative; whereas some may dramatize symptoms, others are passive in response to their symptoms and conditions. Health professionals also have values and norms that direct their lives and guide their practice; however, health professionals cannot assume that their particular way of viewing an illness, issues of prevention, or the importance of carrying out treatment recommendations are shared by all patients.

Gaining an appreciation of patients' life situations helps health professionals better identify and understand patients' beliefs, perspectives, and priorities. Only with this type of information will the health professional be able to devise an effective teaching plan that is suited to the individual. Conducting patient teaching based on the values and needs of the health professional, rather than on those of the patient, can result in patients rejecting information as well as recommendations given. Once this has occurred, it is difficult to reinvolve patients.

Health professionals' knowledge of psychosocial issues can be incorporated into patient teaching so that factors influencing patients' receptiveness to information and their ability and willingness to follow recommendations can be taken into consideration. Health professionals may recognize the need to gather additional information. Discovering additional psychosocial factors may serve as a prompt to refer the patient to another health professional or agency for assistance, or the services of other health professionals may be incorporated to help meet patient needs. Outcomes and expectations for patient teaching need to be negotiated between patients and health professionals with the establishment of new goals and expectations tailored to meet patients' individual needs.

The greater the health professional's understanding of psychosocial factors, the greater the chance that such information can be incorporated into a more effective teaching interaction. As a result, there is an increased probability that the patient's ability to follow recommendations will be enhanced. Effective patient-centered patient teaching uses creative techniques in which psychosocial factors are identified and incorporated. Each patient is an individual; consequently, there can be no generalization about specific factors that affect all patients. The health professional must become skillful, confident, and adept in assessing patients' needs and factors that have an impact on the degree to which they are willing or able to follow recommendations.

THE PATIENT AS AN INDIVIDUAL

Patients come to the patient teaching situation with different levels of knowledge and skill as well as different beliefs about their illness. In addition to assessing an individual's level of knowledge and skill, it is important to assess attitudes, perceptions, and past experiences of patients as they relate to their current health status. Just as all patients are unique individuals, the presentation of the same type of acute or chronic condition is highly variable in different patients, and consequently so are their reactions to it.

A variety of factors determine each patient's reactions not only to symptoms and illness, but also to patient teaching and recommendations provided. Because of this variability, health professionals sometimes find it difficult to know how to approach patient teaching so that it is most effective. The better able health professionals are to tailor patient teaching to the individual patient, the greater the likelihood that patients will be able to follow recommendations given. Recognizing the individual needs and priorities of each patient helps health professionals to present information in a way that is meaningful to the individual and will enhance their ability to follow recommendations. Unless health professionals understand the patient's perceptions of his or her condition and treatment, the effectiveness of any patient teaching intervention as well as the level of adherence with any treatment advice given will be seriously compromised (Gerteis et al., 1993).

Each patient has their own personality, individual method of coping with stress, a variety of past experiences, and a system of beliefs about the world. Recognizing the individual needs and priorities of each patient helps health professionals alter their approach to patient teaching as well as the information given. Recognizing factors that can influence patient receptiveness to patient information increases teaching effectiveness.

For example, how patients perceive manifestations of a condition and the impact it has on them may vary with their developmental stage in the life cycle. A skin lesion experienced by an adolescent may be devastating because of their sensitivity about appearance, but a skin lesion in an older adult may be of concern because they fear it could be cancer. The lesion may be similar and both patients may consult with a health professional about the lesion, but each comes with a different concern and different expectations for outcomes. How the health professional approaches the individuals in both instances can affect effectiveness of patient teaching. Even if the lesion is similar in both cases, the teaching approach will be different because each patient has different priorities and concerns.

Consideration must also be given to patients' past experiences and expectations. Attitudes, values, experiences, and life stresses all help formulate patients' beliefs about health and illness and, to a large extent, their receptiveness to information and acceptance of treatment recommendations (Rankin, Stallings, & London, 2005). For instance, a pregnant teenager whose mother had no prenatal care and no resulting complications from pregnancy may see little need for regular visits to the physician during her own pregnancy. The patient who is accustomed to receiving antibiotics routinely for sore throats regardless of the cause may have some difficulty understanding why the physician is only giving instructions about gargling with salt water.

The way individuals perceive their condition and symptoms, and the degree to which they act on seeking information or following recommendations are also unique to each individual and their beliefs about health and illness (Mechanic, 1961). Some believe that health and illness are predetermined and that they have little control over health outcomes. They may assume a "what will be, will be" attitude, feeling they have little control over whether they develop an illness. In some instances, they may not believe they are susceptible to the disease in question, and that they will be immune to consequences of their behavior, even though those behaviors have been shown to contribute to the development of disease. For instance, an individual may scoff at preventive practices such as stopping smoking because they saw their grandfather smoking all his life and still living to a ripe old age.

Another critical factor to consider in patient teaching is the meaning patients attribute to their condition. How the patient assesses the symptoms and/or consequences of a disease or health behavior in terms of significance and importance all play a part in the degree to which patients receive information and incorporate recommendations. Despite a patient's knowledge or skill acquisition, medical management and patient teaching may be extremely difficult if he or she has not accepted the condition or its seriousness, if he or she views it as a means of controlling others or of punishing themselves or others, or if he or she has a variety of other detrimental feelings about their condition.

To illustrate the importance of meaning associated with a particular condition, take the case of Mrs. Yablonski, who was seen in the neighborhood health clinic because of severe hypertension. The clinic nurse, aware of the importance of patient teaching, spent considerable time with Mrs. Yablonski, explaining hypertension, the particular treatment prescribed, how the medication was to be taken, and the possible consequences of not taking it properly. Being very conscientious, the nurse evaluated Mrs. Yablonski's understanding of her condition and treatment recommendations, and was delighted to find that she was able to describe her condition and treatment in detail, as well as why the medication was important, and what might happen if her condition was left untreated. No other barriers to following recommendations, such as inability to purchase the medication, were identified. The nurse felt that the teaching session had been effective and felt certain that Mrs. Yablonski would be extremely dedicated to following recommendations.

Mrs. Yablonski was seen at the clinic weekly for blood pressure checks, but each week her blood pressure remained elevated. The physician at the clinic continued to add antihypertensive medications to her treatment regimen, until at last it was decided that she should be referred to a nephrologist for further evaluation. Mrs. Yablonski had been at the referral center for about a week when the nephrologist called her physician, saying that all her tests had been negative and that her blood pressure was currently being controlled on one medication. Upon questioning Mrs. Yablonski closely, the nephrologist had found that she had not taken any of the medication prescribed by her physician. When Mrs. Yablonski returned to her regular physician, he questioned her, puzzled as to why she would deliberately not take her medication when she had understood the possible consequences of stroke and even death from her lack of adherence with the regimen. Mrs. Yablonski replied that she viewed her hypertension as deserved punishment for indiscretions she had committed in the past and therefore was accepting the consequences as "payment" for her previous behavior.

Mrs. Yablonski's severe guilt, as described in the example, would warrant counseling and therapy that were beyond the scope of patient teaching. However, had either the physician or nurse been aware of Mrs. Yablonski's attitudes about her condition earlier, appropriate referral for counseling could have been made, and an exposure to a potentially dangerous situation could have been avoided. In addition, a needless expenditure of time, effort, and money could have been saved. Had the physician or nurse developed a relationship with Mrs. Yablonski that enabled her to share her feelings, the situation also might have been avoided. By referring Mrs. Yablonski to the appropriate health professional for the help she needed, the patient teaching intervention might have had a more successful outcome.

In this instance, Mrs. Yablonski's attitudes, not her level of knowledge, were the determinant of the degree to which she followed the physician's recommendations. Had her attitudes and the meaning she attributed to her condition been identified, counseling and support could have been recommended that could help her resolve her feelings, and consequently could have made patient teaching efforts more effective.

SOCIAL INFLUENCES

We are all part of a social group, whether it consists of family, friends, culture, or a religious group. Each group establishes its own norms or values to which individuals within the group are expected to subscribe and adhere. Deviation from these values or norms can be the source of ridicule from the group or, in some cases, even expulsion. Consequently, when conducting patient teaching, it is also important to consider the patient's system of social support, the attitudes and beliefs of the patient's social group, and cultural and religious influences that may impact on patient's receptiveness to information or ability or willingness to follow recommendations.

Social groups provide a sense of self and give individuals a framework within which to interpret various aspects of life and ways of responding to a variety of events. Values of health and health care, the meaning of illness, and which treatments are deemed acceptable or unacceptable are learned within the social group.

Patients and health professionals frequently come from different social groups and therefore may have different values, beliefs, and assumptions. Those differences may emerge not only with regard to reactions and interpretations of various life events but also with regard to health and health care in general. If health professionals make the assumption that everyone subscribes to the same values they do, or if differences in values between health professionals and patients are not identified, there is a basis for misunderstanding as well as a barrier to communication.

The influence of social groups is extremely relevant to patient teaching. Without an understanding of the influence of these groups, health professionals can spend much effort conducting patient teaching that is irrelevant, or at times offensive, to patients who have values different from their own. Patients will not only be unwilling to follow recommendations that conflicts with their own beliefs or values but may also be alienated from consulting with the health professional in the future. Consider the case of Mrs. Taylor.

Mrs. Taylor had just delivered her fifth child. The postpartum unit of the hospital had established a regular patient teaching session for all patients who had delivered. Part of the program consisted of a module on contraception. The nurse proceeded to teach Mrs. Taylor about contraception according to the teaching protocol. She observed that Mrs. Taylor appeared to be more withdrawn as the teaching went on. The nurse interpreted this to mean that she was tired and concluded the session, asking Mrs. Taylor if she had any questions about the information. She also mentioned that she would come back at a later time to continue the teaching session. Mrs. Taylor replied that she had no questions and that it would not be necessary for the nurse to return. Puzzled, the nurse left the room, charting that Mrs. Taylor was uncooperative and resistant to patient teaching. Had the nurse taken some time before the teaching session began to gather some information about Mrs. Taylor as an individual, she would have learned that the woman was a devout Roman Catholic who was very much opposed to birth control. Not only had the nurse not considered the patient's needs when conducting the teaching intervention, she had created a barrier to further teaching as well. The nurse's time was wasted, and the opportunity for future teaching was lost.

Other instances of the influence of social groups may be illustrated by various patients' use of folk remedies or folk healers. Folk remedies endure in various areas of the United States because they are well-known, trusted, accessible, and inexpensive. Advice about folk remedies passed down through generations by trusted individuals is often perceived as more helpful than prescribed medical treatments. Recommendations may be distrusted when given by a health professional whom the patient does not know, and with whom he or she has insufficient rapport. In other instances, prescribed treatments may be expensive and/or distasteful and may not give the immediate results the patient expects.

In some cultures, folk healers are still intermingled with modern medicine. It does little good to try to discredit folk remedies or the advice of folk healers that has been given to the patient. The folk healer may be a trusted part of the patient's healthcare system. Efforts to discredit such healers or the advice given by other trusted members of the patient's social group may only alienate the patient, who may distrust the health professional in the first place. It may be far better to identify the folk remedies tried by the patient or recommended by the folk healer and add medical technology to them rather than demanding that the patient abandon them altogether. At times, the consequences of folk practices may be somewhat difficult to deal with, especially if they can cause harm. Such a situation is illustrated in the case of Mr. Romaro.

Mr. Romaro, a patient of Filipino-American background, was seen at a family practice center for epigastric pain. After a number of diagnostic tests, the physician diagnosed him as having an ulcer and immediately prescribed a regimen of medication and a restricted diet. Mr. Romaro was referred to the dietitian for diet counseling, during which the diet and its purpose were explained. Sometime later, the patient returned to the clinic with severe worsening of symptoms. On evaluation, the physician indicated that surgery might be necessary and admitted Mr. Romaro to the hospital for further observation. The dietitian who had conducted the original diet teaching visited Mr. Romaro in the hospital. In the course of the conversation about the extent to which he had followed the prescribed diet and treatment regimen at home, Mr. Romaro revealed that he had not taken the medication and had disputed the dietitian's advice to avoid spices in his food. In the Filipino culture, spices were actually considered to have healing properties. Obtaining a variety of spices from his grandmother, the patient had proceeded to spice his food liberally. When his condition became worse instead of better, he attributed the worsening to the prescribed treatment and discontinued it.

Such situations are indeed difficult to work with. In this case, the patient's beliefs and folk remedies were the cause of potential harm. Had the dietitian recognized these beliefs in the initial teaching interaction, they could have at least been considered. The situation might have been different had the dietitian been alert to the possibility of culture differences rather than conducting teaching in a standardized manner. The dietitian might have taken the time to ask Mr. Romaro about his beliefs and perceptions. The dietitian might have said: "I know very little about the Filipino culture. I find sometimes even when Americans are born in this country, the traditions of our heritage, of our grandparents and great-grandparents, are still important to our own lifestyle. Are there any special things that we've talked about with regard to your diet that are contrary to any of your cultural or personal beliefs?" Additional information about multicultural issues is addressed in Chapter 7.

To discount patient beliefs completely only creates a barrier to establishing trust in the future. To correct erroneous beliefs or to criticize advice given the patient by well-meaning friends or relatives destroys trust and rapport. In such instances, it is far better for health professionals to identify the beliefs and health practices of patients, and to work within the patient's framework to build a stronger relationship for the future. Rather than arguing with beliefs, the health professional will be more successful and effective if the patient's beliefs are considered and incorporated into the teaching plan.

Social influences also impact patients' feelings about appearance. In the United States, being slender is considered an attractive attribute. Many take the saying, "You can never be too thin or too rich," quite seriously. It is quite easy for health professionals to assume that all patients view obesity as undesirable, not only in terms of appearance, but also in terms of health. Not all cultures hold similar views, however. In many cultures, eating occupies a central role in life. Overweight may actually be viewed as attractive, with obesity a sign of health and prosperity. In some cultures, food may be equated with love and affection.

In these instances, talking with patients about weight control and its importance may disavow their own perceptions and beliefs and set the stage for failure. If health professionals view obesity as a health threat, it is far more important in the initial teaching session for the professional to assess what eating means to the individual and to begin working with the patient at that level. If the patient's beliefs about weight appear firmly ingrained, it may be better to begin talking with them about other means of prevention or other aspects of the medical regimen than to attack their basic views. On the other hand, if the patients see eating as a source of comfort and solace or a way of dealing with stress, health professionals may gradually incorporate their views into the discussion, helping them recognize other ways of coping and reducing stress.

The patient's family and peer group are important social groups that have considerable influence over the patient's ability and willingness to carry out medical recommendations. Even if the patient has sufficient knowledge, skill, motivation, and attitude to carry out the treatment recommendations, the patient's family or peer group can have a profound impact on the extent to which he or she actually follows health advice. It would seem, for instance, that a patient who has solicited advice about weight control, been counseled accordingly, and appears to have an understanding of the diet regimen would have an excellent potential for success. Surely, the healthcare professional would have every reason to believe that teaching would be effective. However, if the family considers obesity attractive and criticizes the patient's efforts to lose weight, without additional counseling and support, the patient may fail to reach his or her goal. In many instances, the health professional's best teaching efforts are undermined if the family does not understand the condition for which the patient is being counseled, or the importance of treatment itself, if medical recommendations conflict with their beliefs.

On the other hand, family and friends can also be a great support and can reinforce the patient's effort to maintain the prescribed treatment or recommendations. Families who offer support of the patient in following a treatment regimen are tremendous aids in helping the patient adhere to recommendations.

The importance of understanding the individual patient and the significance of the influence of the social group, especially family or peers, can be illustrated by the case of Ms. Elkins, a 19-year-old female, who was diagnosed with insulin-dependent diabetes at the age of 14. Her diabetes had been fairly well controlled, and Ms. Elkins appeared to manage her diet and insulin quite well on her own throughout high school. She had adapted well to her condition and seemed to have an excellent understanding of diabetes and the importance of diet and the accurate administration of insulin. She also was shy and withdrawn, having few friends and dating very little during high school. When she went to college, she had found it extremely difficult to meet and interact with new people. Much to her delight, during the second semester at college, she met a young man who appeared to be interested in her. They began to see each other on a regular basis and eventually talked of plans to marry.

Upon coming to college, Ms. Elkins had immediately established herself with the University Health Service and had regular follow-ups for her diabetes. Although her diabetes continued to be well controlled for the first 8 months, at one visit to the health service, her blood glucose levels were significantly elevated. The nurse reviewed Ms. Elkins' activity levels and found them to be no different. Her skill at drawing up the insulin and injecting it was observed, and she performed these procedures correctly. Her understanding of her diet was excellent. All levels of knowledge and skill appeared adequate. Because Ms. Elkins had apparently accepted her diabetes, there was no reason to suspect that her fluctuating sugar levels were caused by denial or maladaptation to the disease. The physician, puzzled by the changes in her condition, placed Ms. Elkins in the health service infirmary to stabilize her blood sugar levels. During visiting hours, the nurse observed that a young man had come to visit who appeared quite important to Ms. Elkins.

After the visitor left, the nurse began talking to Ms. Elkins about the young man. In the course of conversation, the nurse learned that the man, now Ms. Elkins' fiancé, believed very strongly that illness was a state of mind and that most illnesses could be overcome by force of will. He felt that with the proper attitude, Ms. Elkins could gradually be weaned off insulin and could live a life free of medication. Because of his importance to her and her fear of losing him, Ms. Elkins periodically skipped her insulin dose or decreased the amount. The nurse, now aware of the problem, arranged to have Ms. Elkins' fiancé come to the infirmary early the next day for a joint teaching session with her. In the session, rather than confronting his beliefs directly, the nurse talked about the role of stress in disease and acknowledged that there were still many things that were unknown about the interaction of body and mind and the development of disease. The nurse continued that although emotions could still influence the course of disease, the mind alone could not always help a process that had already begun. She then began to describe the disease process of diabetes, explaining why insulin was important in its treatment. Ms. Elkins fiancé had had limited previous understanding of diabetes. Neither had he had a firm understanding about the role of insulin and the consequences of non-adherence to the prescribed dosages. He was encouraged to help Ms. Elkins become emotionally strong and calm to help reduce the chances of her developing complications. He was also helped to understand that taking insulin was a very important part of helping Ms. Elkins reach this goal.

The beliefs, attitudes, and values of a variety of social groups have a tremendous impact on patients and must be taken into consideration in planning and conducting patient teaching. Just as it is important to consider these variables, and especially those related to the patient's social group in terms of culture or ethnic background, it is also important not to overgeneralize about the patient's social group. Even within the United States, there may be differences between groups of the same ethnic origin, depending on where in the country members were raised. Likewise, there are differences between persons of various ethnic backgrounds who were raised in the United States and those raised in the country of origin. As with all social groups, each member is still an individual, with a personal makeup and past experiences that make him or her different from every other member of the group. Each patient must still be considered uniquely individual. The key is to gather information about each individual to determine his or her values, beliefs, or perceptions and to translate those values, beliefs, or perceptions into patient teaching.

ENVIRONMENTAL FACTORS

A variety of factors within patients' environments can also influence how effective patient teaching will be. Factors such as patients' geographic location, their living arrangements, financial status, daily schedule, or type of employment can all influence the extent to which they are willing or able to carry out recommendations. Factors that facilitate or impede patients' following recommendations may include the physical environment, the work environment, their schedules, or the personal lifestyles they have adopted. Even when patients have sufficient and appropriate knowledge, proficient skills, appropriate attitude, and strong support, unless obstacles within the environment that may interfere with adherence to recommendations are identified, patient teaching may still be less than effective.

When environmental factors contribute to nonadherence, the issue may not be a function of unwillingness or inability to follow recommendation, but rather a result of lack of knowledge of how changes could be made so that the recommendations could be followed. In these instances, part of patient teaching must be directed toward helping patients devise a plan whereby recommendations can be followed despite environmental limitations.

Such was the case of Ms. Knoll, an elderly patient who lived alone in the same farmhouse where she had been born. Because of symptoms she had been experiencing, she sought advice from the physician practicing in a small town several miles from where she lived. After examining Ms. Knoll, the physician ordered a variety of tests, one of which necessitated the collection of a 24-hour urine specimen that would have to be refrigerated. The physician carefully explained the tests to Ms. Knoll, how she should prepare for them, and why they were being ordered.

In concluding patient teaching, the physician asked Ms. Knoll if she felt she would be able to carry out the preparations for the tests, or if she felt there were any problems that would make preparations difficult for her. Ms. Knoll replied that she felt there were several problems. First, transportation was difficult for her because she did not drive and was, therefore, dependent on her niece or neighbors to take her places. Although they had always been very willing to help her, the tests were scheduled at such an early time that she was reluctant to ask them. She continued that she had never had electricity put into her farmhouse and, consequently, had no means of refrigerating the urine specimen even if she was able to collect it. After the physician was made aware of Ms. Knoll's situation, the physician began to help her find alternatives and resources that would enable her to have the tests. Because environmental factors were identified early, diagnostic procedures and understanding subsequent treatment were not delayed, and the physician's original efforts at teaching were not wasted.

Patients must sometimes be helped to identify strategies that would enable them to follow recommendations. Telling a person who has had a myocardial infarction to avoid going up and down stairs can be unrealistic for the patient whose bedroom and only bathroom are on the second floor. Patients' ability and willingness to follow recommendations will be much greater if the health professional identifies environmental restrictions and teaches patients how to modify their environment appropriately.

Other barriers that may affect adherence may arise from patients' work or home environments in terms of lifestyle or responsibilities in their daily lives. For example, it is unrealistic to expect a prenatal patient with symptoms of preeclampsia to maintain full bed rest when she has several other preschool-aged children at home as well. To maximize the possibility that she will adhere to advice, the health professional must explore with the patient the possibility for provision of childcare during the day while her husband is at work. Likewise, a patient whose occupation involves considerable bending and stooping may not be able to follow advice to avoid bending and stooping altogether.

It may be far more profitable, in terms of effectiveness and efficiency, to teach the patient proper body mechanics when stooping or bending, or to help the patient identify alternative methods for accomplish tasks, which may minimize bending and stooping.

THE NATURE OF TREATMENT RECOMMENDATIONS

At times, even though the patient may be receptive to information and may fully intend to carry out recommendations, factors in the recommendations may become cumbersome, noxious, or burdensome in other ways that eventually impact on adherence. The nature of treatment recommendations alone can interfere with a patient's ability and/or willingness to comply with the prescribed treatment. Complexity of the treatment regimen, frequency, and duration of treatment have all been linked to adherence (Dunbar-Jacob, Burke, & Puczynski, 1995; Wing et al., 1986). The more treatments or medications prescribed, the more adverse the effect on patient adherence (Vollmer, 1998). Adherence with the treatment recommendations also decreases with the length of time it must be carried out (Rosenstock, 1988). Although side effects may not affect patient adherence in all instances, from a practical standpoint, it makes sense that a patient experiencing unpleasant side effects from a medication or treatment may be prone to discontinue the regimen (Spiker, 1991), and in some patient populations, side effects can be a major contributor to nonadherence (Harris, 2008). In other instances, patients may be unable to take medications in their prescribed form. For example, a patient may have difficulty swallowing pills but be able to take a liquid form of the medication. If the patient's inability to take the medication in pill form is not identified, however, the patient may elect to discontinue the medication without telling the health professional.

In areas of diet, exercise, or other lifestyle changes, patients may find the regimen too difficult, too time consuming, or too unpleasant to follow. Health professionals can greatly enhance the chances that patients will follow recommendations by exploring their perceptions of the recommendations and their ability and/or willingness to carry them out.

INFLUENCE OF DIFFERENT PERSONALITY STYLES

Personality has been defined as the underlying cause of individual behavior and experience within a person (Cloninger, 2008). Each patient has a unique personality style, which includes a combination of traits and characteristics that determines how they interact with others, how they respond to experiences, and how they make decisions. These characteristics can predispose individuals to certain emotional states, affect their reaction to various situations, determine coping strategies for stress, and subsequently affect behavior (Lazarus, 1966).

Although a number of individual factors affect patients' receptivity to information and the degree to which they will adhere to treatment recommendations, their basic personality plays a large role as well. The outward manifestations of personality in terms of behavior are a reflection of the individual's internal mental state. Individual personality characteristics give individuals some degree of consistency and predictability regarding their behavior. Personality traits, to some extent, determine which aspect of illness individuals may find anxiety provoking and which techniques they will employ for coping with their anxiety.

Some personality traits exhibited by patients can be very frustrating for the health professional unless they are recognized as such and consequently taken into consideration when working with patients. The more aware health professionals are that some behaviors patients exhibit relate not only to their reaction to illness but also to their basic pattern of behaving in a nonillness state, the better they will be able to tailor their teaching methods to the individual patient so that it will be most effective.

Take, for example, Ms. Lee. Although she frequently demanded information, direction, and support from Dr. Franklin, she rarely followed the recommendations given. She appeared to be impulsive and unpredictable, praising Dr. Franklin's teaching efforts on some occasions and devaluing them on others.

Patients such as Ms. Lee can be very demanding and produce feelings of anger and frustration in the health professional who is trying to conduct patient teaching. This type of behavior may, however, merely be a reflection of the patient's basic personality style and its manifestation as a reaction to illness. Ms. Lee, in demanding information and support, may be expressing a need for security and reassurance that Dr. Franklin will continue to be there for her. Ms. Lee's case illustrates potential conflict that many patients experience in which they desire the health professional to rescue them and, at the same time, fear that the health professional will desert them.

Luckily, Dr. Franklin took time to look at Ms. Lee's behavior objectively, rather than personally, and, in an attempt to discover techniques that would help him to work more effectively with Ms. Lee, he discovered that by using gentle but firm limit-setting, Ms. Lee responded by becoming more cooperative and easier to work with.

Another personality type may be illustrated by the example of Mr. Boyce, who had been diagnosed as having hepatitis. The nurse, Mr. Morgan, became increasingly annoyed when trying to conduct patient teaching with Mr. Boyce, who seemed preoccupied with trivial details, seeking more and more information and, at the same time, being rigid and indecisive. Mr. Boyce became extremely upset at any variation in routine and became very demanding in his expectations of Mr. Morgan. In discussing his difficulty in working with Mr. Boyce with his colleagues, it became evident to Mr. Morgan that Mr. Boyce was desperately struggling to maintain a sense of control in light of an illness he viewed as threatening. With this insight, Mr. Morgan changed his approach to Mr. Boyce, offering a more methodical approach to patient teaching and engaging Mr. Boyce in fuller participation.

Mr. Williams illustrates yet another example of personality style. He seemed very flamboyant with exaggerated emotions. He had been scheduled for coronary artery bypass surgery. The nurse, Ms. Applebaum, had been assigned to conduct the preoperative teaching. It became very difficult for Ms. Applebaum to conduct the teaching session because Mr. Williams seemed to have little interest in understanding the procedure, stating very dramatically that he just wanted to have the procedure done and over with. Ms. Applebaum talked with Mr. Williams' family physician in an attempt to gain some insight into Mr. Williams' reaction that might enable her to conduct patient teaching more effectively. She discovered that Mr. Williams appeared to need much attention and reassurance of his physical prowess. Consequently, when she returned to the teaching situation, she offered reassurance regarding his postoperative course and offered him an opportunity to express his own fears about the procedure and consequences.

Some patients are, by nature, suspicious and mistrustful. When such individuals become ill, these traits may become exaggerated so that every question, procedure, or recommendation is closely scrutinized, and motives of the recommendations questioned. Although such hypervigilance on the part of patients can be annoying to health professionals who, during patient teaching, are asked to justify everything, by attempting to understand patients' viewpoints, being supportive, and keeping some interpersonal distance, health professionals can maintain objectivity and conduct patient teaching more effectively.

PATIENTS' SELF-VIEW

Patients' psychological makeup is multidimensional, and various dimensions impact how patients view themselves in the context of health and illness. The more health professionals know about individual patients, the more this knowledge can be used to customize patient teaching. When patient teaching is tailored to the individual patient, the more likely it is that the intervention will be effective. Learning about how to best approach individual patients does not always have to be a time-consuming process. Considerable information can be gained from simply listening closely to patients' statements and observing their behavior.

Self-Identity

How individuals view themselves is linked to various factors; however, one factor is their self-identity, or how they categorize or define themselves in a broader context. Individuals may have several categories of self-identity, such as cultural identity, religious identity, gender identity, family role identity, or occupational identity, to name a few. Whether the patient's self-identity is as a professional, homemaker, neighbor, or a number of other labels patients may use in their own self-description, it is important for health professionals to know what the patient's self-identity is and to utilize this information in patient teaching. If, for example, the patient's self-identity is tied to his or her role as a business executive who is capable of handling considerable responsibility and making decisions, placing them in a dependent, passive role during patient teaching would most probably decrease the likelihood of teaching effectiveness and may even alienate the patient. Or, if a patient's identity is strongly linked to cultural heritage, regardless of citizenship, knowledge of the patients self-identity can help the health professional utilize that information in how they conduct patient teaching. For instance, a patient appearing to be from the Pacific Rim, but who was born and educated in the United States and speaks perfect English, may still have a strong cultural identity based on the heritage and influence of their parents and grandparents, with associated customs or taboos.

Self-Esteem

Another factor involved in how individuals view themselves is their self-esteem, or how much they like themselves. Self-esteem is linked to the individual's sense of self-worth and value, or how positively or negatively they view themselves in relationship to others (Blascovich & Tomaka, 1991) or how well patients like themselves and feel that others like them. Although research studies have shown little association between self-esteem and health behavior (Baumeister et al., 2003), the relationship between self-esteem and psychological well-being—including depression, anxiety, and alienation (Blascovich & Tomaka, 1991)—have definite implications for patient teaching. Individuals' degree of self-esteem determines how much confidence they have in themselves and their abilities, as well as how capable they believe they are in handling certain situations and performing certain tasks (Bernard et al., 1996).

Illness alone can lower an individual's self-esteem. When individuals already have low self-esteem, illness may contribute to lowering self-esteem further. Individuals with low self-esteem may have little confidence in their ability to learn new material or new skills and may seem overdependent on others. When health professionals are aware of and sensitive to a patient's lack of self-esteem, they can use this information in the patient teaching situation to make the intervention more effective.

Take, for example, Mrs. Sanders, a 78-year-old woman who had broken her hip, had surgical repair, and had done well in the postoperative period. The nurse, Ms. Friedman, in preparation for Mrs. Sanders' discharge, came to her room to begin patient teaching about her management at home. Although Mrs. Sanders was alert and seemed capable of understanding the information, she told Ms. Friedman that she must wait until her daughter arrived because she probably would not be able to comprehend the directions anyway. When Mrs. Sanders' daughter came, Ms. Friedman proceeded to give them both the information but found that Mrs. Sanders repeatedly made self-deprecating remarks, such as, "I'm just too stupid to understand" and, "I never could do anything right."

After the teaching session, Ms. Friedman spoke with Mrs. Sanders' daughter and learned that Mrs. Sanders had always been self-critical and had a poor opinion of herself and her abilities. Ms. Friedman used this information in her next teaching session with Mrs. Sanders, making a special effort to compliment Mrs. Sanders and to reinforce her performance. In so doing, Ms. Friedman was attempting to build Mrs. Sanders' self-esteem and also her self-confidence, both of which would be necessary if she was to participate in her own self-management at home and if the patient teaching intervention was to be effective.

Self-Efficacy

Self-esteem is linked to self-efficacy, the degree to which an individual believes they have control over events in his or her life. Some people believe that most of what happens to them is determined by outside forces, and that they have little control over their own destiny. Such individuals usually have a fatalistic view, which may be demonstrated by statements such as, "I suppose I'll try to follow the recommendations, but no matter what I do, it probably won't do any good anyway. Some things are just meant to be." Other people believe that they have considerable control over their lives and believe that their own actions can, at least in part, determine their destiny. Statements such as, "Even though it's hard to stay on a low cholesterol diet, I know if I want to be around to see my grandchildren grow up, I'd better stick to the diet" are indicative that the patient believes that his or her actions do, at least to some degree, have a relationship to health consequences.

Self-Concept

Self-identity, self-esteem, and self-efficacy are all linked to the individual's self-concept. Self-concept involves not only how individuals view themselves but also their perception of how others view them. Self-concept can have an impact on both the individual's receptivity to patient teaching as well as their willingness to follow recommendations. Self-concept is usually consistent with an individual's attitudes, experiences, and behaviors. If information presented to the patient, or the recommendations given, are in conflict with the individual's self-concept, his or her level of involvement in patient teaching and level of adherence will likely be affected. Take for example, Mr. Jones. Mr. Jones had been a powerlifter since high school, winning many regional and state championships. He continued in college and as an adult, competing in various weight lifting events. Mr. Jones viewed himself as strong and proficient, as did many of his friends and colleagues. At age 30, on the way to a competitive weight lifting event, Mr. Jones was in a motor vehicle accident, which resulted in severe musculoskeletal injury. After an extended period of hospitalization, the physician advised Mr. Jones that because of his injuries he would need to end his career as a weight lifter, but prescribed a course of rehabilitation that would enable Mr. Jones to regain mobility and function for most day-to-day activities. Rather than fully participating in rehabilitation in order to get back to normal as soon as possible, Mr. Jones became fearful, angry, and frustrated, refusing to participate in many of the rehabilitation activities. His self-concept as a strong, capable man had been firmly entrenched in weight lifting. Without that activity, his self-concept had been shattered. Consequently, his altered self-concept caused significant setback in the rehabilitation process.

Whether or not health professionals share their patients' views, ignoring their views or attempting to argue with them about their views makes the patient teaching interaction less than effective. A better approach is for health professionals to use this knowledge to make the teaching interaction more effective. If, for example, an individual believes that he or she has little control over his or her health, rather than making the patient more dependent, or arguing and barraging the patient with statistics regarding risk behavior, the health professional will probably be more effective in identifying some immediate concerns, establishing some short-term goals, and helping the patient experience some control and results from accomplishing the goals.

PATIENTS' ADJUSTMENT TO ILLNESS

The onset of chronic illness can have major impact on physical, psychological, social, economic, and recreational aspects of an individual's life. Illness usually elicits some type of response in patients. These responses, which are highly individual, are influenced not only by the personal experiences and beliefs of the individual, but by those of others and of society at large. Patients differ remarkably in their perceptions of, and reactions to, what may appear to be similar medical conditions. Although some patients react mildly to a disease or condition that might devastate others, others may react with significant emotional and physical discomfort to conditions many people would consider minor. Individuals also vary on how susceptible they believe they are to disease and illness and, consequently, on how they perceive advice about preventive health measures.

Obviously, a variety of psychosocial factors determines individuals' reactions to illness and, consequently, their reactions to recommendations and advice given. Each patient's perspective on health, illness, and medical care itself is based on their self-identity, self-esteem, self-efficacy, and self-concept, as well as their developmental stage and life situation. Before health professionals can conduct meaningful patient teaching resulting in positive patient teaching outcomes, there must be a clear understanding of patients' perceptions about their illness, its meaning, and what they have as goals for the future.

When individuals become ill, their view of themselves changes. Patients' reactions to the fact that they are ill or could be ill involve their attitudes toward illness, how they interpret symptoms of illness, and their attitudes about health care. Their perspectives will determine how willing or able they are to listen to health recommendations and to follow them.

Health professionals frequently assume that patients seeking health advice are motivated to follow recommendations in order to get well or stay well. However, if patients believe that no matter what they do they cannot get well, it is unlikely that they will follow recommendations they consider to be of no benefit. In other instances, health professionals may assume that the reasons patients are seeking health advice is because of the symptoms they present. This may not always be the case. Symptoms patients present may be an entrée to access health advice for other issues that the patient may feel reluctant to bring forward, or other issues may overshadow the concern patients have for presenting symptoms. Recommendations given for conditions or symptoms that are not of primary concern to the patient have less chance of being followed accurately.

For example, Mrs. Connors sought help from her physician with regard to weight control. She was referred to a dietitian for dietary counseling and regular follow-up visits to monitor her weight loss. Mrs. Connors failed to keep her follow-up appointments. When she was next seen by her family physician several months later for an unrelated problem, it was noted that she had failed to lose any weight. Had the physician and dietitian listened closely to Mrs. Connors' needs, they might have recognized that although weight loss was Mrs. Connors' presenting problem, her concern about her blood pressure actually seemed more pressing. Mrs. Connors' unspoken concern was her blood pressure because she had a friend who had recently suffered a stroke. Consequently, Mrs. Connors had done extensive reading on the subject and discovered that obesity was linked to high blood pressure and stroke. After visiting the physician, however, and finding that her blood pressure was normal, it was no surprise that she did not comply with the physician's or dietitian's recommendations. In Mrs. Connors' view, because her blood pressure was normal despite her obesity, the recommendations for weight loss made little sense.

Health professionals may assume that patients who are sick are naturally motivated to follow recommendations that will help them to get well. Patients' response to illness and their associated behaviors, however, may not always be consistent with this philosophy. How individuals respond to illness is dependent not only on their personal characteristics and life situation, but on the reactions of others.

Although there are a number of explanations that have been developed to try to explain patients' reaction to illness, Parsons introduced the concept of the *sick role* in 1951. Parsons noted that the sick role itself is of a mixed nature, and described the sick role with the following characteristics:

- Individuals are not viewed as being in power to overcome being sick by themselves; some therapeutic process is necessary for patients to recover.
- While patients are ill, they are not expected to function in their normal role or to perform their regular obligations.
- Patients are expected to want to get well.
- Patients are expected to seek help for their illness and to cooperate with health professionals in their attempts to get well.

Although there are a number of other explanations of why people behave as they do when confronted with illness, some aspects of this model may apply to certain individuals. People who are ill are generally excused from social responsibilities. For instance, people are usually not expected to come to work when they are sick; individuals are excused from school because of illness; an individual would not usually be expected to host a social event or attend a meeting when they are ill. Although people are excused from activities when they are ill, they are also usually expected to take some responsibility for their recovery, such as seeking medical treatment or engaging in behaviors that will help them recover. Most people do not want to be sick and most do not view the sick role as a positive role to occupy. Therefore, many patients will be self-motivated to get better and will be encouraged by others to participate in activities that facilitate their recovery. For some individuals, however, if they are dissatisfied with the social role they occupy, they may view the sick role as preferable. These patients may be less motivated to follow recommendations that would help them recover and return to their former social role and obligations. In these instances, illness legitimizes a dependency that they enjoy, or brings them attention they desire from others. In these instances, a patient's motivation to retain his or her sick role may be greater than the motivation to get well. Although he or she may engage in the socially acceptable behavior of seeking medical advice, he or she may sabotage the treatment plan by not following recommendations. In some instances, patients may vacillate between their wish to be independent and get well and their wish to remain ill and be taken care of.

In the framework of the sick role model as described by Parsons, not fully participating in efforts to get well is socially unacceptable. Consequently, nonadherence may not be easily recognized and can be subtle. Take, for example the case of Mrs. Jensen, a part-time seamstress who had begun experiencing numbness and tingling in her thumb. Her physician diagnosed mild carpal tunnel syndrome, prescribed anti-inflammatory medications and wrist splints, and encouraged her to modify her sewing activities so as not to aggravate the condition further. Mrs. Jensen filled her prescription, and from all indications appeared to be taking her medication as recommended. She always appeared at the physician's office wearing the wrist splint and told the physician she had given up her part-time seamstress position. Mrs. Jensen's family pitched in, helping her do housework, and neighbors brought food over frequently so Mrs. Jensen would not have to strain her hand by cooking Although from all outward appearances it appeared that Mrs. Jensen was fully participating in her treatment, she continued to sew in her spare time, an activity she did not inform her physician of, nor an activity of which her family was aware.

Illness itself may be used for coping with personal problems. Mr. Wilson had recently graduated from college with a degree in secondary education. Shortly after taking his first job in a secondary school, he developed flu symptoms and severe congestion. Consequently, he was advised to stay at home for several days. Although Mr. Wilson sought medical care, received a prescription for medication, and had been advised to rest at home, he continued to appear at school, walking there in bad weather, staying for a few hours, and then returning home. He neglected to pick up his medication at the pharmacy until several days after his visit with the physician, saying that he was too ill at the time to go to the pharmacy. The symptoms became progressively worse; Mr. Wilson continued his routine of performing his tasks at school in a perfunctory way and then returning home. He continued to seek medical care for his continuing symptoms. After several visits to the health clinic, the nurse began to note that although Mr. Wilson appeared consistent in keeping his appointments, he did not appear to be following any of the other recommendations that, presumably, would help him recover at a more rapid rate. In talking with Mr. Wilson before the appointment, the nurse questioned him about his job. Through their discussion, the nurse noted that although Mr. Wilson stated that he was happy with his work, he also appeared rather vague and uncomfortable when talking about how he perceived his level of performance. Through further discussion with the physician, the patient later revealed that he was quite unsure of his ability to perform in the classroom setting. Because of his illness, expectations about his performance were lowered, both by students and his peers. In addition, Mr. Wilson was actually somewhat martyred by coming to school despite his illness.

Health professionals may not be able to immediately determine patients' levels of motivation to get well or to remain sick. Although there may not be a conscious motivation on the part of the patient to stay in the sick role, it behooves health professionals to be aware of the possibility and how, in turn, the impact such unconscious motivation can have on patient teaching and adherence. Astute observation and deduction can help health professionals identify patient motivation level, and give the health professional the opportunity to begin open discussion of patients' feelings and fears, so that other ways in which patients needs can be met can be determined.

Patients' responses to illness may also relate to their life circumstances. Economic consequences of illness, both acute and chronic, can have an impact on patient receptivity to patient teaching and, subsequently, on adherence with recommendations. Although many occupations include fringe benefits of paid sick days, or even time off with pay to keep medical appointments, other occupations have no such benefits. In the latter instance, days taken off from work because of illness or for follow-up visits to the physician may result in decreased income. Unfortunately, many people in these employment situations may also be part of a socioeconomic group that can least afford to take days off without pay. In such cases, no matter how complete patient teaching is about the necessity of staying home or of returning for a follow-up visit, the likelihood of adherence with such recommendations is slight.

Awareness of these factors by health professionals may help them to modify the teaching plan to maximize the patient's ability to follow recommendations under the given circumstances. For instance, it may be sufficient for the patient to call the health professional with a progress report rather than returning for an office visit. Or, if the patient cannot remain at home for a week, the provision of rest periods during the working day may be sufficient. If rest or follow-up visits are crucial, the health professional may refer the patient to a community agency where financial assistance for such expenses may be available. It is essential, in any case, that the problem be identified and addressed if patient teaching is to be effective.

Economic consequences of illness may, on the other hand, in some cases cause a reverse reaction by the patient. If patients receive financial benefits as long as they are ill, and especially if the opportunity for satisfactory employment is slight, they may be less likely to follow recommendations that help them return to health and optimal functioning if their benefits will be diminished or eliminated as a result.

Economic factors may also affect patients' willingness to follow preventive health practices, especially if patients do not view the benefits of the prescribed recommendations as being worth the cost. For example, people with limited economic resources who have no perceived illness may choose not to follow their physician's recommendations to return for an annual physical. Women with limited financial resources may neglect mammography because of the cost. Patients being treated for strep throat or a urinary tract infection may not return for a follow-up visit because of the cost, even though its importance has been explained to them. Awareness of patient's financial concerns enables the health professional to problem solve with the patient to reach alternatives. When patients' concerns are identified and considered, the health professionals may also weigh the benefit of making recommendations they know the patient will not be able to follow.

Reactions to illness are also dependent on the meaning the patient attributes to the condition. For instance, in some cases, the patient may believe that the illness is a punishment for a transgression earlier in their life. If they believe the illness is a punishment for their transgression, they may be less likely to follow recommendations to aid in recovery or management of their condition if they believe recommendations interfere with punishment that is "deserved."

Such was the case of Mr. Anderson, who was diagnosed with non-Hodgkin's lymphoma. After diagnosis he refused any treatment saying to the nurse, "I knew it would catch up to me eventually. I cheated on my wife the first year we were married, and I've been cheating on her ever since. She's a good woman. I don't deserve her. This is now my comeuppance." In other instances, patients may experience guilt because they perceive their behaviors as contributing to their illness. This was true of Mr. Taylor who developed chronic obstructive pulmonary disease after years of heavy smoking. He refused most patient teaching, and became increasingly nonadherent with treatment recommendations, stating "I brought this all on myself. I should have given up smoking years ago, just as my physician and family asked me to do. I've made my bed. Now I guess I'll have to lie in it."

TEACHING PATIENTS HOW TO COPE WITH ILLNESS

Illness can alter an individual's identity, distort thinking, and disrupt the way patients view themselves and the world, creating a sense of vulnerability. Illness shatters the patient's magical belief that they are immune from illness, injury, or even death. Some patients may react with superstition, grasping at straws, searching for ways in which they can again feel they have control. Patients may lose a sense of security and of cohesiveness. They may become frustrated and angry at their sense of helplessness or loss; some become self-absorbed, others more dependent. While some patients may draw on hidden resources of strength and courage, others become more demanding, clinging, or regressed. Some patients may react with rebellion against medical advice. Life may become a maze of inconveniences, hazards, and restrictions. With others, recommendations may be adapted into their regular way of life.

One goal of patient teaching is to help patients to reorganize, make necessary changes, and maximize their resources. This requires a nonjudgmental attitude on the part of the health professional, along with an effort to understand patients and their reactions. If health professionals are unable to empathize with patients and their reactions, such nonacceptance may well in itself push patients into nonadherence.

For example, Ms. Capanio, at age 20, was diagnosed with diabetes. Despite extensive patient teaching sessions with the dietitian, she continued having difficulty following the prescribed diet. During teaching sessions, the dietitian observed that Ms. Capanio showed little interest in the diet instructions. Rather than criticizing Ms. Capanio for her lack of interest or for failure to follow the diet, the dietitian hypothesized that she was having difficulty adjusting to the dietary restrictions, and that she may be having difficulty accepting the condition in general. The dietitian demonstrated an understanding of Ms. Capanio's feelings by taking time to listen to her expound on the difficulties she was having with the recommendations and allowing her to vent feelings. Such actions showed acceptance of, as well as interest in, Ms. Capanio as a whole. Such an atmosphere is more conducive to working with patients to institute behavior change than one created by an adversary relationship. The latter may result in rebelliousness or rejection by patients, limiting the chances to achieve the level of adherence desired.

Illness often creates a sense of uncertainty and unpredictability. Patient teaching can help to restore a sense of control, reducing the patient's sense of powerlessness. By helping the patient understand manifestations of the condition and its treatment, and identifying issues the patient is facing, the patient and health professional work together toward initiating strategies that facilitate adjustment. In order to best help patients cope, health professionals need some understanding of various strategies and methods patients use to cope with the stress they are experiencing as a result of their condition and their attempts to adapt to it.

UNDERSTANDING PATIENT COPING STRATEGIES AND METHODS OF ADAPTATION

Stress is a normal part of life even in healthy individuals, and anxiety is a normal reaction to stress. Stress cannot be easily quantified and may be defined differently by each person. In order to cope with stress, individuals mobilize a set of psychological strategies, which are used to decrease the impact of the stressful situation (Billings & Moos, 1981; Krohne, 1993; Lazarus & Folkman, 1984). Each individual has his or her own unique way of dealing with stress through coping strategies, which have been learned and developed over time. Coping is complex and multifaceted (Livneh & Cook, 2005). Individuals use these coping strategies to manage, tolerate, or reduce stress and to restore equilibrium. In illness, stress may be more pronounced and related to biological, psychological, social, cultural, or environmental factors. A patient's ability to cope is dependent on the effectiveness of coping strategies, the patient's perceptions of the impact the condition has on various areas of his or her life, and the degree of threat the condition represents to the individual. Potential threats of illness as perceived by the patient may involve those to life or well-being; to comfort; to independence, privacy, autonomy, and control; to identity and self-concept; to future plans and goals; to social and family relationships; and to economic well-being (Falvo, 2009).

When confronted with illness, patients usually revert to the predominant coping strategies that they have used effectively to cope with stress in nonillness situations. There are times, however, that stress becomes so great that old coping strategies are no longer effective, or old coping strategies are no longer appropriate to the situation. In these instances, new coping strategies must be developed. Effective use of coping strategies reduces anxiety, helps patients attain emotional equilibrium, and helps patients avoid incapacitation from fear, anxiety, or other emotions that interfere with their progress toward goals. Although use of coping strategies can be helpful, overuse can have the opposite effect, immobilizing the individual. Coping is effective and adaptive when it helps individuals reduce stress and help reach their goals. It is ineffective and maladaptive when it inhibits the individual from reaching goals, or contributes to negative health consequences.

How well individuals have coped with stress in the past will determine to some extent how they will cope with the stress of illness. Many people take their health and body for granted, as well as their continued ability to perform daily activities and social roles. When people are ill—whether the illness is acute or chronic, a result of trauma, or a slow progressive disease—their lifestyle is interrupted, and varying degrees of stress are experienced.

Coping can help patients adjust to their condition and follow recommendations; however, coping can also be detrimental to positive patient teaching outcomes. The health professional's awareness of patient coping strategies can promote and foster those that contribute to positive outcomes and help patients develop new strategies to replace those that are no longer effective in their current situation.

Denial

Denial is a coping strategy used to negate the reality of a situation. In some instances, denial can be useful as a protective device to prevent the patient from experiencing overwhelming stress. For instance, in the event of a sudden, catastrophic event that the individual finds devastating, denial of the seriousness of the event and its implications can reduce anxiety, enabling the individual to adjust to the reality of their situation at their own pace. Extended or overuse of denial can also have negative effects and become dangerous if it prevents the patient from seeking medical care or following advice that is crucial to recovery or palliation of a condition.

An example of the negative effects of denial as a coping strategy can be illustrated by the case of Mr. Jacob, who had consulted a physician because of what he considered indigestion. After examination, the physician concluded that Mr. Jacob's symptoms were the result of coronary artery disease. The physician recommended cardiac catheterization and also recommended that Mr. Jacob schedule an appointment with the nurse for a patient teaching session about heart disease as well as about the procedure. Mr. Jacob failed to make the appointment for patient teaching and did not have the cardiac catheterization. He confided to his wife that the physicians were just out to make money, and that he was not going to have any expensive tests just to prove he had indigestion. Mr. Jacob had experienced such anxiety at the potential diagnosis and procedure that he unconsciously implemented denial as a coping strategy. To have attended the teaching session or to have had the procedure would have been admitting that the possibility of the diagnosis existed.

As illustrated above, denial can have an impact on patient teaching efforts as well as on adherence. When confronted with patients who are using active denial as a coping strategy, forcing the patient to acknowledge facts only increases their stress and anxiety, and thus strengthens denial. Health professionals should not actively engage in challenging the patient, but should rather assess the level of patient anxiety and seek other means to help reduce anxiety, so that the patient is able to relinquish their false beliefs.

In other instances, patients may exhibit ambivalence about learning more about their condition. They may adopt a "What you don't know won't hurt you" attitude, consequently resisting patient teaching. To force information upon the patient is of little benefit. A more efficient approach at this point is to determine what information is essential for the patient to have, proceeding to deliver it in bits and pieces, and monitoring patient acceptance along the way.

At the other extreme, some patients cope with anxiety about their illness by wanting to know every detail of their condition and its treatment. The use of this coping strategy can help reduce anxiety by reducing patients' fear of the unknown and by helping patients feel as if they are in control of their condition. This type of reaction can, quite naturally, be beneficial to patient teaching. Health professionals should not only provide initial information to patients in this situation but also make sure that continuing information is provided about their illness and progress.

Determining how patients are coping with their condition can help the health professional judge how much and what type of information may be the most useful for the patient at that particular time. By remaining open, supportive, and empathetic to patient feelings, the health professional will gain the opportunity to continue to monitor and be available to the patient in the future. Gradual provision of information when the patient is ready to receive it can reduce patient anxiety, and create increased receptiveness to additional information and incorporation of the information into their life.

Compensatory Strategies

Illness can cause alteration in an individual's activities or areas of function. When this occurs, individuals may mobilize strategies to compensate for real or imagined limitations experienced due to illness by becoming stronger or more proficient in another area. For example, Ms. Lawrence had enjoyed dancing as a creative outlet of self-expression; however, after developing emphysema, she was unable to maintain a level of physical activity that would enable her to participate in dancing. Instead, she developed writing skills as a means of self-expression, thus increasing self-satisfaction without requiring excessive physical strain.

Although use of compensation as a way of coping can be highly constructive, it may also be destructive and detrimental. For instance, Ms. Kapur felt unattractive after having a radical mastectomy. She compensated for her perceived unattractiveness by becoming promiscuous. Another example of the detrimental use of compensation is the case of Mr. Atkins, a cardiac patient who was no longer permitted to smoke but compensated by eating excessively.

Providing patients with information alone about their condition and treatment in each of these instances is insufficient if patient teaching is to be effective. Recognition of patients' reactions can, however, be the first step in helping them learn to cope with their feelings about their condition and treatment, and can subsequently increase the potential effectiveness of future patient teaching. Through patient teaching, health professionals can help patients learn ways to maximize existing skills or to develop new skills to replace those lost because of their condition. In the instance of Ms. Lawrence described earlier, the health professional helped her explore other activities, which helped her to find another creative outlet for the one she had lost.

Taking time to understand the patient's reactions helps the health professional establish an alliance and atmosphere of collaboration in which issues that may serve as barriers to reaching treatment goals, or may be detrimental to the patient's health status can be addressed. In the cases of Ms. Kapur and Mr. Atkins described above, regardless of the health professional's view, it is the patient's perceptions, values, and judgments that are the issue. Whether or not the health professional believes that Ms. Kapur is unattractive or that overeating is as detrimental as smoking is of little consequence. It is the patient's perceptions and beliefs that determine behavior. Consequently, awareness of these factors can help the health professional develop strategies and interventions to address them.

Benign Forgetfulness

Some patients may cope with stress experienced as a result of their condition by subconsciously expelling disturbing facts or situations from their minds. Benign forgetfulness can be beneficial in helping patients reduce anxiety, as was the case of Mr. Goldberg, a patient who had experienced serious burns and was treated in the regional burn center. After leaving the hospital, and in preparation for future reconstructive surgery, Mr. Goldberg forgot the severity of pain he had experienced during dressing changes, and instead remembered the kindness of the hospital staff and the positive aspects of rehabilitation. In this instance, forgetting the unpleasant part of his experience contributed to his willingness and ability to continue to progress with rehabilitation and treatment recommendations.

As with most coping strategies, benign forgetfulness can be positive and help patients cope with stress and adjustment to their condition, but in some instances it can also interfere with adjustment and subsequently with adherence. For example, Mr. George, who consistently experienced periodic chest pain and shortness of breath "forgot" about his symptoms when he went to see his physician and consequently failed to report them. Ms. Carlon consistently "forgot" her dental appointment for a root canal.

Benign forgetfulness can take considerable energy, and while it can be helpful, it can also be potentially harmful. Recognition of the patient's excessive use of this coping style can help the health professional either reinforce its use when it is helpful, or mobilize a process to enhance more realistic confrontation of the problems or issues at hand when its use is detrimental. When benign forgetfulness is used in a productive manner, such as in the case of Mr. Goldberg, facilitation of this coping style can help the patient achieve more positive health outcomes. If the health professional recognizes that a patient appears to be a "chronic forgetter," and that such behaviors are detrimental to his or her care, intervention may be necessary. Rather than approaching the patient in an accusatory way, the health professional may spend some extra time talking with the patient about his or her feelings concerning the condition and treatment. Through a relationship of trust and mutual respect, the health professional will be better able to help the patient identify and disclose feelings, making a problem-solving approach more likely.

Avoidance

Some people use avoidance as a strategy to cope with their illness. Avoidance involves removing oneself emotionally or physically from a situation that is anxiety producing. If the situation is potentially dangerous, then avoidance or withdrawal from the situation is, of course, constructive. For example, Ms. Little had been in recovery from alcohol dependence for 2 years. She received an invitation to attend a reunion of her "drinking buddies" who she knew still abused alcohol, and many of whom were still alcohol dependent. She knew that most of them continued to be in denial of their substance abuse and dependence and that they would place extreme pressure on her to join them in drinking. Although she had faith in her ability to resist the temptation to drink again in most situations, she feared her ability to resist in the situation with her former friends. Consequently, she declined their invitation and avoided the activity.

A less constructive use of avoidance as a method of coping may occur in cases in which individuals refuse to learn needed behaviors because of fear of failure. Such was the case of Mr. Carter, who had recently experienced an above-the-elbow amputation as the result of a farming accident. Although the prosthetist continued to attempt to work with Mr. Carter, and show him how the prosthetic device could be used to increase function, Mr. Carter refused to learn to use the prosthesis, fearing that he would appear silly or would be unable to perform the activities adequately.

Avoidance may be used emotionally as well as physically. Emotional avoidance may also have positive and negative aspects. In some instances, emotional avoidance may be a necessary part of helping patients cope with stresses experienced because of their illness. For instance, Ms. Angeles was diagnosed as having a meningioma of the temporal lobe of her brain. Although the physicians explained that the surgery posed some risk and loss of function as a result of removal of the meningioma, Ms. Angeles remained calm, avoiding thoughts of any potential negative effects, and focusing only on positive outcomes. Emotional avoidance may, however, interfere with patients' health care and treatment, as well as their receptiveness to patient teaching. Mr. Markel underwent surgery for removal of his pancreas after being diagnosed with pancreatic cancer. After surgery, when the nurse attempted postoperative teaching regarding insulin administration, as well as teaching him about the enzymes he would need to take daily, she noted that he was inattentive and often changed the subject. The nurse suspected that the Mr. Merkel felt overwhelmed by the diagnosis as well as the treatment, and was avoiding learning the information as a way of coping with his anxiety. Through this realization, the health professional was better able to employ strategies to help Mr. Merkel cope with his anxiety, thus increasing the probability that the teaching would be effective.

Role Modeling

Role modeling as a coping strategy consists of internalization of attributes of another into an individual's own behavior or attitudes. Role modeling can, of course, have positive and negative consequences depending on the behaviors or attitudes the patient chooses to model. When the patient models behaviors and attributes of others who are managing their illness and treatment successfully, use of role modeling is positive. Health professionals may foster this type of role modeling for patients to help them adjust to their illness by doing such things as asking a patient with an ileostomy who is now leading an active life to visit a hospitalized patient with a new ileostomy. Role modeling may have a negative effect, however, if patients are exposed to others with similar conditions who have not adjusted well to their illness, or are managing their illness in a maladaptive way, such as a patient on dialysis who is nonadherent to dietary recommendations between dialysis treatments. In these instances, the patient may incorporate the negative attitudes or behaviors expressed by these individuals. In this case, role modeling would be detrimental to the adjustment of the patient. In patient teaching, knowledge of this method of coping can be facilitated by providing role models that help the patient achieve positive health outcomes. Knowledge of role modeling as a strategy patients use for coping can also help the health professional identify those instances in which negative effects emerge.

Regression

In regression, individuals revert to immature behavior that was part of their behavioral repertoire at an earlier stage of development. It is used to some degree by most persons when ill, whether the illness is acute or chronic, major or minor. Most people, even when only ill with the flu, exhibit more child-like behaviors, such as a short temper, excessive emotionality, or dependency, than they may normally exhibit in their adult roles. Regression, especially in the early phases of illness, may even be necessary to eventual recovery. For instance, patients with a new myocardial infarction, as part of treatment, may need to regress to a more dependent role, giving up some of their responsibility and allowing others to take care of them. In such instances, regression is important to avoid relapse. As recovery begins, however, the health professional may need to encourage the patient to become more independent. Patients who use regression on an ongoing basis establish maladaptive adjustment patterns to their illness that can have a negative impact on their ability to function as well as to follow recommendations. Awareness of a patient's use of regression as a coping strategy can help the health professional adapt teaching accordingly by anticipating potential problems with patient receptivity to information or problems that may interfere with the patient following recommendations.

Blaming Others

When an individual's thoughts, impulses, or ideas produce stress or are unacceptable to the individual, he or she may cope by attributing his or her thoughts or feelings to others, or blaming individuals for his or her condition. For example, Mr. Mason sustained an injury to his spinal cord resulting in paraplegia. The injury occurred in a car accident in which Mr. Mason was driving while intoxicated. His wife was in the car, but had not been drinking. She was uninjured. Mr. Mason exhibited hostile behavior toward his wife every time she came to visit, telling her that had she had distracted him in the car and consequently blamed her for the accident and his injury.

In another instance, Ms. Andrews sustained an injury that caused her to limp and use a cane. She had negative feelings and views about people with a disability prior to experiencing her injury. Instead of recognizing her own feelings about people with disability, however, she ascribed negative feelings to others, believing that everyone looked down on her now that she appeared disabled, regardless of whether or not negative behaviors were actually exhibited by others. As a result, during a teaching session in which the physical therapist was monitoring ambulation with a cane, Ms. Andrews exploded by saying, "You don't think people with a limp like mine have much worth in the world, do you?" If the physical therapist had been unaware of the reason behind Ms. Andrews' statement, he could have been bewildered or defensive. However, because he recognized the reaction as a coping strategy, he was able to explore Ms. Andrews' feelings and help her learn how to cope more effectively.

If the health professional is aware of the patient's anxiety and feelings, patient teaching can be better adapted to first cope with the patient's feelings, then proceed to teach the patient about their condition or treatment. For example, in the preceding situation, rather than responding to Ms. Andrews' statement with a comment like, "How can you possibly accuse me of such a thing when I've spent so much time trying to help you?" the physical therapist may offer a response such as, "No, I don't feel that way, but I'm wondering why you asked. Tell me a little more about your question."

By encouraging patients to talk about their feelings, health professionals demonstrate acceptance as well as gain insight into patients' feelings and behavior. To pursue patient teaching without first gaining more information about patients' statements sets a precedent for less-than-desirable outcomes.

Again, although adherence cannot be guaranteed by helping patients cope with their feelings, the more accepting patients are of their own conditions, and the more they feel the health professional is accepting of them and willing to listen to their concerns, the greater the possibility is that patient teaching will be effective.

Patients may also blame their own nonadherence on others, stating that family members are uncooperative or unsupportive of their treatment. Because this may be true in some instances, health professionals should assess the validity of patients' statements before drawing conclusions. If it is found that, in fact, the patient's family appears supportive and actively encourages the patient to follow recommendations, then the use of blaming as method of coping by the patient may be suspected. The health professional can then incorporate interventions into patient teaching by which the patient is gradually helped to cope with anxiety and to accept responsibility for his or her own actions.

Self-Blame

Anger may be a reaction experienced by patients when they develop a chronic illness or disability. Rather than expressing anger toward others, however, individuals may cope with their feelings of anger by turning them inward and blaming themselves. For example, Mrs. Sherman developed significant hearing loss after experiencing a blow to the head when she fell during a rock climbing trip with her husband, an activity she never enjoyed and only reluctantly participated in. During her aural rehabilitation, her husband became very impatient with her hearing loss and was relatively unsupportive of her attempts to compensate for her hearing loss with alternative means of communication. Instead of becoming angry with her husband, Mrs. Sherman frequently made statements such as, "I have no patience. I'm so selfish. I expect entirely too much from my husband. It must be so difficult for him to have to live with me now. If I only had been paying more attention, I never would have fallen. I brought all of this on myself, and now he has to suffer because of my stupidity."

Health professionals who are alert to cues such as those demonstrated by Mrs. Sherman can help patients recognize and express those feelings, thereby offering the opportunity to discuss problems that may interfere with patient teaching or their following recommendations.

Rationalization

Rationalization consists of providing false reasons, which are socially acceptable to explain what is often considered unacceptable behavior to offset negative feelings or consequences. This method of coping enables people to invent excuses for not doing things they know they should have done, as well as helps to soften disappointment if desired goals were not met. Rationalization can affect patient teaching as well as adherence. For example, when Mr. Giovanni, who has diabetes, went off his diet, he rationalized, "I've been following my diet very well, so I deserve a little break. It won't hurt to cheat every now and then."

Appointments for various diagnostic procedures may be missed for reasons such as, "They probably wouldn't find anything wrong, anyway, so it's better that I gave up my space for the test to someone who really needs it," or, "There's no reason to spend the extra money for a mammogram, since I have no family history of cancer. I'll use the money I would have spent had I kept the appointment to support the local food bank."

Rationalization as a method of coping can also play a positive role in adjustment to illness. For example, when a chronic illness limits the amount or type of activities in which a patient may participate, statements such as, "I've really had more time to get to know my family since I've been ill and haven't been able to run around doing all the things I used to do. All the other things I used to do were pretty meaningless, anyway," or a statement such as, "I never really enjoyed running in competition anyway. Just watching as a bystander is much more pleasant" may illustrate examples of rationalization as a method of coping that can be reinforced.

Reinforcing the positive use of rationalization can enhance effectiveness of patient teaching. In instances in which rationalization produces negative outcomes, health professionals might direct teaching efforts toward helping patients discuss their feelings about their condition, gradually helping them accept a more realistic view of their condition and treatment.

Hiding Feelings

At times, patients react to their illness or to those around them by behaving in a way that is opposite to their actual feelings or thoughts. For instance, the patient using this method of coping may appear to be excessively cheerful and unconcerned about the illness and its implications while actually feeling very frightened and sad. In other cases, patients may be especially charitable to family members or individuals around them when they are really feeling hostile and resentful. Hiding feelings as a coping strategy can be of value in adjusting to illness if it helps the patient maintain behavior that is socially acceptable. It is detrimental to the extreme that it is self-deceptive and prevents the patient from recognizing and dealing with actual feelings that, if hidden long enough, may result in additional stress.

Through accurate assessment and understanding of patient behavior, health professionals can individualize patient teaching so that it is better suited to the individual needs and reactions. Whether this involves referral to another professional or merely encouraging patients to verbalize their feelings, by recognizing the impact of patients' reactions to their condition, health professionals are in a better position to alter the approach during patient teaching, which in turn makes patient teaching more effective by increasing the chances of adherence.

Redirecting Emotions

Most people, at one time or another, as a method of coping, redirect emotion from the person or situation originally provoking the emotion to an individual or object that seems less threatening. Take the example of Mrs. Garcia. Mrs. Garcia came into the hospital for a hysterectomy because of fibroid tumors. During the routine preoperative exam, the physician also found a lump in her right breast. Upon biopsy, the lump was found to be malignant and a mastectomy was performed. Mrs. Garcia was angry with the physician for giving her an unfavorable diagnosis, and one she had not expected. Rather than venting anger at the physician, Mrs. Garcia became very disagreeable and hostile to the nurse who attempted to teach her about self-care at home. Rather than directing her emotion to the physician, who was actually the source of her anger, Mrs. Garcia expressed anger toward the nurse, a person she felt was less intimidating and less threatening.

Although redirecting emotions can be valuable in the sense that it allows the individual to release strong emotions without threat of retaliation from individuals who may be perceived to be more powerful, those people at whom anger is directed may become alienated. Because she recognized Mrs. Garcia's behavior as a reaction to stress, rather than becoming angry in return, the nurse attempted to encourage Mrs. Garcia to express her feelings. She discontinued further teaching until Mrs. Garcia was more receptive to the information she planned to give her.

Excess Activity

Some people react to illness by engaging in activities that distract them from thinking about their condition, or by thinking about things other than the issue at hand. Although this coping style can be positive if used in a constructive way (dwelling on symptoms or implications of disease to the point of inactivity is not therapeutic), its overuse prevents people from dealing realistically with their feelings about their condition and the limitations that may be imposed by it. Such was the case of Mr. Hester, recently diagnosed with diabetes. Mr. Hester's insulin was to be regulated on an outpatient basis. He was also to return as an outpatient for regular patient teaching sessions. At the outpatient visits, Mr. Hester always seemed extremely pressed for time. He frequently seemed preoccupied with other commitments during the sessions. Both the physician and the nurse noted that Mr. Hester appeared to be overextending himself. When Mr. Hester had an appointment for patient teaching, he often called saying that he had a pressing commitment that kept him from attending. If he arrived, he seemed preoccupied throughout the visit, saying that it would have to be short because he had numerous other appointments to keep. He failed to read most of the materials about diabetes given to him, saying he had been too busy even to glance through them.

The physician and the nurse questioned Mr. Hester about how he might be able to arrange some of his other activities to allow more time for his scheduled appointments. He replied simply that there was no other way to arrange the schedule of an extremely busy man. Aware of the possibility that Mr. Hester might be anxious about his condition and using excess activity to escape facing his feelings, the physician and the nurse used each contact with Mr. Hester to allow him to express some of these concerns until gradually he became aware of his behavior as a method he had been using to avoid dealing with his diabetes.

Diverting Feelings

One of the most positive and constructive of all methods of coping can be the diversion of unacceptable feelings or ideas into socially acceptable behaviors. Patients with a chronic illness or traumatic injury, for instance, may have particularly strong feelings of anger or hostility about their diagnosis or the circumstances surrounding their injury. If the energy of their emotions can be diverted into positive activity, however, the result can be quite beneficial. An example of such a diversion may be the case of Mr. Meyer with Parkinson's disease. He has strong feelings about having the condition but directed his strong emotion into a positive activity. He worked relentlessly to establish a local Parkinson's disease support groups for patients and their families, participated regularly in fund-raising activities for research on Parkinson's disease, and often appeared as a guest speaker at public and civic events about Parkinson's disease.

Health professionals who notice this method of coping during patient teaching can facilitate positive outcomes through its use. Patients may be encouraged to participate in teaching activities directed to other patients with their condition or they may be asked to serve as role models for those with similar conditions, discussing common areas of concern and offering suggestions and support.

As with all other methods of coping, indiscriminate use or misuse of diversion can be very negative. Ms. Lankford, after experiencing a spinal cord injury resulting in paraplegia, began going to casinos to gamble; soon, her gambling turned to excess and she accumulated massive debts. Before health professionals facilitate the use of diversion by patients as a coping method, they should carefully assess the patient's attitudes and knowledge base to be sure that diversion is being used in a positive way and that the patient actually is serving as the positive role model, and is not detrimental to the patient's well-being.

HELPING PATIENTS COPE

Reactions of patients to disease, illness, or disability are variable. Methods of coping discussed in this chapter are common behaviors learned and used by all individuals to some degree to adjust and adapt to the stress of daily life. Such methods of coping, because they are part of everyday life, are normal and desirable. In illness, individuals may use the same methods for coping with stress that they used in their healthy state, or coping patterns may become more pronounced. The danger emerges when use of coping methods is excessive and prevents the individual from adapting or reaching their potential, or when their use is detrimental to their health or well-being.

In the case of an individual with illness, overuse of coping methods can interfere with medical care or treatment. It is not within the role of most health professionals conducting patient teaching to attempt to drastically alter patients' methods of coping. In order to facilitate patient teaching effectiveness, however, it is important for health professionals to be aware of different coping methods so they are better able to understand the behavior of individual patients, anticipate potential barriers to effective patient teaching, and work toward solutions to overcome barriers or problems. The better able health professionals are to view the situation from the patient's perspective, the less likely they are to avoid or dismiss the challenging patient. By understanding patients' perceptions of health and illness, health professionals are better able to empathize and be more sensitive to the patients' needs, thus conducting patient teaching accordingly. By understanding patients' coping methods, health professionals are better able to encourage patients to express their feelings and to encourage and motivate them to follow recommendations.

Allowing patients to express their fears and feelings in a nonjudgmental, empathetic atmosphere, along with developing a sensitive teaching plan based on patients' needs, can reduce patient anxiety, help them to adjust to their condition, and maximize the probability that they will adhere with recommendations.

Patients' anxieties or other concerns can interfere with the effectiveness of patient teaching. Timing of patient teaching is important, especially to the patient's readiness to learn. Early after diagnosis of serious illness or injury, for example, patients may focus only on the restrictions imposed on them by their illness. They may see few positive aspects in information offered during patient teaching. Although at this stage, patient teaching may not have an immediate impact, it is important for the health professional to meet with the patient to begin to establish a relationship. This early intervention should be directed toward laying a foundation for effective teaching later. Initially, patients may have little awareness of the implications of their condition and their reactions to their condition may be minimal. Building rapport with the patient during the early stages of the patient's illness helps to establish a relationship that will be better able to withstand possible later reactions of anger, frustration, or depression that patients may exhibit.

As patients eventually begin to recognize the impact of their condition on their lifestyle or on longevity, or when they begin to realize the extent of loss or limitation, they become anxious—not necessarily in proportion to the seriousness of the illness. During this phase, anxiety may interfere with learning. Instead of bombarding patients with extensive information at this time, it may be far more productive to effective teaching outcomes to assist them to express their fears, questions, and concerns. Acceptance of patient fears and concerns rather than offering superficial reassurance helps to build trust and rapport, which can later facilitate patient teaching. Such phrases as, "Oh, I'm sure everything will be fine," or, "Lots of other people have your condition," are likely to be rejected by patients and can establish barriers that interfere with further teaching effectiveness.

To help patients cope with their anxiety, any number of combinations of the coping methods discussed in this chapter may be used. If methods of coping are severely impaired so that they are interfering with medical care or the individual's ability to function, referral to other health professionals for in-depth counseling may be indicated. Such suggestions may, however, be met with resistance if offered by a health professional who has not established a trusting relationship with the patient. Blind persistence at patient teaching at this stage is a waste of time for both health professional and patient, and may also interfere with the possibility of patient teaching effectiveness later. It may be more important during this time for the health professional to gradually provide realistic information in a supportive manner, giving the information with sensitivity, but also not reinforcing the patient's false beliefs.

Patients who accept their condition and subsequent limitations may become depressed as they acknowledge perceived losses. The health professional conducting patient teaching should not equate this reaction with a lack of motivation or with an inadequate teaching plan or strategy. It is more productive at this point for the health professional to accept the patient's right to grieve, at the same time establishing short-term teaching goals that continue to move the patient forward. To discontinue efforts toward patient teaching totally or to provide only sympathy at this point may encourage the patient to assume maladaptive patterns of behavior that are not consistent with independence and positive health outcomes.

By accepting, acknowledging, and helping patients work through their initial reaction to illness, health professionals also help people adjust to new limitations or special treatment recommendations that may be associated with the illness. Effective patient teaching is dependent on patients reaching this point.

Although there is no way to accurately identify individual methods of coping, health professionals should be aware of their existence and explore possibilities. Rather than using a method of coping, the patient may be reacting to other environmental factors or to a differing belief system. Only through continued observation, assessment, and information gathering, can health professionals gain additional insight into patients' behavior. Behaviors of health professionals are important in facilitating this process. Facilitative behaviors for the health professional are illustrated in Table 4-1.

Table 4-1   Facilitative Behaviors

---

1. Recognize that coping styles are defenses patients use to protect themselves from threat, either real or imagined.

2. Recognize that patients' reactions to their conditions and recommendations will be determined by a combination of personal characteristics, learning history, and current circumstances.

3. Avoid stereotyped approaches to patients or to the content of information presented. Even patients with the same conditions do not adapt and react in the same way.

4. Set aside assumptions, and perform a careful assessment of the present beliefs, reactions, and circumstances of each patient.

5. Recognize that timing of the teaching intervention is important to the patient's readiness to learn and to work toward established goals. If a good relationship has not previously been established, suggesting that the patient change may lead to rejection of other education efforts.

6. Lay the foundation for effective teaching later with empathetic understanding.

7. Acknowledge and accept patients' fears, frustrations, and other reactions in an understanding way.

8. Give sensitive support that recognizes the stress patients feel.

9. In instances of denial or other coping styles that appear to be having a detrimental effect, gently and gradually confront the patient with reality.

10. Avoid agreeing with patients' statements that do not appear to be an accurate representation of fact; do not reinforce patients' negative beliefs.

11. If the coping style is not interfering with the patient's condition or treatment, leave it alone.

ENHANCING PATIENT ADHERENCE

Many variables impact an individual's ability and readiness to follow health-care recommendations and the impact of nonadherence varies in its magnitude of seriousness. Some acts of nonadherence may be trivial, but others can have significant impact on patients' health, well-being, and overall quality of life. The purpose of effective patient teaching is to help patients understand the purpose and importance of recommendations and to facilitate their ability to make informed choices. In order to be effective, patient teaching must be patient-centered, and based on individual patients needs, circumstances, and goals. Effective patient teaching is conducted in a nonjudgmental atmosphere of respect and support. Effective patient teaching facilitates patient adherence.

Facilitation of patient adherence, in this sense, should not be confused with coercion. Rather, increasing a patient's ability and willingness to follow recommendations should be directed to understanding the patient's supports and barriers to following recommendations as well as understanding and accepting patient goals. By listening to patient concerns, and understanding the patient's unique perspective and experience, health professionals begin to establish an atmosphere of collaboration and partnership. Health professionals conducting patient teaching should present themselves to patients as consultants rather than authoritarians, never criticizing patients' efforts or criticizing their failure to follow recommendations as expected. Patients may have their own reasons for not following recommendations. By providing empathy and support, as well as feedback and guidance, health professionals help patients to consider recommended changes and enhance their ability to follow them.

Understanding patient resistance, lack of motivation, and nonadherence can help health professionals become more effective in helping patients achieve health-related goals. One model that may provide insight into more effective ways of providing patients with the assistance needed to help them achieve their goals is the Stages of Change model (Miller, Sovereign, & Drege, 1988; Prochaska, DiClemente, & Norcross, 1992; Rollinick, Kinnersley, & Stott, 1993; Kushner, Levinson, & Miller, 1998), as discussed in Chapter 3. The model proposes that there are predictable stages of change and by understanding which stage of change the patient is currently experiencing, interventions appropriate to that stage can be instituted to motivate the individual to change. Even when change has been accomplished, change must be maintained. Patient teaching directed toward offering continued support, encouragement, and reinforcement can help patients maintain the changes they have made. Continued feedback about patient progress in maintaining their behavior is, in itself, reinforcing.

Effective patient teaching demonstrates respect for patients, their views, and their values. Effective patient teaching focuses on helping patients make informed decisions based on individual needs and circumstances. Health professionals should engage in ongoing examination of patients' feelings and experiences related to their illness and the recommendations. Listening to patients', and offering them support can help to empower them so that they are active and engaged in the patient teaching process and are participants in reaching positive health outcomes in accordance with their goals.

REFERENCES

Baumeister, R. F., Campbell, J. D., Krueger, J. I., & Vohs, K. D. (2003). Does high self-esteem cause better performance, interpersonal success, happiness, or healthier lifestyles? *Psychological Science in the Public Interest, 4*(1), 1–44.

Bernard, L. C., Hutchison, S., Lavin, A., & Pennington, P. (1996). Ego-strength, hardiness, self-esteem, self-efficacy, optimism, and maladjustment: Health-related personality constructs and the "Big Five" model of personality. *Assessment, 3*(2), 115–131.

Billings, A. G., & Moos, R. H. (1981). The role of coping responses and social resources in attenuating the stress of life events. *Journal of Behavioral Medicine, 4,* 139–157.

Blascovich, J.. & Tomaka, J. (1991). Measures of self-esteem. In J. P. Robinson, P. R. Shaver, & L. S. Wrightsman (Eds.). *Measures of personality and social psychological attitudes (*Vol I. pp. 115–160). San Diego, CA: Academic Press.

Cloninger, S. (2008). *Theories of personality* (5th ed.). Saddle River, NJ: Pearson/Prentice-Hall.

Dunbar-Jacob, J., Burke, L. E., & Puczynski, S. (1995). Clinical assessment and management of adherence to medical regimens. In P. M. Nicassio & T. W. Smith (Eds.). *Managing chronic Illness: A biopsychological perspective.* Washington, DC: APA.

Falvo, D. (2009). *Medical and psychosocial aspects of chronic illness and disability.* Sudbury, MA: Jones and Bartlett.

Gerteis, M., Edgman-Levitan, S., Daley, J., & Delbanco, T. L. (Eds.). (1993). *Through the patient's eyes: Understanding and promoting patient-centered care.* San Francisco: Jossey-Bass.

Harris, B. (2008). Psychopharmacology. In P. G. O'Brien, W. Z. Kennedy, & K. A. Ballard (Eds.). *Psychiatric Mental Health Nursing: An Introduction to Theory and Practice* (pp. 89–108). Sudbury, MA: Jones and Bartlett.

Krohne, H. W. (1993). Vigilance and cognitive avoidance as concepts inn coping research. In H. W. Krohne (Ed.), *Attention and avoidance: Strategies in coping with aversiveness* (pp. 19–50). Seattle, WA: Hogrefe & Hububer.

Kushner, P. R., Levinson, W., Miller, W. R. (1998). Motivational interviewing: What, when and why. *Patient Care, 32*(14), 55–56, 58, 64, 66, 69–72.

Lazarus, R. S. (1996). *Psychological stress and the coping process.* New York: McGraw-Hill.

Lazarus, R. S., & Folkman, S. (1984). *Stress, appraisal, and coping.* New York: Springer.

Livneh, H., & Cook, D. (2005). Psychosocial impact of disability. In R. M. Parker, E. M. Szymanski, & J. B. Patterson, (Eds.). *Rehabilitation counseling: Basics and beyond* (4th ed. pp. 187–224). Austin, TX: Pro-ed,

Mechanic, D. (1961). The concept of illness behavior. *Journal of Chronic Diseases, 15,* 189–194.

Miller, W. R., Sovereign, R. G., & Drege, B. (1988). Motivational interviewing with problem drinkers: II. The drinker's check-up as a preventive intervention. *Behavioral Psychotherapy, 16,* 251–268.

Parsons, T. (1951). *The social system.* New York: Free Press.

Prochaska, J. O., DiClemente, C. C., Norcross, J. C. (1992). In search of how people change: Applications to addictive behaviors. *American Psychologist, 47,* 1102–1114.

Rankin, S. H., Stallings, K. D. & London, F. (2005). *Patient education in health & illness* (5th ed). Philadelphia: Lippincott Williams & Wilkins.

Rollnick, S., Kinnersley, P., & Stott, N. (1993). Methods of helping patients with behavior change. *British Medical Journal, 307,* 188–190.

Rosenstock, I. M. (1988). Enhancing patient compliance with health recommendations. *Journal of Pediatric Health Care, 2,* 67–72.

Spiker, B. (1991). Methods of assessing and improving patient compliance in clinical trials. In J. A. Cramer & B. Spiker (Eds.). *Patient compliance in medical practice and clinical trials* (pp. 37–56). New York, NY: Raven Press.

Vollmer, S. (1998). Compliance: a physician's problem. *Family Practice Recertification, 20,* 91–108.

Wing, R., Epstein, L., Nowal, M., & Lamparski, D. (1986). Behavioral self-regulation in the treatment of patients with diabetes mellitus. *Psychological Bulletin, 99,* 78–89.

CHAPTER 5

Patient Teaching Through the Lifespan: A Developmental Perspective

LIFESPAN DEVELOPMENT

Knowledge of lifespan development is integral to effective patient teaching. Because the focus of attention in patient-centered teaching is the patient, rather than the disease, knowledge of lifespan development is fundamental for patient teaching to be effective. In order to fully understand the nature of issues, reactions, or concerns patients bring to the patient teaching interaction, their situation must be considered in the context of their stage of life. Knowledge of behavioral changes from conception to old age enables the health professional to view patient issues from a developmental perspective. This allows patient teaching to be altered in accordance with the patient's developmental stage and the specific issues that may be associated with their present point of development. Knowledge of lifespan development enables health professionals to use strategies appropriate to the individual, rather than conducting all patient teaching the same way, regardless of the patient's age or life stage.

Each stage of life has its own particular stressors or issues apart from those experienced because of illness. When people become ill, they experience additional stress. A patient's reaction to illness and the type of stress experienced may vary according to his or her developmental stage. The proper approach to patients differs at particular phases of development. For instance, children obviously differ from adults—not only physiologically, but in their reactions to illness. Just as treatment of illness differs in accordance with the patient's age, patient reactions and information needs and, consequently, the approach to patient teaching also differs at various developmental phases. Because patient reaction to illness differs at various life stages, the approach to patient teaching cannot be the same for patients who are at different stages of development, even though their conditions may be similar. Teaching a child with cancer is certainly different from teaching an adult with cancer. In most instances, language ability differs as well as the ability to understand concepts surrounding the condition and its treatment. The person who has a myocardial infarction at age 40 will require a different teaching approach than a patient who has a myocardial infarction at age 80. Lifestyle, responsibilities, and attitudes are different in middle age than at older age. These contrasts affect not only patients' reactions to their condition but also their reactions to and motivation for carrying out recommendations.

The approach to teaching patients about prevention or providing them with information about potential problems they may encounter also varies with age. Prevention teaching for a toddler, for instance, may involve talking with the parents about child safety, whereas prevention teaching for adults may range from awareness of health risk factors to stress reduction. An understanding of lifespan development helps health professionals to recognize specific patient needs at various life stages, enabling them to give support in accord with particular needs. Using a developmental approach to patient teaching can help health professionals understand and anticipate patients' reactions to illness, alter the approach to patient teaching in accordance with individual needs, and identify patient teaching needs related to a particular life phase, all while teaching about a specific disease entity.

Because all aspects of development are related, each life stage must be understood within the context of the patient's past experience and system of social support. Lifespan development is a continuing process without clear lines of demarcation between life stages. For purposes of discussion in this chapter, life stages will be delimited by category; however, phases of development for each individual, of course, are not separated nearly so clearly.

MODELS OF LIFESPAN DEVELOPMENT

There are a number of models of human development over the lifespan based on different theories and beliefs of researchers who have studied systematic age-related changes in behavior or functioning over time. For the most part, theories fall into three broad categories of models (Broderick & Blewitt, 2006):

1. Stage models in which individuals are viewed as sharing some common behavioral characteristics during different stages of life, which change as the individual moves through different life stages.
2. Incremental models in which behavioral changes occur as a gradual, step-by-step process throughout the lifespan.
3. Multidimensional models in which behavioral changes are the result of reciprocal interactions between internal characteristics of the individual and external characteristics of his or her environment.

Although no one theory or model of lifespan development has been accepted as the defining theory of behavioral change over a lifetime, most theories characterize development as incremental; not a stepwise progression, but rather a progression that continues from birth to death (Broderick & Blewitt, 2006). A lifespan approach to development emphasizes potential for change throughout an individual's life.

As individuals progress through life, development and change are not isolated from the influence of family, social network, and culture. Individual environments include material objects, expectations regarding gender- or age-related behavior, social structures, and behavior-guiding beliefs. Consequently, a lifespan development approach to patient teaching must also consider developmental issues in the context of the individual's social, cultural, and physical environment.

Although there are many ways of viewing development, depending on the particular theoretical approach, there are some commonalities on which most individuals studying development agree (Poole, Warren, & Nunez, 2007). One such commonality is the belief that development is gradual and incremental. A second commonality is the idea that influences help to shape future behavior, with current functioning built on previous functioning. A third commonality is that environmental influence on behavior may vary with time and context. For instance, although environmental influences shaped the individual's development at one point in his or her life, these influences may be altered when the individual finds himself or herself in a different situation at a different life stage.

PATIENT TEACHING WITH PARENTS AND CHILDREN

Teaching the Prenatal Patient

During the embryonic period, the individual is vulnerable to many hazards that influence development and health potential, not only in utero, but also over a lifetime. Because growth and development of the fetus are so dependent on the mother's health and well-being, the prenatal period is an extremely crucial time. Although health professionals obviously cannot deal with the fetus directly, effective teaching of the prenatal patient holds paramount importance for the well-being of the fetus. Consequently, in order to be effective, patient teaching during the prenatal period must consider not only the information that is critical to relay at this time, but also the mother's reaction to pregnancy. Her reaction may influence both her receptiveness to information and her ability or willingness to follow given recommendations.

Pregnancy, even if planned and wanted, can be stressful. A variety of physical and emotional changes are part of pregnancy. In addition, parents gain awareness of the considerable change in lifestyle and increased responsibility that will likely result after birth of the child. Health professionals should be aware of potential stressors associated with pregnancy as well as factors in patients' individual life circumstances that may be sources of support or that could cause additional stress. In this way, patient teaching can be adjusted in accordance with patients' specific needs.

Most parents have some ambivalence toward pregnancy and parenthood during the prenatal period, no matter how much the pregnancy is desired, especially if it is a first pregnancy. Having total responsibility for another human being may seem like an awesome task. The realization that parenthood means giving up certain freedoms and fantasies may also cause expectant parents to reflect on their own past, present, and future goals and aspirations. Although such ambivalence is natural, normal, and usually resolved, not all expectant parents recognize it as a normal phenomenon. Consequently, such feelings may cause them considerable guilt. Awareness of the potential for patient anxiety or guilt enables the health professional to promote discussion that encourages patients to share their feelings. Health professionals can relieve stress by helping parents express their feelings about the pregnancy and by offering reassurance, guidance, and support. Helping expectant parents prepare for their role as parents can also help reduce stress and help new parents develop confidence in their ability to assume their new role. During patient teaching, in addition to preparing them for the physical care of their infant, encouraging parents to discuss their feelings, and offering reassurance and practical advice, not only helps them develop confidence in their ability as parents, but it also creates an open atmosphere in which they feel comfortable addressing other feelings and concerns should they arise.

Stress may also be generated from the unknowns associated with pregnancy. Expectant parents vary in their sophistication and knowledge about pregnancy, labor, and delivery. Health professionals can do much to alleviate stress by teaching prospective parents about the emotional and physical changes to be expected during pregnancy and about what to expect during labor, delivery, and the postpartum period.

It should not be assumed that a patient who has had multiple pregnancies has little need for patient teaching or that stressors are not associated with her pregnancy. Individual responses to each pregnancy, as well as life circumstances, should always be considered and addressed. If there are other children in the family, patient teaching may also involve teaching parents how to talk with their children about pregnancy and birth, as well as helping the children prepare for the addition of a new family member.

Although health professionals may have more contact with the prenatal patient herself, the impact of other people in her life should not be underestimated. Including the expectant father in patient teaching promotes a feeling of inclusion for him in the prenatal and birthing process. It can also do much to reduce stress between the couple if there is a common understanding of changes to be experienced and what to expect. Not all prenatal patients have a partner supporting them through pregnancy. In such instances, health professionals must be aware of the additional stress this may cause and its impact on the patient's health behavior, as well as other potential sources of social support that may help the patient in carrying out the recommendations made in patient teaching.

Many parenting behaviors are learned from family members, friends, or other social contacts outside of the healthcare system. These individuals provide information as well as moral support and may even share care of the infant. An awareness of the patient's social network and their involvement in the pregnancy and future care of the infant helps the health professional identify and address any issues that may arise from involvement of family or friends. Whereas strong social networks can increase parents' satisfaction with parenting and help the parents gain confidence in their ability to care for their infant, not all social interactions are welcomed by the patient, and can be a source of stress. By identifying patient feelings about the degree and quality of social support they experience, the health professional is able to provide guidance and support as needed.

Just as it is important for the health professional to have an awareness of the patient's social support, it is equally important to be aware of lack of social support. Decreased access to supportive and competent social networks have been found to predispose to patient sense of isolation, lack of parenting skill, and the potential for abuse (Osofsky & Thompson, 2000). Knowledge of a patient's level of social support can help health professionals anticipate potential problems, offer support and guidance, and incorporate supplemental information about parenting skills in patient teaching interventions. It also allows the health professional to direct the patient to appropriate referral sources that may also be a source of support.

The approach to prenatal patients and significant people in their lives by the healthcare professional should be open-minded and have no preconceptions. Health professionals should be aware of parental attitudes about pregnancy and be alert to potential adjustment problems. When developing a patient teaching plan, health professionals should also be aware of a patient's current life situation, knowledge level, misinformation, and any other barriers that may affect the patient's receptiveness to information and ability or willingness to carry out recommendations.

Common informational content areas for most patients in this life phase are the normal emotional and physical changes associated with pregnancy, such as sexual activity during pregnancy, preparation for the newborn, diet counseling, preparation for parenting, and what to expect during labor, delivery, and postpartum. As with all patient teaching, more than this content must be considered. Especially in this phase of lifespan development, patient teaching may need to include a high degree of emotional support and awareness of barriers interfering with adherence to those recommendations that are crucial not only to the patient's own health, but also to the growth and future development of her infant.

Patient Teaching with Parents when Children are Patients

When the patient is a child, he or she should be included as much as appropriate for his or her age level in the teaching process. The fact remains, however, that in most instances it will be the child's parents who will supervise the degree to which recommendations for preventive health practices and/or treatment recommendations are followed. The health professional's ability to work effectively with parents is crucial to the effectiveness of the patient teaching interaction.

Health professionals conducting patient teaching must establish rapport not only with the child as the patient, but with the parents as well. Not only must the child's learning readiness be assessed, so must the parents'. In preparation for patient teaching, the health professional should assess the quality of relationship between parent and child and take the relationship into account during teaching interactions. Although some parents are open and honest with their children, and foster independence, others do not. Some parents provide structure and guidance while allowing their children the latitude to make some choices of their own, whereas other parents are rigid and controlling, allowing their children little freedom of thought or expression. In other instances, parents provide little structure or guidance, practice little rule enforcement, and essentially abandon the child emotionally. Therefore, the approach the health professional takes to patient teaching in each of these instances will differ.

Child-rearing practices can be a source of conflict and controversy. Rather than being critical, health professionals should use the relationship between the child and parent to its maximum advantage for patient teaching to be most effective.

In addition to the parent–child relationship, the degree of parent involvement in patient teaching depends not only on the cognitive ability and learning readiness of the child but also the ability of the parents to grasp the concepts. This ability can be hampered by parents' limited intellectual ability, their own degree of emotional maturity and responsibility, and, in some instances, their level of anxiety. Some parents, although concerned and well meaning, may have difficulty understanding information presented or directives that are to be carried out. In this instance, health professionals should alter their approach to patient teaching to meet the parents' as well as the child's ability to understand. When patient teaching is directed toward helping parents and the child learn how to manage a chronic condition, health professionals should be sensitive to the parents' perception of the child's condition, as well as the child's reaction, and deal with their concerns and anxiety as much as possible.

Patient Teaching with Children as Patients

Although patient teaching with children usually involves the parent or caregiver as a recipient of information as well as the child, health professionals should keep in mind that under these circumstances, the patient is still the child. Consequently, health professionals should direct patient teaching to the child in an age-appropriate manner.

When initiating patient teaching with the child, health professionals should introduce themselves to the child as well as to the parents or caregiver. To place the child at ease and to build rapport, health professionals should engage in friendly conversation about topics of interest to the child. When talking with children, health professionals should make an effort to speak with them at eye level. Children, just as adults, should be allowed the opportunity to express their concerns, as well as to ask questions.

Because health recommendations given to a child necessitates involvement and cooperation of a caregiver, health professionals should, as much as possible, present information in such a way as to establish a "team effort" involving parent or caregiver, child, and health professional. Having an understanding of development of children at different ages and what generally can be expected behaviorally and cognitively at each stage will assist the health professional to tailor patient teaching to best meet the individual child's needs.

AGE-SPECIFIC PATIENT TEACHING OF CHILDREN

Infancy

During infancy, patient teaching about the infant's health and care is, of course, directed toward the parent or caregiver. In most cases, patient teaching during infancy involves little time spent teaching about illness, unless there are congenital problems or other issues that arise. Considerable time is spent teaching the parents about development and about aspects of prevention and child care. In addition to helping parents learn what they should expect from their infant developmentally during the first year of life, teaching about issues of prevention such as infant safety and the importance of immunization are vital parts of patient teaching.

Infancy is a time of rapid growth and development (Gabbard, 2004). New parents may misinterpret many normal aspects of infant development and may view these changes as a deviation from the norm. Helping parents gain awareness of developmental milestones can help reduce parental anxiety and enable them to gain increased confidence. Parents with little experience in child care may also experience insecurity in their ability to care for their infant. Much of this can be alleviated by encouraging them to express their concerns, informing them of what to expect, and helping them gain the knowledge and skills that will enhance their self-confidence.

Infant development, although occurring at a rapid rate, does not occur at the same rate for all infants. Unless new parents are aware of this, they may experience anxiety when comparing their infant to other infants who may be developing more quickly. Teaching parents about normal infant development, as well as the range of individual differences, can relieve unnecessary anxiety and increase parents' enjoyment in watching their infant reach various milestones.

As the infant develops more physical skills, the importance of exploration of self and the environment becomes paramount in stimulating further infant development. Patient teaching may also involve increasing the parents' awareness of the importance of stimulation for their infant. Parents may be taught means of providing stimulation at home, such as holding and talking to the infant, or hanging colorful mobiles above the crib.

An infant's psychosocial development consists of building a basic trust that his or her needs will be met. Parents should be helped to understand the importance of consistency in meeting their infant's needs, but at the same time they should be helped to learn how the infant's schedule can gradually be adjusted to the parents' schedule as well.

If patient teaching is to be effective, health professionals must consider affective as well as cognitive and psychomotor aspects of patient teaching. Parent strain has an impact on the health and well-being of the infant as well. Health professionals who are alert to clues indicating potential stressors can alleviate strain by providing anticipatory information that may help prevent problems from occurring. In other instances, if problems already exist, the health professionals can work with parents to find alternative solutions to reduce or alleviate the problem.

In the context of family relationships, the health professional may need to reinforce the importance of the couple finding alone time for themselves. If there are other children in the household, the health professional may reinforce the importance of spending time with and giving other children individual attention as well. In the same vein, talking with both parents can be an opportunity to emphasize the need for the new mother to have some time alone away from the baby. Assessing the new mother's emotional, as well as physical status, can alert the health professional to potential areas of stress that can cause additional problems. Strain can be ameliorated if health professionals address specific issues that arise, and reassure the parents that feelings of frustration in caring for a newborn are normal, and experienced by many new parents.

Being aware of the insecurity of new parents, sibling rivalry, and other sources of parental stress helps health professionals form an approach based on patients' individual needs. Supplemental information can be given as needed to alleviate stress and enhance the parents' ability to carry out recommendations.

The Toddler

Like in infancy, development proceeds rapidly in the toddler years. Consequently, health professionals have numerous topics of patient information that can be shared with parents. Information can be given during any contact with parents and child. Unless an illness exists, much patient teaching at this life phase, in addition to milestones of development, include aspects of prevention and safety.

Because many behavioral changes occur during this developmental phase, an important part of patient teaching during this stage may be helping parents learn what to expect and how to respond to some of new behaviors the child may be exhibiting. For instance, during the toddler stage, children can rapidly acquire language skills. Health professionals can help parents foster this aspect of development by encouraging them to talk with, as well as listen to, their child.

The toddler stage is also a time of increased autonomy, when toddlers recognize themselves as individuals different from their mothers. Their newfound independence may be asserted through negativism, frequently referred to as the "no" stage. Children in this stage may have difficulty making up their minds and may be prone to temper tantrums. Such behavior can be a source of irritation for parents, especially if they fail to realize that such behavior is common to children in this age group. Health professionals can teach parents about normal development by helping them learn what behavior to expect as well as by teaching them what steps to take to handle their toddler's behavior. Teaching parents how to use appropriate and consistent techniques of discipline and limit setting, without being overly restrictive, is an important aspect of patient teaching in this phase.

Another important aspect is child safety. As the toddler becomes more mobile—not to mention more curious and more interested in exploring his or her environment—the risk of accident and injury increases. The health professional should make the parents aware of potential safety hazards, and help them learn ways in which they can reduce risk of injury by child proofing their home.

The toddler stage is also characterized by toilet training. Toilet training is commonly an emotional process in which parents place considerable pressure on themselves and their child to perform. By teaching various ways to implement toilet training and by emphasizing individual rates of development, parents may be helped to accomplish the task with considerably less stress both for themselves and for their child.

Although most patient teaching will still be directed to the parents, children in the toddler stage are capable of some degree of understanding the procedures they may experience. Health professionals should establish rapport with the child through simple patient teaching that can also enhance cooperation from the child. The health professional's approach to the child should be warm and matter-of-fact. Although children at this age are able to comprehend more words, they are still unable to reason, and may take things literally. Consequently, explanations given to toddlers should be simple and accurate with no analogies.

Early Childhood

Preschool children continue to develop their own identities and expand their world through involvement with others outside the family unit. In previous stages, although the child might have played alongside another child, there was little actual interaction between the two. In the preschool phase of development, children begin to interact with each other in cooperative play. During this phase, the child also engages in imaginary play and may develop imaginary playmates.

Health professionals' interaction with preschool children and their families may be sporadic, occurring only when there are medical problems or during standard child checkups. Every interaction is an opportunity to teach parents not only about their child's condition, illness, or medical recommendations if the child is ill, but about health promotion and prevention, as well as to offer guidance and reassurance.

Children in early childhood begin to develop a gender identity in which they distinguish themselves as a boy or girl and become aware of differences in the opposite sex. During this phase they also develop increased sexual curiosity, resulting in questions or in behaviors such as masturbation. A child's sexual curiosity may bring about anxiety in parents who do not know how to respond to their child's questions or who question whether their child's sexual curiosity and behavior are normal. Health professionals can facilitate the parents' understanding and acceptance of their child's sexual curiosity by reassuring them that such interest and activities are normal parts of development and by teaching parents ways to respond to their child's questions by using simple, straightforward responses that are presented in a relaxed manner.

In recognizing approaches to children at this age, health professionals facilitate communication between parent and child as well as their own relationship with the children. Children have a vocabulary of approximately 2000 to 2500 words by the time they are 5 years old. Teaching children about procedures to be performed should, therefore, become a routine part of the interaction with children as patients. Although the preschool child has developed a fairly extensive vocabulary, they may be unable to recognize someone else's point of view. Consequently, at this developmental phase, explanations should focus on simple facts rather than attempting to reason with the child as to why he or she should follow a recommendation or have a procedure performed. Because children at this phase fantasize, they are quite vulnerable to fear of pain and bodily harm. It is important to acknowledge children's fears and help them to express their fears openly while providing reassurance. At the same time, however, it is important that explanations continue to be honest with no false promises that could erode the child's trust in the future.

Middle and Later Childhood

During this phase of development, health professionals are increasingly able to establish a one-to-one relationship directly with the child as a patient. At this stage, although there will still be some input from parents, children are capable of reporting symptoms fairly accurately. They are able to reason, are more autonomous than at previous stages, and are emerging as more distinct individual personalities.

Later childhood brings about great changes as the child expands their world through school and broadening social relationships, in which they develop a greater sense of personal responsibility and reliability. Although there has been a gradual expansion of their world since birth, during this phase of development, children begin to establish their self-concepts as members of a world larger than their own family. As they become exposed to more people through school experiences and other activities, they begin to compare the values of their family with others in the outside world. As a result, they begin to form their own values. Throughout this phase of development, children decrease their dependence on family, becoming more social beings by learning how to handle strong feelings and impulses appropriately. During later childhood, the child enlarges the extent of intimacy beyond family, to include a special friend, forming special groups, cliques, or clubs.

Although children in later childhood may still engage in some magical thinking and may experience a need for some ritualistic behavior, they are capable of concrete, logical reasoning. Including children in patient teaching, especially about procedures, becomes even more important as they increase their ability to comprehend. Health professionals should explain procedures, as well as the reasons for them, in a simple, logical way and with confidence and optimism, although explanations should also be realistic in helping the child understand what to expect.

Health professionals will, of course, still spend considerable time teaching parents. In addition to teaching them about the child's illness and treatment plan, parents may also be encouraged to foster the child's independence and to praise his or her accomplishments. During middle to late childhood, children develop physical prowess; however, their ability to make sound judgments lags behind, and as a result, the potential for injury is high (National Center for Injury Prevention and Control, 2003). Consequently, considerable patient teaching might be devoted to teaching about safety issues and how to prevent injuries.

Specific problems arising during this phase of development that may come to the health professional's attention are behavior disorders, hyperactivity, learning disorders, and enuresis. Any of these problems may cause stress for the child as well as the family and may require extensive teaching to enhance both the parents' and child's understanding of the condition and the methods to be used in dealing with it.

In all stages of childhood, when patient teaching is provided because of illness, it is important to keep the child's developmental stage in mind, and to encourage parents to foster the child's normal development despite limitations that may be imposed by illness.

Adolescence

Adolescence is a phase of development that marks a transition cognitively, socially, and physically from childhood to adulthood. Understanding characteristics of the adolescent phase of lifespan development is crucial in order for patient teaching to be effective. Adolescence is a time of marked change. Adolescents are in the process of forming their own identity, emancipating themselves from their parents, and adapting to a rapidly changing body. Because adolescents are capable of abstract thought and reasoning, they are capable of comprehending most explanations given as part of patient teaching.

Although the adolescent's family may still be included in some aspects of patient teaching, the adolescent alone is the major focus of patient teaching because at this stage they have considerable independence and are, consequently, in more control of the degree to which recommendations will be carried out. Considerations of the family and solicitation of its support in helping the adolescent patient following recommendations is important; however, building a relationship with the adolescent and facilitating the relationship between the adolescent and his or her family is perhaps more important now than at any other time in order to increase the likelihood of adherence with recommendations.

Patient teaching needs of the adolescent are wide and varied, and extend beyond the teaching that may be involved when there is illness or injury. Although adolescents have increased potential for abstract thought and the ability to reason, they lack life experience and may have difficulty making rational decisions. Consequently, teaching and guidance regarding a number of issues has increased importance. Adolescents have difficulty imagining that they can become sick or injured and subsequently have increased potential for engaging in risky behavior, which may make them more vulnerable to injury and accidents, experimentation with drugs or alcohol, and sexually transmitted diseases and unwanted pregnancy (Centers for Disease Control and Prevention [CDC], 2006).

Because of adolescents' strong need for peer acceptance and support, health recommendations that they view as interfering with their concept of themselves as independent beings, or that they feel would set them apart from their peers, may be less likely to be followed. In addition, as part of their need to establish themselves as independent individuals, adolescents may rebel against authority and become disillusioned with parents or other authority figures. This can also interfere with adherence to health recommendations— whether those recommendations are related to management of disease, recovery from injury, or preventive health measures.

Rapid body changes that occur during adolescence can bring about a strong preoccupation with body and appearance. Sexual adjustment is an important part of adolescent development. During this time, adolescents experience a strong desire for sexual exploration and to express sexual urges. Sources of information available to them about sexual issues may be weak and misleading, obtained from movies or peers, rather than reliable sources. Parents may not know how to talk with their adolescent child about sexual matters, and sex education in schools, if existent, may be inadequate. Although discussion of sexual issues with adolescents has been feared by some to promote sexual activity, comprehensive information about sexual issues has not been found to increase adolescents' sexual activity, but has been found to decrease it (McElderry & Omar, 2003; Weaver, Smith, & Kippax, 2005). Consequently, sexual health issues are an important part of patient teaching during adolescence. Teaching adolescents about sexual issues requires a special sensitivity and understanding. Regard for the adolescent's modesty and privacy is important in providing an atmosphere of openness and trust so these issues can be addressed.

Adolescents' tendency to engage in risk-taking behaviors, their lack of experience, and their tendency to become distracted contribute to a higher rate of injury during this life phase. For instance, vehicle accident rates for adolescents are higher than for any other group (National Highway Traffic Safety Administration, 2006). In addition, because of the adolescent need to be part of a group, difficulty with judgment, tendency toward risk taking, and the potential for drug and alcohol use during adolescence increases dramatically (Substance Abuse and Mental Health Services Administration, 2004). Patient education programs that simply provide factual information about the dangers of drugs have shown little impact on drug use, and have actually been found to increase drug use in some instances because of curiosity arousal (Botvin & Griffin, 1999). More effective patient teaching about substance use includes addressing many other issues in the adolescent's life that may contribute to drug use. Patient teaching should include helping adolescents to learn life skills that help them achieve positive goals, and help them learn how to resist peer pressure to use substances or take risks (Montoya, Atkinson, & McFaden, 2003; Robertson et al., 2003).

Numerous other issues are potential topics of patient teaching during adolescence. For instance, adolescents develop at different rates that can cause stress and concern. Teaching adolescents about individual differences and offering reassurance to those adolescents who mature either "too late" or "too early" in comparison with their peers can help them increase self-esteem, and adjust in the transition to their next phase of development.

No matter what the topic, the likelihood that patient teaching will be effective is higher if an atmosphere of trust has been established by respecting adolescent needs and showing empathetic understanding. Patient teaching should take on the form of guidance, not lecturing. Adolescents should be treated neither as adults nor as children; however, as with all patients, the approach to patient teaching should be modified to meet the specific needs of the individual.

Although the family of the adolescent should also be considered and included in patient teaching when appropriate—especially when illness or injury are involved—a health professional who wants to gain credibility with an adolescent must establish himself or herself as an advocate of the adolescent rather than as a representative of the parents. Although much patient teaching is conducted directly with the adolescent, health professionals may also provide guidance and support to family members, and help them to understand adolescent behavior. Parents should be encouraged to set realistic limits for adolescents while, at the same time, fostering their independence. Adjustment to an adolescent's gradual independence may be difficult for parents, who must now also begin to redefine their role as parents. Patient teaching with adolescents can be enhanced if health professionals can identify potential sources of stress in the family and support parents in their own readjustment. Because of the ambivalence of the stage between childhood and adulthood, health professionals should be aware of the importance of considering both adolescents and their parents when conducting patient teaching.

When conducting patient teaching with adolescents about illness or injury, the same characteristics of this stage of lifespan development that impact issues of prevention may also impact an adolescent's receptiveness to information and adherence with recommendations for management of his or her condition. Adolescents need to establish themselves as independent individuals; the need for peer inclusion, as well as changing body image and belief in immunity from consequences of behaviors, may impact the effectiveness of patient teaching. The consequence of nonadherence is, of course, a result of the seriousness of the illness or condition for which the adolescent patient is being treated. In any instance, health professionals who are concerned about effective patient teaching must consider and include issues that are part of this stage of development, altering their approach to meet the adolescent patient's needs.

TEACHING ADULTS THROUGHOUT THE LIFESPAN
Young Adulthood

Because developmental changes are individual, occur gradually, and continue throughout young adulthood, moving from adolescence to adulthood is not clearly demarcated. Challenges associated with this stage of lifespan development include selecting and building a career, adjusting to work life, establishing relationships, establishing and maintaining a home, and perhaps beginning a family. All of these challenges may provide opportunities for patient teaching. Awareness of change occurring in the patient's life, and his or her reaction to it may provide cues that specific aspects of patient teaching should be initiated. For instance, when a patient engages in an intimate relationship, there may be a need for patient teaching about contraception or safe sex practices. If a patient becomes pregnant, prenatal teaching, newborn care, and numerous other topics related to child care need to be covered during the next years of interaction. Although many challenges associated with young adulthood can be happy events, they can also be a source of stress. Recognizing potential stressors, assessing the level of stress the individual is experiencing and their reaction to it, provides the health professional with information that not only helps him or her determine the approach to patient teaching, but information that helps determine specific content areas that may need to be addressed. Identifying the significant people in the patient's life can also help the health professional determine the degree to which these relationships are available as support for carrying out recommendations, or the extent to which they may hinder the individual's ability or willingness to adhere to recommendations. Health professionals should refrain from making assumptions. Questions about patients' significant others should be approached in a direct, neutral, and sensitive way. Not all patients have positive or supportive relationships with family or friends, even when they are present. Likewise, not all patients live in a traditional, nuclear family setting. A variety of living arrangements, alternative lifestyles, and close family bonds may be present even though the relationships are not legalized by marriage, adoption or guardianship, or are not determined by heredity.

Data suggest that 4 to 9% of the population is in same-gender relationships (Harrison & Silenzio, 1996). Although an increasing amount of individuals are more open now about being in a same-gender relationship, there are still many individuals who remain reluctant to acknowledge their preference or their relationship because of fear of discrimination or, in some instances, fear of physical or emotional abuse (Greco & Glusman, 1998). Consequently, patients may not always be forthcoming about sexual preferences. Making assumptions about individuals' lifestyle or sexual preference, or who they consider as their major source of emotional support without checking with patients themselves not only serves to alienate patients, but can also cause missed opportunities for patient teaching.

Patients with same sex preferences have the same patient teaching needs in all aspects of their lives as do individuals who are in traditional relationships. Pregnancy, parenthood, job stressors, sexual issues, prevention practices, or illness management are situations that offer potential patient teaching opportunities for all patients, regardless of sexual orientation. All patients should be approached in an open, nonjudgmental way that helps the health professional build rapport and trust with the patient. As with all patients, frank and open discussion helps health professionals determine patient teaching needs. Patients who trust their health professional are more likely to follow given recommendations (Greco & Glusman, 1998).

Although individuals can become ill at any age, the leading causes of death, illness, and disability in young adulthood are related to behavior (Hoyert, Kung, & Smith, 2005; Poole, Warren, & Nunez, 2007). For instance, in young adults, vehicle accidents are often associated with speeding and alcohol use, and a number of chronic illness are associated with smoking, lack of exercise, and poor diet (Marks et al., 2000). Obesity has become an increasing problem in all age groups, and places young adults at risk for many chronic conditions including high blood pressure, heart disease, diabetes, and arthritis-related disabilities (Poole, Warren, & Nunez, 2007).

Health promotion issues, although often neglected, may be especially important to address during young adulthood. Stress may contribute to further illness and poor coping practices such as alcohol or drug use. Much of the individual's future health may be determined by health practices established now. Helping patients learn to cope with stress, talking with them about health risk factors, and helping them establish good health practices may all be important in preventing many of the health problems that may otherwise occur in the future.

Patients' cultural and economic circumstances may determine their ability to follow recommendations regarding healthy lifestyle. In addition, some environments are more stressful than others. For instance, violence is one of the major threats to health during young adulthood (CDC, 2006). Although no one is immune to being a victim of violence, rates of violence tend to increase for groups with lower socioeconomic status (Reiss & Roth, 1994). When conducting patient teaching about prevention, it is important that the health professional be sensitive to the patient's particular life circumstance and conduct patient teaching in the context of the individual's particular situation.

Knowledge of all aspects of an individual's life helps health professionals determine the type of patient teaching most relevant to the patient's circumstances as well as helping to identify supports and barriers to their following treatment recommendations. Financial constraints, family responsibility, cultural differences, and work schedule may all be common factors in this stage that can influence an individual's ability to adhere to recommendations.

Middle Adulthood

Just as adolescence is the link between childhood and adulthood, midlife is a transition period between young adulthood and the later years. During these years, many individuals have reached the peak in their career. They may also begin to reexamine and question former goals and values as well as their perceived degree of achievement. During this personal assessment, people may begin to modify aspects of their lives that they consider unsatisfactory. They may begin to adopt a new life structure that is perceived as a solution to the dissatisfaction they may be experiencing.

Physical changes of aging may begin to be more apparent. Individuals may begin to notice some decrease in physical stamina, changing hormonal levels for women result in menopause, and vision and hearing acuity may begin to decrease. In addition, individuals become more aware of their own vulnerability to certain illnesses during middle adulthood. Discussion of hormone replacement therapy and calcium supplements may be particular patient needs for women who are concerned about the potential for developing osteoporosis. Cholesterol levels and the potential for developing heart disease may also be of concern to patients. The need for routine screening, such as mammography or colonoscopy, for early detection of cancer may be issues included in patient teaching. Teaching about basic practices in health promotion and their role in disease prevention may be even more relevant at this life stage. In addition, individuals may develop issues or questions about their own sexuality as they age. Sensitive and open discussion can help individuals address their concerns regarding these issues. Patient teaching about physical changes and management can help individuals make adjustments to changes they are experiencing, and incorporate behaviors that will help them maintain their health.

Those in the middle adult phase of lifespan development, if in a family group, may find themselves reappraising not only their marital relationship, but the relationship with their children as well. As their offspring begin to leave home and establish their own families, parents need to adjust their roles. At the same time, people in middle adulthood may grow increasingly responsible for their parents, whose own health may be failing. Recognizing their own physical changes, their parents' declining health, and their own goals and values, middle-aged people may become especially aware of their own mortality. This realization may either motivate the individual to follow recommendations more closely or, if the prospect of mortality is especially threatening, to deny illness or abandon health promotion and prevention practices.

Depending on the individual's situation, there may be many areas of stress and a variety of reactions that can contribute to illness behavior as well as act as barriers to effective patient teaching and, consequently, barriers to recommendation adherence. Health professionals should be aware of potential problems and approach patients with a nonjudgmental attitude. In addition to teaching about specific medical recommendations, teaching should also include health risk factors, stress reduction, and identification of misconceptions or misinformation that may be present. Misconceptions regarding physical changes such as menopause and other changes may be especially prominent. Helping people in midlife cope with stress can enhance teaching and enable patients to live happier, healthier, and more productive lives. As with all other life stages, the health professional should be aware of potential sources of stress associated with this age as well as particular circumstances of the individual's life and how these factors may impact the type of patient teaching required. The health professional should also consider how these factors impact the patient's ability to follow recommendations.

Later Adulthood

Although many older adults remain healthy and active in later life, the incidence of chronic diseases increases with age for many people. As a result, much patient teaching may revolve around illness and disease with aspects of prevention being neglected. Health professionals may have had little formal training regarding approaches to the older adult, and may therefore be uncomfortable with patient teaching. Attitudes of health professionals as well as inadequate understanding of later life stages may well be the greatest barriers to effective patient teaching for this group. Working with older patients may elicit fears in health professionals of their own aging and death; therefore, interaction with older patients may be avoided. Health professionals may believe myths about aging and approach older adults with those stereotypes rather than approaching them as individuals. Patient teaching with older patients can, however, be of great benefit to the patient and rewarding to the health professional as well.

Many older patients may be coping with various degrees of loss. Older adults may be facing retirement and adjustment to a new lifestyle. Others may retire and return to the workforce after they have left a career. Retirement may be a source of satisfaction or anxiety, depending on the circumstances. Economic issues, health issues, individual factors, and family issues all contribute to the degree of stress or satisfaction an individual experiences.

Family situations also vary greatly in older adulthood. Individuals may have lost a spouse, may have never married, or may be divorced. They may be active with their partner or friends, or they may be the sole caretaker of an ill spouse or partner. They may have adult children they are close to or from whom they are estranged. Grandchildren may be a joy and diversion, or may be the source of stress if the patient needed to assume the responsibility for their care.

As individuals age, they may also experience increasing losses such as friends or their own physical capability. As individuals reach the later stages of this phase of lifespan development, physical decline becomes more rapid. Depending on the degree of loss present, there may also be decreased independence, with resulting loss of self-esteem and self-satisfaction.

Health professionals conducting patient teaching with patients in later adulthood should realize that individuals are diverse and this group can include healthy, alert individuals who may have some physical limitations, but still enjoy life and continue to have an interest in learning how to stay active as long as possible, manage their condition, and prevent further disease, complications, or disability from occurring. Health professionals should approach each patient without stereotypes or preconceptions. As in all other life stages, not all changes of aging occur at the same rate, and not everyone in the same age group has the same experience or life circumstances. Aging should be viewed as a multidimensional process in which the individual's function and health status are related to multiple factors. When conducting patient teaching, the health professional should treat older adults as individuals and with the same interest and respect as any other patient with whom patient teaching is being conducted. For instance, health professionals should not use first names in teaching interactions with older adults unless invited to do so. Patient teaching with older adults should be conducted with the same conviction with which it would be delivered to patients at any other age.

When conducting patient teaching with individuals who have altered hearing acuity, health professionals should position themselves close to the patient and speak clearly and concisely, remembering that raising the loudness of the voice does not necessarily contribute to the listener's better hearing. Patient teaching should be realistic but hopeful. Pat phrases, such as, "What do you expect at your age?" or "You'll live to be 100," are inappropriate and should be avoided.

Patient teaching need not be confined to illness with older individuals anymore than it is with younger patients. Issues to be addressed in addition to those that deal with specific illness or treatment recommendations might include sexuality, exercise, nutrition, and a variety of other topics that are oriented toward prevention of illness or disability and toward the enhancement of the quality of life.

Barriers to independence should be assessed to help the patient find ways to maximize strengths and independence. Older patients should be helped to learn how to make optimum use of their skills and functions. Because of problems that may exist in this life phase, health professionals should be especially aware of adherence problems due to misunderstanding, physical limitations, or financial barriers. Health professionals may be able to enhance patient ability to follow medical recommendations by providing information, considering patients' individual needs, and building an awareness of community services and resources that can help them follow given recommendations.

A LIFESPAN PATIENT-CENTERED APPROACH TO PATIENT TEACHING

Knowledge about lifespan development has obvious relevance for health professionals conducting patient teaching. In order to conduct effective patient teaching, patients must be understood in the context of their particular situation and circumstances. This includes not only physical, psychosocial, and social circumstances, but also the particular stage of life they are experiencing along with the specific challenges related to that stage.

Throughout life, people experience challenges at different stages that lead to a variety of changes. These challenges, and resulting changes, influence an individual's attitudes, perceptions, actions, and behaviors. Although developmental changes may be more apparent in childhood, such changes occur in adulthood as well. Knowledge of changes that can occur at various points during the lifespan enhances the health professionals' ability to teach effectively, as well as helps them identify topics that may be presented to patients along with specific recommendations related to the patient's illness. Opportunities for patient teaching exist regardless of illness or injury. Examples of health-related topics that may be covered at various life stages are illustrated

Table 5-1 Patient Teaching Issues Through the Lifespan

Prenatal Period	Normal changes associated with pregnancy, both emotional and physical; sexual activity during pregnancy; preparation for the newborn; diet counseling; preparation for the role of parenting; process and procedures during labor, delivery, and postpartum
Infancy	Normal infant development; individual differences; immunizations; infant stimulation; infant feeding; safety issues; teething; family interactions
Toddler	Child development; safety; toilet training; discipline and setting limits; nutrition
Preschool-aged Children	Importance and role of play; dealing with sexual curiosity and questions; general health practices; school adjustment; sleep problems
Adolescence	Normal development patterns and individual differences, emotional and physical; sex education; skin problems; nutrition and other health practices; safety; drug and alcohol use
Young Adult	Stress reduction; health maintenance and promotion; intimate relationships and adjustment; prenatal teaching; child-rearing practice
Middle Adulthood	Physical changes, such as menopause; health risk factors; changes in family relationships; stress reduction; health promotion
Later Adulthood	Adjustment to retirement; nutrition and exercise; adaptation to loss; modification of environment to promote independence as necessary; sexuality

in Table 5-1. The list, although not all-inclusive, points out a variety of topics that may be discussed whether or not the patient is seeking advice for a health problem.

During early phases of the life cycle, most patient teaching is conducted with parents rather than children themselves. As the individual moves through the life cycle, more interaction will obviously occur directly between the patient and the health professional. Although health professionals should always approach each patient as an individual, knowledge of general human characteristics at various stages of development can be helpful. Table 5-2 offers suggested approaches for use with patients at various stages of development to make the teaching interaction more effective.

Table 5-2   Patient Teaching Approach Through the Lifespan

Lifespan Phase	Approach of Health Professional
Prenatal	Parents: Use an open-minded approach with no preconceptions; nonjudgmental; give emotional support to both parents; work within parents' framework
Infancy	Parents: Foster security by giving positive feedback regarding parents' ability to care for the child; no nagging or lecturing; take what may appear to be small problems seriously
Toddler	Parents: Use a nonjudgmental approach; continue support and positive reinforcement Patient: Encourage child in warm, matter-of-fact manner; use no analogies when giving explanations; give explanations in accurate, simple terms
Preschool-aged Children	Parents: Provide guidance and encouragement Patient: Encourage child to express fear; give no false promises; explain procedures before doing them
Later Childhood	Parents: Give continued guidance and support Patient: Give explanations in simple, logical way; approach child in confident, optimistic manner
Adolescence	Patient: Treat neither as adult nor child, but rather modify approach depending on expectations and reactions; demonstrate empathetic understanding and respect; show regard for modesty and privacy; identify and dispel misconceptions; provide guidance regarding sexual issues as appropriate Parent: Provide guidance and support to help parents understand adolescent behavior; encourage parents to set realistic limits; support parents in their own readjustment
Young Adult	Patient: Use an empathetic, nonjudgmental attitude
Middle Adulthood	Patient: Use an empathetic, nonjudgmental attitude
Later Adulthood	Patient: Approach patient as unique, not stereotyping because of age; keep awareness that aging is multidimensional in which multiple factors affect functioning; capitalize on patients' strengths; refrain from using first names unless invited to do so; speak clearly and concisely; avoid patronizing

REFERENCES

Botvin, G. J., & Griffin, K.W. (1999). Preventing drug abuse. In A. J. Reynolds, H. J. Walberg, & R. P. Weissberg (Eds.), *Promoting positive outcomes* (pp. 197–228). Washington, DC: Child Welfare League of America.

Broderick, P. C., & Blewitt, P. (2006). *The life span: Human development for helping professionals* (2nd ed.). Upper Saddle River, NJ: Pearson/Merrill Prentice Hall

Centers for Disease Control and Prevention. (2006). Health topics. Retrieved June 27, 2009, from http://www.cdc.gov/HealthyYouth/healthtopics.

Gabbard, C. P. (2004). *Lifelong motor development* (4th ed.). San Francisco: Benjamin Cummings.

Greco, J. A., & Glusman, J. B. (1998). Providing effective care for gay and lesbian patients. *Patient Care, 32*(12),159–162, 167–168, 170.

Harrison, A. E., & Silenzio, V. M. B. (1996). Comprehensive care of lesbian and gay patients and families. *Primary Care, 23,* 31–46.

Hoyert, D. L., Kung, H. C., & Smith, B. L. (2005). *Deaths: Preliminary data for 2003.* National Vital Statistics Reports, 53(15).

Marks, D. F., Murray, M., Evans, B., & Willig, C. (2000). *Health psychology: Theory research and practice.* Thousand Oaks, CA: Sage.

McElderry, D. H., & Omar, H. A. (2003). Sex education in the schools: What role does it play? *International Journal of Adolescent Medicine and Health, 15,* 3–9.

Montoya, I. D., Atkinson, J., & McFaden, W. C. (2003). Best characteristics of adolescent gateway drug prevention programs. *Journal of Addictions Nursing, 14,* 75–83.

National Center for Injury Prevention and Control. (2003). Childhood injury fact sheet. Retrieved June 26, 2009, from http://www.cdc.gov/ncipc/factsheet/children.htm

National Highway Traffic Safety Administration. (2006). Saving teenage lives, Section I: Introduction: The need for graduated driver licensing. Retrieved June 26, 2009, from http://www.nhtsa.dot.gov/people/injury/newdriver/SaveTeens/sect1.html

Osofsky, J. D., & Thompson, M. D. (2000). Adaptive and maladaptive parenting: Perspectives on risk and protective factors. In J. P. Shonkoff & S. J. Meisels (Eds.), *Handbook of early childhood intervention* (2nd ed., pp. 54–75). New York: Cambridge University Press.

Poole, D., Warren, A., & Nunez, N. (2007). *The story of human development.* Upper Saddle River, NJ: Pearson/Prentice Hall.

Reiss, A. J. Jr., & Roth, J. A. (Eds.). (1994). *Understanding and preventing violence, Vol 3: Social influences.* Washington, DC: National Academy Press.

Robertson, E. B., David, S. L., Rao, S. A., & National Institute on Drug Abuse. (2003). *Preventing drug use among children and adolescents: A research-based guide for parents, educators, and community leaders* (2nd ed.), Bethesda, MD: National Institute on Drug Abuse.

Substance Abuse and Mental Health Services Administration. (2004). *Results from the 2003 national survey on drug use and health:. National findings.* Office of Applied Studies, NSDUH Series H-25, DHHS Publication No. SMA 04-3964.

Weaver, H., Smith, G., & Kippax, S. (2005). School-based sex education policies and indicators of sexual health among young people: A comparison of the Netherlands, France, Australia and the United States. *Sex Education, 5,* 171–188.

CHAPTER 6

The Family, Patient-Centered Teaching, and Patient Adherence

ROLE OF THE FAMILY

Patients rarely exist in a vacuum. Family, friends, and other relationships a patient may have all play an important role in the patient's life and health. A patient's significant other affects not only the patient's health behaviors, but also his or her ability to cope with illness and the degree to which they adhere to recommendations (Mannes et al., 1993). Patient beliefs and attitudes about health, lifestyle, and health care begin at home with the family (Lipkin, 1996). Many of the health practices and beliefs patients hold stem from what they have been told, have experienced, or have observed as part of their family system. It should be obvious then, that the family has considerable influence on a patient's health practices and, consequently, should be an important aspect of effective patient teaching in healthcare settings.

As a patient's primary support system, family can affect a patient's decision making about health and health care. Families often help patients make decisions about how and when to enter the healthcare system, whether entry involves emergency care or care for acute or chronic disease, or for general health maintenance (Reust & Mattingly, 1996). Families may also influence the extent to which patients follow recommendations. These influences can affect whether or not patients take their medication, follow the prescribed diet, have recommended diagnostic tests or surgical procedures, or even determine end-of-life decisions or nursing home placement (Jecker, 1990). Family members may also assist by providing the patient with functional support in which they help the patient carry out certain tasks as part of the treatment recommendations, or provide emotional support (Shirey & Summer, 2000). Understanding how family contributes to patient ability or willingness to follow recommendations given by health professionals can be a valuable asset in conducting patient teaching.

Although consideration of the individual is important in patient teaching, the patient's family is also of central importance if teaching is to be effective. Consequently, not only should patient teaching be patient-centered, it should also be family-focused (Clark & Dunbar, 2003). For the individual patient, the family constitutes the social context in which illness occurs. Illness and treatment affect the family as well as the patient. When a family member becomes ill, the illness alters the context of daily living and requires additional time and energy from family members. Illness can disrupt employment or school patterns of family members and cause financial hardships. In addition, illness and treatment can enhance or threaten family relationships, or alter the roles its members play (Reust & Mattingly, 1996).

Likewise, the family contributes to the health and health behavior of the patient. The happiness and health of each individual family member depends, to a significant degree, on the nature of his or her interaction with other members in the family unit. How a family functions influences the health of its members as well as how an individual reacts to illness. Teaching the patient without considering the family may result in less-than-adequate adherence with recommendations. Family functioning, family support, problem solving, communication, and self-efficacy all contribute to and influence the degree of assistance and support the patient receives (Dunbar et al., 2008). The ability of the health professional to teach the patient how to maintain or restore health depends on his or her insight into the patient's relationship with family members, as well as other family issues. Consideration should be given to the extent to which family members can help the patient in terms of offering assistance, support, and encouragement. The health professional should attempt to include the family in patient teaching. For instance, what good does it do to teach a middle-aged man about his diet if his wife does all the cooking and is excluded from patient teaching about dietary restrictions? Likewise, it may be difficult for a husband to be supportive of his wife's blood pressure treatment program if he does not understand the reasons for the recommendations and the consequences of not carrying them out.

It is important to consider the influence of family members on the patient's health behaviors, and to include them in patient teaching as appropriate; however, it is also important to not make assumptions. The health professional should remember that not all patients want their families involved, and even when they do, not all families can meet expectations of health professionals. Not all patients receive the support and encouragement needed from their families and not all families have the emotional stability to cope with long-term illness. If the relationship between family members was not stable before the patient's illness, or if the relationship was strained, the additional stress of illness may cause even more problems. In other instances, family members may have conflicting obligations. They may have other responsibilities to fill in addition to their roles within the patient's family unit, and some roles and obligations may conflict with the patient's needs. For example, children of an older patient may have families of their own. Although they may feel concern and responsibility for their aging parent, the health professional cannot realistically expect that they will sacrifice their own family to help their aging parent carry out all treatment recommendations.

Long-term illness, even in the most stable of family units, is bound to bring about changes in family relationships. Illness itself changes the patient's role within the family. Such change naturally produces some disequilibrium within the family structure until adjustment occurs. For instance, if the head of the household and chief breadwinner has been the husband, a disabling illness that prevents him from working may change his role in the family. His wife may have to assume the role of chief breadwinner while he assumes the role of a dependent. If the health professional does not recognize this change, what the change might mean to the patient and family, and how it might affect the patient's willingness and ability to carry out the recommendations, the effectiveness of patient teaching may be diminished.

When teaching the patient and family, it is important for health professionals to identify patterns of relationships and to be alert to attitudes of family members. Health professionals may also be able to identify resources within the family group and help family members mobilize their resources to help the patient.

When gaining support from family members to facilitate the patient's ability to follow recommendations, health professionals must also remember that family members are just that—family members—and not health professionals. The purpose of involving families in patient teaching is to gain their support by helping them to be better informed, not to prepare them as spies to monitor the patient in the health professional's absence.

When conducting patient teaching with the patient's family, it is important for health professionals to be aware that the same barriers that may interfere with effective teaching with the patient can also exist with individual family members. Family members have their own personality style, coping methods, values, beliefs, and other psychosocial variables that must be considered. For instance, illness in a family member tends to raise the anxiety of those who are close to the patient. Anxiety may be misinterpreted by the health professional as lack of interest or as reluctance on the part of the family member to provide the patient with help and support. In other instances, a family member's method of coping may be to deny the seriousness of the patient's illness or the importance of following recommendations. The more health professionals can be aware of these reactions and help family members deal with their feelings, the more effective the health professional will be in teaching family members about the patient's condition and treatment, as well as in mobilizing their support.

Although it is important to understand how devastating illness can be to a patient, it is also important to understand that illness causes strain on the family as well. If the family is already under stress, illness will probably subject both patient and family to additional emotional pressures. Information about the family function, stress, transition, and expectations can be invaluable in developing the most effective teaching plan for patient and family alike. Although the major focus of the health professional's attention is on the patient, the impact of the family on the patient's receptivity to information, as well as ability and willingness to follow treatment recommendations, must also be considered.

FAMILY STRUCTURE AND STYLE

Commonly, most health professionals think of family in terms of the nuclear family—a group in which there are parents and children—or in terms of the extended family—which includes parents, children, grandparents, aunts, uncles, and the like. Today, family extends beyond the traditional family boundaries and includes those individuals who the patient looks to for assistance and support, and considers emotionally close and most influential in their life, regardless of whether legal or blood ties exist. People's emotional effects on one another need not be limited to blood relations. If perceived this way, a family might include two people living together with or without sexual attachment, single-parent families, remarried families with children and/or stepchildren, and a host of other family forms. Rather than viewing the family in only the traditional manner, expanding the definition of family may be important when developing a teaching plan for the patient.

The family is the social network in which each individual has a specific role and from where the patient derives at least some of his or her identity. It is also the network with which the patient has strong psychological bonds. The family influences health behavior through interactions and reactions, through past experiences and attitudes, and through the family's relationship to the community in which its members live. For example, an individual whose family is in a socially isolated, rural area will probably hold different attitudes and perform different practices of health and illness behavior than individuals whose families live in a suburban metropolitan area. The child whose father is a physician will probably have different reactions and attitudes toward health and health care than the child whose father is a farmer.

Not all families function the same way, nor do all families have the same structure or style. As each individual in the family unit goes through his or her own stages of development, the structure, composition, and role of the family change. As a result, the family as a whole goes through different stages of development. Just as illness may have a different impact on individuals at different phases of development, so may it have a different impact on families at different developmental stages. For instance, illness of a spouse or partner in a newly formed family union without children has a different impact than it might have for a middle-aged couple with children they are sending to college, and would have yet a different impact for a couple in old age. Awareness of the impact at different family developmental stages helps the health professional approach patient teaching in a way that maximizes the potential for effective patient teaching.

Determining who the patient looks to for support in the family can be accomplished by talking with the patient and by observing family interactions. Who does the patient talk about most? What is the patient's reaction when talking about his or her family and the individuals in it? Who comes to visit the patient in the hospital? Who accompanies the patient in an outpatient setting? What is the interaction between the patient and individual family members like? What sources of stress were family members experiencing prior to illness as a result of their developmental stage?

Illness in a newly formed family, for example, may cause additional strain because of economic considerations, interruptions in career development, and/or adjustment to the new relationship itself. If the patient is a young child, there may be additional strain to the family if there are other children whose needs also must be met. Illness in the middle stage of family life, when adolescents are attempting to emancipate themselves from family ties at the same time their parents are experiencing their own midlife transitions, may place further strain on what already is a tumultuous time for the family. Illness in either parent or child may interfere with the mutual weaning process that should be occurring at this stage. Illness in later age may not only have an impact on grown children, but may also occur when the older couple had anticipated a time of enjoyment together and are less able to care for each other as a result of their own physical limitations that may be associated with aging.

Health professionals will be more effective in patient teaching if they are able to identify the family's predominant lifestyle and find ways to sustain and incorporate recommendations into it rather than trying to impose a different pattern. For instance, some families exhibit a high degree of structure, while others exhibit little structure and appear to be in a constant state of chaos. When aware of the system by which the family operates, health professionals can work within the system rather than trying to fight it. Again, the most effective patient teaching is that which fits into the patient's frame of reference and with which the patient feels most comfortable.

If health professionals can identify relationship patterns and attitudes within the family unit, these factors can be incorporated into patient teaching. These factors can then at least be considered when estimating the patient's potential for following recommendations. An example of family influence is illustrated by the following case.

Mrs. Roberts was pregnant with her first child. She and her husband lived in the same small community in which they had grown up, and their extended family was quite large. Mrs. Roberts regularly attended prenatal classes offered at the local hospital. At one session, the topic was breastfeeding versus bottle feeding. The pros and cons of each were discussed. It appeared to Mrs. Roberts that there were obviously more benefits to the infant from breastfeeding than bottle feeding.

At her next prenatal visit, she discussed breastfeeding with her physician, and it was agreed that she would breastfeed her infant. After the birth of her baby, Mrs. Roberts had considerable difficulty breastfeeding. After 2 weeks, she visited her physician, stating that she would have to bottle-feed instead. She was obviously upset, perceived herself as failing, and worried that the transition from breast to bottle would affect her infant. The nurse in the physician's office took time to talk with Mrs. Roberts about her feelings and discovered that Mrs. Roberts' mother and mother-in-law had both been quite opposed to her breastfeeding, feeling that in their day breastfeeding had been done out of necessity. They were anxious for their children to have it easier than they did and strongly encouraged the use of modern conveniences—in this case, premixed formula. In addition, Mr. Roberts had concerns about breastfeeding and the effect it would have on his wife's figure. He also perceived breastfeeding as imposing severe limitations on his wife's ability to be away from the baby for any length of time.

Mrs. Roberts had little support or encouragement from family members in her efforts to breastfeed. Under the circumstances, even the best information about breastfeeding was bound to be less than effective in helping her attain her goal. The family's influence might have been identified earlier and Mr. Roberts might have been included in more of the patient teaching, which might have addressed many of his fears. The nurse, knowing the attitudes of the couple's mothers, might also have provided more individual support and suggestions to Mrs. Roberts. Not surprisingly, the family's attitudes and support, or lack thereof, have a far greater impact on the degree to which patients follow health advice than mere information presented by a health professional. These influences must be considered if teaching is to be used effectively to help patients follow recommendations.

The family may also influence the patient's beliefs about the severity of various illnesses and the benefits and costs of treatment. If family members fail to realize why a certain medicine is ordered to treat a specific disease, or fail to see the cure or effects they had expected of treatment, their attitudes may be a direct barrier to patient adherence.

FAMILY AND ILLNESS

Illness disrupts the family. Each individual within a family—whether child or parent—plays a certain role that the family incorporates within its basic everyday function. When a family member becomes ill, other members must also alter their lifestyle and make some allowances for role changes for the individual who is ill, as well as changes in their own functioning. The illness of an individual within a family may cause all other members to experience some degree of strain, whether the illness is acute or chronic. A child who is ill with otitis media and is up most of the night, or who must stay home from school, requires parents and perhaps even other children to reorganize some of their regular activities. If a husband who is the breadwinner suffers a myocardial infarction, his wife may have to return to work to supplement, or bring in, income for the family. A grown child whose aging parent becomes chronically ill may need to alter daily living patterns to accommodate care of the parent.

The extent of disruption of a family, of course, is dependent to some extent on the seriousness of the illness. It is also dependent on the family's level of functioning before the illness, on socioeconomic considerations, on the emotional dependency of others, and on the extent to which the role of the person who is ill can be absorbed by other family members. The dynamics of the family or other close personal relationships that existed before illness affect family relationships after illness (Badr & Acitelli, 2005; Palmer & Glass, 2003; Pierce & Lutz, 2009). In some instances, major illness brings a family closer together; in others, even a minor illness causes significant strain. When conducting patient teaching, health professionals should assess the impact of illness on the family because the group's reaction can have a significant influence on the patient's motivation to recover and cooperate with the recommended treatment.

As previously mentioned, health professionals can gain this type of information by talking with, listening to, and observing the patient and family and then altering teaching accordingly. Take, for example, the health professional teaching the wife of a patient with a recent amputation about stump care. The health professional may note the wife's reluctance to look at the stump or touch it. The professional may also notice the wife grimacing when procedures in stump care are discussed. At this point, an alteration in patient teaching may be needed. The health professional may need to take time to talk privately to the wife about her feelings. If the wife's feelings cannot be altered, then the health professional may have to develop alternative methods to help the patient with stump care at home. In any case, the health professional should be aware that the wife's attitude can affect the degree to which the patient is willing to follow recommendations.

In this context, it is important for health professionals to identify the meaning of the illness not only to the patient but also to the family. The family's perception of illness is often more important than the type of illness for which the patient is being treated. The following two cases illustrate this point.

Michael was a 4-year-old boy with asthma and many allergies. Although Michael's mother brought him to the health clinic when he had asthma attacks and had received patient teaching about how to clear the home of many of the allergens thought to precipitate his attacks, and about what to do to lessen their severity, Michael continued to have frequent attacks. During one visit, the physician began to question Michael's mother about the changes she had made in the home to help reduce allergens in the environment. Many of the recommendations had not been followed for a variety of reasons, none of which seemed substantial to the physician. Michael's mother concluded by saying, "Well, if I wasn't working, I'd have time to do all the things I need to do. Our child's health is suffering because my husband insists I supplement our income. I never wanted to work outside the home. Now we're seeing what the consequences are."

The physician gained some insight into the meaning of Michael's asthma attacks. The boy's attacks provided his mother with an excuse to stay home as well as leverage to quit her job. Although her feelings were no doubt unconscious, they appeared to be a strong contributing factor in Michael's continued illness through lack of adherence with the recommendations provided. Through identifying the meaning of Michael's illness to his mother, the physician was able to take a different approach to patient teaching and to begin to help Michael's parents start to discuss openly some of the issues that were interfering with their son's treatment.

In a second case, Mr. Arnett, a 65-year-old retired businessman with arteriosclerosis, had had a mild stroke with some residual paralysis. Both Mr. and Mrs. Arnett received extensive teaching about his care and rehabilitation, ways to prevent complications, and information about arteriosclerosis itself. Upon follow-up visits, the nurse noted that although Mr. Arnett appeared to be progressing well physically and his degree of adherence with recommendations appeared excellent, he seemed somewhat sad and withdrawn. Observation of the interaction between Mr. and Mrs. Arnett alerted the nurse to the possibility that their relationship had become somewhat strained. Further investigation indicated that Mrs. Arnett demanded that her husband comply rigidly with every recommendation and enforced many of them quite literally, to the point where Mr. Arnett had very little freedom to live his life to its full potential.

After talking with the couple in several consecutive visits, the nurse learned that Mrs. Arnett felt that Mr. Arnett's illness was a great threat to his life. She feared being left alone and became so frightened at the possibility that she had virtually made him a prisoner of health advice. After Mrs. Arnett's beliefs were revealed, the nurse was able to help her establish priorities in carrying out the teaching recommendations, demonstrating which were crucial and where there could be more flexibility.

In other instances, illness may place individuals in a new family role that they prefer over the old role. For example, a patient who has craved dependence and attention in the family, rather than functioning in an independent role, may have less incentive to get well. On the other hand, if the illness of a dominant person within the family enables another family member to assume the more authoritative role they desired, there may be less support and encouragement to help the patient become well.

THE FAMILY MEMBER AS CAREGIVER

When the patient experiences a chronic illness or one that requires extended care, family members may need to assume the role of primary caregiver. In some instances, family members accept this role out of love. In other instances, it is out of a sense of duty or obligation. The individual's primary motivation for assuming the role of caretaker will affect his or her approach to the role of caregiver as well as his or her receptiveness to patient teaching. Family members who assume the role of primary caregiver face multiple problems, issues, and concerns. Although providing the role of caregiver can have many positive aspects, including a sense of enrichment, pride, and a strengthened relationship between caregiver and patient, it can also have negative aspects such as stress, strain, burden, and burnout.

When a family member becomes the primary caregiver, the health professional has an important role in extending patient teaching to include the caregiver, and to assess his or her feelings and adjustments to the role. By being alert to the effects of caregiving on the individual, the health professional can offer support and reassurance if the impact of the role is perceived positively, or teaching and support about techniques or resources for coping with stress or avoiding burnout if the impact is perceived negatively. Caregiving has been associated with depression (Chumbler et al., 2004; Family Caregiver Alliance, 2006) as well as a variety of other health problems (Halm & Bakas, 2007; Mausbach et al., 2007; Plowfield, Raymond, & Blevins, 2000). In addition to teaching the family member who is acting as caregiver about the patient's condition and treatment recommendations, the health professional can also include patient teaching that will help the caregiver maintain his or her own health.

Although not all family members providing care experience stress, many do (Pierce & Lutz, 2009). The degree of strain experienced depends on the type and intensity of care needed, the personal characteristics of the caregiver, the amount of support available to the caregiver, the relationship between the patient and family member, financial burden, and competing obligations the family member may be experiencing. Caregivers who have a higher sense of self-efficacy and sense of personal mastery have been shown to experience fewer untoward effects (Chumbler, Rittman, & Wu, 2008; Mausbach et al., 2007). Consequently, patient teaching with the family member acting as caregiver helps him or her gain the knowledge and skills required to carry out recommendations. It also offers support and reassurance and can help improve health outcomes not only for the caregiver, but for the patient as well.

THE HEALTH PROFESSIONAL AND THE FAMILY

Family members cope with and adjust to the patient's illness in different ways, depending on a variety of factors. Family members have different knowledge levels, different emotional states, and different concerns. Patient teaching efforts will be more successful if health professionals are able to recognize the impact that illness has on the family and take steps to incorporate and individualize this information as they include the family in patient teaching. By considering the needs and circumstances of family members when conducting patient teaching, the health professional can begin to enlist the family as a system of support to help the patient adhere to recommendations and achieve his or her health goals (Berry, 2007).

Gathering information about family structure, reactions, and interactions does not have to be time-consuming. Much information about the family can be gathered through simple observation. Who appears the most concerned and interested in the patient? What types of interactions are observed among family members? Who talks to whom and in what way? What is the family's general lifestyle? What activities appear important to them?

Health professionals should also be alert to family reactions to learning about the patient's condition and treatment. Do family members appear apprehensive about learning skills to be used in caring for the patient at home? Is there virtually no response from family members in patient teaching interactions? What stresses are present in the family? How has the family coped with stress in the past? How are they coping now?

When conducting patient teaching that includes the family, health professionals should identify conceptual problems through appropriate data gathering. The meaning of the patient's illness to the family may be assessed by asking members what they consider to be the major problems. Health professionals should develop sensitivity to reactions and behaviors associated with different areas of patient teaching by observing verbal and nonverbal indications. Does the family appear responsive to patient teaching? Is there dominance of conversation by one family member? Are there numerous disruptions of patient teaching from the family?

When including the family in patient teaching, health professionals should use open and factual terminology and use a calm and supportive approach with no unwarranted optimism or pessimism. Various goals in patient treatment should be discussed so the family, as well as the patient, knows what to expect. Although patient responsibility for carrying out treatment recommendations should be clearly established, the importance of the family's supportive role should also be stressed. If the patient has a chronic illness, or requires ongoing medical intervention, it should be noted that just as patient teaching and feedback should be ongoing, so should be teaching with family members. Proficiency in self-care skills and illness management evolves over time. Learning how to make recommendations fit into the patient's daily life not only requires problem solving with the patient, but input from family members as well (Dickson & Riegel, 2009).

If particular problems are uncovered, they should be discussed along with ways they might be solved or at least alleviated. Families themselves can be helped to generate options. Family values should be accepted rather than criticized. Family members should receive help in recognizing and expressing their own feelings. Only after health professionals have identified feelings and problems within the family can help be given to the family in working toward solutions. Is lack of family support a barrier to patient adherence? Can the lack of support be changed through intervention? If not, can the health professional provide additional support or refer the patient to other sources of support? Can the health professional help the family identify outside resources that will increase the patient's potential for following recommendations?

Health professionals should also be aware of the tendency of family members who are anxious and under stress to misunderstand or misinterpret what they are told. It is not uncommon for people to distort information, turning it into what they want to hear. Such occurrences can cause conflicts between the patient and the family and can contribute to nonadherence. It is often helpful to assess family members' understanding of what they have been told so that any misinterpretation can be corrected early. Although information should be given in a positive way, it is also important that health professionals help family members develop realistic expectations. Giving the patient and the family written information to read at a later time and then having them return to discuss it may be helpful.

Using a family approach to patient teaching in which the family is viewed as the unit of care can help health professionals provide more effective patient teaching (Gotler et al., 2001). Getting to know the patient in the context of his or her family can be important in helping the patient meet his or her health goals. Health professionals facilitate the effectiveness of patient teaching by fostering discussion among family members. If health professionals have continued contact with the patient and the family, they may check on the patient's progress with the recommendations and identify any new problems or strains that interfere with adherence. This helps the patient and his or her family find new solutions and resources to maximize the potential for compliance.

REFERENCES

Badr, H., & Acitelli, L. K. (2005). Dyadic adjustment in chronic illness: Does relationship talk matter? *Journal of Family Psychology, 19*(2), 465–469.

Berry, D. (2007). *Health communication: Theory and practice.* New York: Open University Press.

Chumbler, N. R., Rittman, M. R., Van Puymbroeck, M., Vogel, W. B., & Qin, H. (2004). The sense of coherence, burden, and depressive symptoms in informal caregivers during the first month after stroke. *International Journal of Geriatric Psychiatry, 19*(10), 944–953.

Chumbler, N. R., Rittman, M. R., & Wu, S. S. (2008). Associations of sense of coherence and depression in caregivers of stroke survivors across 2 years. *The Journal of Behavioral Health Services Research, 35*(2), 226–234.

Clark, P. C., & Dunbar, S. B. (2003). Family partnership intervention: A guide for a family approach to care of patients with heart failure. AACN Clinical Issues. *Advanced Practice in Acute and Critical Care, 14*(4), 467–476.

Dickson, V. V., & Riegel, B. (2009). Are we teaching what patients need to know? Building skills in heart failure self-care. *Heart & Lung, 38*(3), 253–261.

Dunbar, S. B., Clark, P. C., Quinn, C., Gary, R. A., & Kaslow, N. J. (2008). Family influences on heart failure self-care and outcomes. *Journal of Cardiovascular Nursing, 23*(3), 258–265.

Family Caregiver Alliance. (2006). *Fact sheet: Caregiver health.* Retrieved July 10, 2009, from http://caregiver.org/caregiver/jsp/content_node.jsp?nodeid=1822

Gotler, R. S., Medalie, J. H., Zyzanski, S. J., Kikano, G. E., & Stange, K. C. (2001). Focus on the family. Part II: Does a family focus affect patient outcomes? *Family Practice Management, 8*(4), 45–46.

Halm, M. A., & Bakas, T. (2007). Factors associated with depressive symptoms, outcomes, and perceived physical health after coronary bypass surgery. *Journal of Cardiovascular Nursing, 22*(6), 508–515.

Jecker, N. (1990). The role of intimate others in medical decision making. *Gerontologist, 30*(1), 65–71.

Lipkin, M. (1996). Patient education and counseling in the context of modern patient-physician-family communication. *Patient Education and Counseling, 27*, 5–11.

Mannes, S. L., Jacobsen, P. B., Gorfinkle, K., Gernstein, F., & Redd, W. H. (1993). Treatment adherence difficulties among children with cancer: The role of parenting style. *Journal of Pediatric Psychology, 18,* 47–62.

Mausbach, B. T., Patterson, T. L., Von Kanel, R., Mills, P. J., Dimsdale, J. E., Ancoli-Israel, S., et al. (2007). The attenuating effect of personal mastery on the relations between stress and Alzheimer caregiver health: A five-year longitudinal analysis. *Aging & Mental Health, 99*(6), 637–644.

Palmer, S., & Glass, T. A. (2003). Family function and stroke recovery: A review. *Rehabilitation Psychology, 48*(4), 255–265.

Pierce, L. L., & Lutz, B. J. (2009). Family Caregiving. In P. D. Larsen & I. M. Lubkin (Eds.), *Chronic illness: Impact and intervention* (7th ed., pp. 191–229). Sudbury, MA: Jones and Bartlett.

Plowfield, L. A., Raymond, J. E., & Blevins, C. (2000). Wholism for aging families: Meeting needs of caregivers. *Holistic Nursing Practice, 14*(4), 51–59.

Reust, C. E., Mattingly, S. (1996). Family involvement in medical decision making. *Family Medicine, 28*(1), 39–45.

Shirey, L., & Summer, L. (2000). *Caregiving: Helping the elderly with activity limitations.* Washington, DC: National Academy on Aging Society.

CHAPTER 7

Cultural Issues in Patient Teaching and Patient Adherence

CULTURE

Individual development within a population is dependent on heredity, the environment to which the individual is exposed, and the society in which he or she lives. Every society has standards to which individuals are expected to conform. The influences of society on an individual are known as culture. Culture comprises many elements, including language, customs, beliefs, traditions, modes of communication, and elements such as tools, art, buildings, science, and technology.

Culture is the characteristic pattern of attitudes, values, beliefs, and behaviors shared by members of a society or population. Members of a cultural group share characteristics that distinguish them from other groups. These characteristics include patterns of communication and interaction that are used to interpret and process messages and to arrive at conclusions. Culture gives individuals a sense of belonging to a group and creates parameters or boundaries within which individuals in the particular culture function.

Culture is learned. Cultural concepts are communicated from one generation to another by specific groups within the culture. Examples of cultural groups are institutions, such as families, social organizations, tribes, or religions. Individuals are socialized within the cultural group or social organization to follow norms or shared values of the culture. Customs, or the habitual practices of the group, regulate the social life within a culture and include specific ways of thinking or behaving that are common to members of that group. All cultures have some taboos, or prohibitive norms. In addition, certain traditions are followed that are important to the culture.

Although many think of culture only in terms of racial background, ethnic identity, or country of origin, cultural variables can also include gender, disability, and socioeconomic status where specific expectations, norms, and values are shared within members of the group. These cultural variables can be expressed within a larger, dominant culture as subcultures, or they can be the dominant culture with which an individual identifies. Subcultures may be based on ethnicity, activity (such as gangs), occupation, sexual orientation, or religion. Each subculture may have its own jargon and rules of acceptable behaviors. Understanding the rules and expectations of subcultures can be just as important as understanding how they relate to larger cultures, and how they are perceived by those larger cultures.

It is important to remember that there is great diversity within cultural groups as well as between them. In some instances, individuals may identify and belong to several groups. Members of various groups may share some aspects of history or tradition, and at times even have a common language, but yet be very different from one another. For example, people of color who may be called "Blacks" collectively may be African American, from Africa, or from the Caribbean, each with their own culture and traditions. Likewise, there are more than 500 different North American Indian tribes and nations, each with tremendous cultural diversity (Andrews & Boyle, 2008). In the same vein, individuals of Asian ancestry may represent cultures from China, Japan, India, Korea, or other parts of Southeast Asia, each with distinct and diverse cultures and traditions. In another example, even though individuals may be classified as Latino or Hispanic, or as Middle Eastern, there are significant cultural variations.

CULTURE AND HEALTH

Cultural factors are an integral part of everyone's life. Attitudes, beliefs, and behaviors in many areas of life are affected by culture. Values, beliefs, and traditions that are observed in various cultural groups have deep roots that affect individual behavior and individual reaction to different situations and events (Cagle & Kovacs, 2009; Washam, 2009). Cultural factors influence personal identity and lifestyle, and are significant variables in health and health status, including views of what constitutes health and how to react to illness (Lewis, 2002). Culture influences the individual's willingness to seek and accept health care, and influences how symptoms of illness and reactions to symptoms are experienced and expressed (Canino & Guarnaccia, 1997; Leong, Wagner, & Tara, 1995), and cultural beliefs can precipitate or aggravate a health condition (Farahani et al., 2007).

Each culture has a belief and value of what constitutes health and illness, how each should be managed, and what priority each has. Every culture has managed to survive in part because it has developed some method to deal with health problems. In doing so, some practices have become deeply rooted in the culture and, although perhaps changed to some degree over time, remain to some extent imbedded in the beliefs and actions of people within that culture.

Culture determines, in part, beliefs about what constitutes illness, when health care should be sought and by whom, and how to behave when sick or injured (Aziz, 2009). To deal effectively with patients, health professionals must understand the impact of culture on patients' health and health care. In some cultures, seeking help from health professionals may be considered a sign of weakness, or it may be viewed only as a last resort. Some cultures have a variety of levels of health practitioners who have different skills that are sought for different perceived needs. For example, in some cultures, when someone becomes ill, a pharmacist may be consulted first for a prescription for the symptoms rather than a physician. In other cultures, women would seek most healthcare advice from older women in the group rather than from another level of healthcare practitioner. Consequently, for individuals from some cultures, seeking care from a physician may not be the first step when illness occurs. Treatment may be sought from other levels of health practitioners first.

CULTURE AS A FACTOR IN PATIENT TEACHING

Patient teaching is often conducted with the assumption that the patient shares the same values, attitudes, and philosophy as health professionals presenting the information. This may not be the case, especially with patients from other cultures. Unless cultural differences are recognized, it is likely that attempts at effective patient teaching will fail. Lack of knowledge or understanding of cultural differences or unwillingness to accept patients' alternative beliefs, values, or attitudes can lead to the inability to empathize or to accept the patient's point of view. These factors can prevent health professionals from being able to conduct patient teaching so that it meets patients' needs, and may interfere with the ability to devise solutions to potential barriers to patient adherence that would be acceptable to all involved. Before trying to change patients' attitudes, beliefs, or health practices, health professionals should first try to understand them, by respecting patients' cultural identity. Health professionals who demonstrate a critical attitude toward patients' behaviors, attitudes, or customs will only alienate patients and discourage opportunity for further patient teaching.

Cultural characteristics of patients obviously have implications for patient teaching. When considering cultural issues and their relationship to patient teaching, it may be easy to focus on language differences that may impede effective exchange of information; however, cultural differences extend beyond language. Culture is a multidimensional concept that affects values, attitudes, and behaviors of individuals within a given group. Every culture has views, practices, and beliefs that relate not only to lifestyle, gender roles, and world view, but also to health and illness. The extent to which patients perceive patient teaching as having cultural relevance for them can have a profound effect on their reception to the information provided and their willingness to follow recommendations. Consequently, inclusion and consideration of cultural factors is critical in patient teaching if it is to be effective.

CULTURE AND ADHERENCE

Culture can have a profound impact not only on patients' receptivity to patient teaching but also on how patients react to recommendations. The degree to which individuals choose to follow health advice, regarding activities related to either prevention of disease or treatment of illness, can be affected significantly by the norms imposed by their cultural environment. Patients from a cultural group that is different from that of the health professional may find the approach to health care or patient teaching incompatible with their own notions of health and illness. Different cultures may have different priorities. Those things highly valued and prioritized by health professionals may be ranked differently by patients from another culture. Although good health and preventive health practices may be valued highly in some cultures, other cultures may view such practices as a luxury, focusing more on economic survival or day-to-day survival, which involves attaining basic necessities such as housing, food, and transportation.

Although each patient must be considered individually, it is also important for health professionals to have an understanding of how a patient's culture may have shaped his or her perspectives regarding health, illness, and treatment and consequently impact on his or her willingness to follow treatment recommendations. Because of past experiences, patients from different cultures may have different views about health and illness than the health professional who is conducting teaching and making recommendations. Incorporating cultural values and practices into patient teaching and incorporating the patient's cultural values and beliefs into recommendations has been found to improve adherence and decrease overall costs for health care (Chang & Kelly, 2007; Leininger & McFarland, 2006).

HISTORICAL INFLUENCES AND CULTURE

When the health professional's culture is different from that of the patient, rather than viewing the health professional as an individual, the patient may generalize from preconceived notions. Historical events may have shaped the patient's views of the health professional's culture, and in turn impact on his or her willingness to accept advice and recommendations from someone from a culture different from their own. Some cultures, for example, have experienced decimation due to war and disease brought on by people from other cultures. In other instances, ethnic minority groups have been relegated to special areas with regulations imposed, experiencing not only prejudice due to cultural differences but also hate because atrocities of war were attributed to the culture as a whole. At different times in history, traditions of various cultures have been undermined, treaties have been broken, and rights have been violated by other cultures. In some cases, cultural groups immigrating to other countries have been used as cheap labor while being denied the right to citizenship. Many culturally different groups have been forced to live in substandard conditions and have often had violence directed toward them by members of different cultures. In still other instances, discrimination based on ethnicity or religion has prevented individuals from receiving the same education, employment opportunities, health care, and living standards as most other individuals living in the same country.

As a result, patients from cultures that have experienced a history of oppression or discrimination may have difficulty trusting the motives and recommendations made by health professionals who are from a culture or ethnic group different from their own. This perception can lead to psychological barriers, which, in turn, affect receptivity to patient teaching and adherence to recommendations, both of which may be viewed as a means of subjugation and social control. The patient may view recommendations from the health professional with suspicion, doubting that recommendations are in their best interest or that they will enhance their well being (Campinha-Bacote, 2009). Consequently, they may be reluctant to follow through with recommendations.

CULTURAL DIVERSITY

As technology has made travel and thus mobility possible for larger numbers of people, few countries remain culturally homogenous. Consequently, many societies have become more pluralistic, and their populations have become more culturally diverse. In the United States, it has been estimated that by 2050, the population will consist of 25% Hispanic/Latino, 14% Black, 9% Asian, and 1% American Indian (Kar, Alcalay, & Alex, 2001). Such cultural diversity has implications for all segments of society, but especially healthcare delivery, and patient teaching in particular. Every patient teaching interaction has a cultural dimension.

Cultural expectations influence individuals' beliefs about the degree of control they have over their lives. Cultural norms may also influence how much personal responsibility individuals take for their health. If, for example, patients believe that the source of illness is spiritual, they may see no need or relevance for information about their condition or treatment.

In addition, some conditions may be thought to be better treated with folk remedies than with remedies prescribed by health professionals. Take, for example, the case of Mrs. Mantea. At an office visit, Dr. Kaster noticed that Mrs. Mantea had several warts on her fingers. Dr. Kaster suggested that the warts should be removed, and that if she would like, an appointment could be made in the next week to have it done. Mrs. Mantea replied that there was no need to go through such a procedure, which may cause pain and scars. Instead, she stated a better solution would be to buy a new silk ribbon and tie as many knots in the ribbon as she had warts. The ribbon, she explained, would then be dropped in the neighborhood, and whoever picked it up would also receive her warts. Under these circumstances, for Dr. Kaster to dispute Mrs. Mantea's remedy or to attempt to discount her belief could reduce his credibility and make future patient teaching attempts less than effective.

The proposed treatment may be unacceptable to Mrs. Mantea because it challenges the effectiveness of a remedy that may have been passed down from trusted generations. In some instances, proposed treatments may clash with cultural norms. Before accepting the treatment, patients from different cultural groups may discuss the recommendations with other members of their culture, seeking group acceptance before adapting to treatment or modifying behavior. In different ethnic communities, the reputation of the health professional frequently travels by word of mouth. Consequently, if the health professional is viewed as one who works within the cultural framework of the patient, credibility will be gained.

Culture is closely allied to the patient's immediate environment and includes all the social, moral, religious, and cultural groups with which the individual comes in contact. Cultural factors influence specific beliefs or interpretations regarding the body, its normal functioning, causes and consequences of illness, help-seeking, treatment, adherence, and many other related issues. Many cultures maintain at least a portion of their own folkways and remedies. To conduct effective patient teaching, health professionals should be prepared to address specific concerns and beliefs of patients from different cultures.

IMMIGRATION

Understanding patients' culture is, of course, important to effective patient teaching; however, when the individual is also a new immigrant, there may be a need for another level of understanding. Immigration is sometimes believed to be motivated because of extreme poverty or political unrest. Although this is true in some instances, an increasingly large number of immigrants are highly skilled workers (Kingma, 2006). Adjusting to a new environment can be stressful even when individuals are moving to new locations within their same country and culture. In the case of new immigrants, exposure standards of the new culture require adjustment and adaptation, especially if the new standards are in conflict with those of their native culture. In addition, new immigrants may have experienced stress throughout the immigration process, which may only add to the stress they experience in their new environment. At times, because of their immigrant status, living and work standards in their newly adopted new country may be considerably lower than they had experienced in their country of origin, further contributing to the stress of their new situation. In some instances, the threat of harm as a result of prejudice, which at time results in violence, may produce significant stress. As a result of these stressors, adaptive coping methods and survival mechanisms adopted by the patient may present considerable barriers to effective patient teaching unless the health professional is sensitive to the origins and meanings of adaptive behaviors and is willing to take them into account when working with individual patients. Even when an individual is born in the same country as the health professional, if he or she is from a different cultural heritage or ethnic origin, the individual may internalize the experience of his or her ancestors and may continue to feel prejudice, whether it is real or imagined (Kaiser Family Foundation, 2001). An understanding of the norms of patients' cultures and the extent of patients' immersion in those cultures are critical to understanding patients' responses to recommendations.

ETHNICITY

Embodied in culture is ethnicity. Although ethnicity is frequently used synonymously with race, it constitutes more than just race. Ethnicity is biological and racial, and although tied to culture, may also be separate. It refers to a common social and cultural heritage passed on to each successive generation (Giger & Davidhizar, 2004). For example, Ms. Liu's ethnic background is Chinese; however, her family had immigrated to another country several generations ago. Consequently, Ms. Liu largely ascribes to and identifies with the culture of the adopted country and is more strongly influenced by the culture in which she grew up and currently lives rather than the culture of her ethnic background. Under these circumstances, for the health professional to assume, without gaining further information, that Ms. Liu holds the same traditions and customs as those of her ethnic background would be as erroneous as assuming that an individual who recently immigrated to the health professional's culture had automatic acceptance and understanding of that culture. Likewise, in some instances, even though individuals have lived within a culture for generations, they may still hold a strong ethnic identity with their native culture, which is separate from the culture in which they now live.

ACCULTURATION

Distinct from ethnicity is acculturation, a term related to the individual's adaptation to the customs, values, and behaviors of a new culture. The degree of acculturation any one individual experiences may be dependent on a number of factors. In some instances, individuals who have immigrated to a new country may reject the beliefs and behaviors of their culture of origin and take on those of the new culture. When this is the case, the individual is said to be acculturated. The length of time in a new country, however, is not an indication of the individual's degree of acculturation. Some individuals may live in a new country for their entire lives but still hold fast to the traditions, values, and beliefs of their own culture.

The amount of acculturation that takes place is affected to some degree by the individual's age at the time of immigration. For instance, children may have a greater tendency to acculturate than older adults (Andrews & Boyle, 2008). Acculturation is also affected by family influences. For example, individuals in a close, socially isolated family may have less exposure to outside influences and thus receive more family support for holding onto traditional values. For example, Mrs. Santos had immigrated to a new country with her family when she was 2 years of age. Her family, however, was quite close and moved to a city community in which many others from Mrs. Santos' own culture lived. Mrs. Santos' family never traveled, and the school she attended was made up mostly of people from her own ethnic and cultural background. Immediately after high school, she married a classmate of her own ethnic background. They settled in the same community in which they had been raised. Although Mrs. Santos has lived in her adopted country nearly 20 years, she continues to ascribe to the traditions and values of her culture of origin.

Education and socioeconomic class also influence acculturation. Those individuals who have broadened their perspectives through education, travel, or wider experiences with others from different countries may acculturate more easily than those individuals who have had little exposure to other cultures. For example, as a child, Mr. Pachesque had been sent to boarding schools located outside his native country. Although during his school years he frequently returned to his country of origin, after completing college he moved to another country to live and has adopted most of the traditions and practices of the new country. Because traditional health beliefs and practices influence health behavior, it is important in patient teaching to assess the degree to which the patient and his or her family adhere to traditional health values and practices and the degree to which the patient has adopted health beliefs and practices of the new culture.

CULTURAL DIFFERENCES AND THE HEALTH PROFESSIONAL

Beliefs of patients from different cultures or ethnic backgrounds and their views about the health professional or health care may have been influenced by their previous experience or expectations because of their minority status. Individuals who have experienced discrimination and hostility may come to expect negative reactions, especially from those perceived as having power or authority. As a result, health professionals of a different culture may have difficulty understanding the patient's apparent hostile or defensive response that would appear to be unjustified. Because of the patient's previous experience, however, expectations may be such that negative meanings are attributed to even the most helpful information. By taking time to investigate patients' previous experiences and by attempting to understand the role these experiences can play in patients' current responses, health professionals begin to build rapport with the patients, a necessary and basic component for effective patient teaching.

The credibility of health professionals is dependent on the frame of reference of patients from a different culture. Understanding the patients' frame of reference may facilitate health professionals' ability to use social influence needed to help patients incorporate recommendations into their own lives. Whether or not patients accept or reject the information given by health professionals will be based on whether they perceive the information as truth, whether in their mind it is an accurate representation of reality, and whether they believe health professionals have their best interest at heart.

When working with patients from other cultures, health professionals must consider more than their patients' cultural background. The culture of the health professional must be considered as well. Both patients and health professionals bring their own cultural values, attitudes, and behaviors to patient teaching interactions.

Cultural differences between health professionals and patients can be a potential impediment to effective patient teaching. Many health professionals hold a cultural perspective that may not be shared by patients from a different ethnic group. Based on one's frame of reference, such differences or diversity can take many forms. The health professional's lack of understanding of specific cultural variables and their impact on patients' lives can create barriers to effective patient teaching and be a source of conflict and misunderstanding. Health professionals' preconceived notion of patients' culture may affect the definition of the problem and assessment of the situation.

Health professionals who are unfamiliar with certain cultural groups and have limited or no experience with members of the patients' culture may hold various myths and stereotypes about the group as a whole. It is important that health professionals avoid projecting their own unconscious myths or stereotypes. Health professionals might hold a pervasive and inaccurate stereotype that individuals from a certain culture are a homogenous group without acknowledging the diversity that exists within all cultural groups. In other instances, myths about a group and its beliefs and practices affect patient teaching.

Myths

Myths are beliefs that are not based on fact. Stereotypes are rigid preconceptions about all people who are members of a particular group. Health professionals unfamiliar with variations within each culture may have a tendency to treat all people within a cultural group as if they were the same, not allowing for individual differences. Rather than forming impressions based on experience with patients as individuals, health professionals may form opinions based on preconceived ideas, myths, and/or stereotypes held for that ethnic group. Consequently, rather than considering individual differences, all incoming information becomes distorted to fit health professionals' own ideas of what the particular ethnic group is like.

Myths and stereotypes that health professionals may have are obviously barriers to effective patient teaching For example, Mr. Perez was a patient of Hispanic background who had been recently hospitalized because of gastritis. He was referred for patient teaching regarding diet. The health professional discussed the possibility that spices may irritate the condition and specified that even though she knew Hispanics liked hot and spicy foods, Mr. Perez would have to become accustomed to a more bland diet. Later, Mr. Perez was asked by another health professional if he had found the patient teaching helpful, he replied, "Not really; where I am from, the foods we eat are only lightly seasoned, and I personally have never cared for spicy food anyway." The health professional conducting the patient teaching had presented information based on stereotype and did not account for individual differences within a culture or differences of various regions or areas within the country from which the culture originated.

Stereotypes

Categorizing individuals into a group perpetuates exaggeration of differences between groups and can minimize distinctions of individuals within the group. There is great intercultural variability among individuals in every cultural group. Variation may occur because individuals have different levels of education, have different socioeconomic status, have different levels of acculturation, and have different values based on generational differences or urban or rural backgrounds.

Cultural groups are represented at all economic and educational levels. The same differences exist between individuals in all cultures. There can be great diversity of thought and behavior within any cultural group. Lumping all persons from one culture together ignores significant differences between groups and violates the patient's identity. Failing to realize that not all individuals from the same culture necessarily ascribe to all of the values, customs, or beliefs of their cultural group can interfere with rapport building, which is necessary for effective patient teaching. In this case, health professionals may fail to individualize patient teaching according to the patient's specific needs, focusing instead on beliefs about the patient's cultural group as a whole. Health professionals must explore their own beliefs regarding certain cultures, separating fact from myth and prejudice, and recognizing differences in priorities and value systems in patients' cultures compared to their own.

REACHING AN UNDERSTANDING OF CULTURAL DIFFERENCES IN PATIENT TEACHING

When conducting patient teaching with patients from a different culture, health professionals may experience feelings of inadequacy, frustration, or resentment. If health professionals know nothing about the patient's culture, some of the patient's behavior or beliefs that are unfamiliar may be viewed as bizarre, uncooperative, or strange, even though in the context of the patient's culture, the behaviors or beliefs are totally appropriate. For example, Ms. Holmes had been a nurse on the diabetic unit for several years and had generally been thought of as having exceptional patient teaching skills. However, she found one patient, Mr. Sayyid, a patient from Afghanistan, extremely difficult to work with. Finally, one day in exasperation, Ms. Holmes stated, "I give up—you can lead a horse to water, but you can't make him drink. I've tried everything, but Mr. Sayyid misses appointments, doesn't appear to have followed through on recommendations we discussed, and at the last session couldn't even remember what we had talked about the session before. He is unmotivated, so until he decides to help himself, there's nothing I can do."

The office nurse, working with Mr. Sayyid's physician said, "Let me talk to him and see what the trouble is." At his next physician's appointment, the office nurse, while preparing him for the exam, said:

> *Nurse*: "You've been going to Ms. Holmes for patient teaching for awhile now, haven't you? How's it going?"
> *Mr. Sayyid*: "Terrible! Ms. Holmes is very nice, but I know she doesn't like me. When I try to explain to her why I can't do some of the things, she says, 'Of course you can; it's easy.' I want to be a good patient and to learn, but it's very hard. She doesn't understand."
> *Nurse*: "Maybe you could give her one more chance."

The nurse then reported back to Ms. Holmes, who had been unaware of her abrupt and insensitive attitude. At the next session, Ms. Holmes said, "You know, Mr. Sayyid, I've been thinking, I really don't know very much about your culture. With all the talking I've been doing, I haven't taken the time to consider that some of the things we're doing may be difficult for you. Tell me a little bit about some of your customs."

Mr. Sayyid seemed pleased and proceeded to explain some basic beliefs and traditions that he held dear. After that, adjustments could be made in his patient teaching plan so that he was better able to follow through with treatment recommendations.

GAINING CREDIBILITY

When developing a relationship with patients from other cultures, health professionals should not assume that patients will automatically accept patient teaching information as accurate or important because of the health professional's qualifications or professional preparation. Although certain credentials may be perceived to indicate a level of expertise and legitimacy, the same credentials or qualifications may not have the same importance in all cultures. More than credentials are needed to establish a relationship between patient and health professional in which open discussion can take place. Building a trusting and open relationship in which such discussion can take place is crucial to patient teaching. Health professionals must be perceived as sincere and genuinely interested in helping patients to obtain their maximal health status. They must also be perceived as trustworthy and accepting rather than condemning, criticizing, or making light of the patients' beliefs or cultural practices.

In some instances, health professionals may avoid conducting patient teaching with patients from other cultures altogether, feeling the situation to be unmanageable. Such a defeatist attitude makes health professionals seem abrupt and distant, further diminishing the opportunity for effective patient teaching in the future. In other instances, health professionals may conduct patient teaching with no alteration or consideration of cultural factors, ignoring, denying, or minimizing differences that do exist.

Even when health professionals are sensitive to cultural differences, they still may not feel they have the knowledge or skills for effective patient teaching with patients from other cultures. In some instances, health professionals may be overly sensitive, so that they are not as direct in the patient teaching interaction as they would be with other patients. Because of their fear of offending the patient in some way, health professionals may not address certain issues or may fail to obtain information that could make the patient teaching interaction more effective. In the same vein, health professionals may not attempt compromises or negotiation, feeling that such efforts may be misinterpreted by patients. At times, health professionals may deny that there are any differences in values or priorities. By acknowledging and understanding differences, health professionals may be able to discuss them with the patient and reach a compromise that would help the patient follow recommendations.

In some instances, health professionals may merely expect that patients will follow directives without examining patients' feelings about the recommendations or assessing whether or not they can be carried out. For example, the concept of prevention may be an unfamiliar concept to individuals in some cultures. In other instances, because of modesty or taboos imposed by the patient's culture, recommendations involving a procedure, such as mammography or Papanicolaou smear, may be viewed as disrespectful or as a violation of privacy. To make patient teaching most effective, it is crucial that health professionals consider specific experiences, beliefs, and values related to the patient's cultural background.

Effective patient teaching demands an understanding of the norms and shared values of patients' culture as well as an understanding that individual differences are present in every culture. Patient behavior should be evaluated within patients' cultural frame of reference. Knowledge of patients' culture gives health professionals a more complete picture of patients' perspectives of their condition and helps health professionals approach patient teaching so that it is best suited to patients' needs.

An understanding of the cultural backgrounds of patients enables health professionals to appreciate attitudes of individuals of different cultures in reaction to hospitalization, dietary restrictions, or other treatment recommendations. In addition, health professionals can become more sensitive to difficulties and fears patients in a new country may have, the frustration those with language difficulty may feel, and the importance and significance of spiritual and religious rituals. Health professionals must show respect for patients' cultural beliefs about illness and provide patient teaching that enhances patients' understanding within their own cultural framework. At the same time, health professionals must make some determinations regarding which behaviors are culturally based and which are unique to the individual.

PATIENT-CENTERED CULTURALLY SENSITIVE PATIENT TEACHING

Cultural differences are too complex and diverse for simple approaches. Cultural patterns are only rough approximations and do not consider individual differences within the culture. There are broad variations of individual behavior within each culture. Although some generalizations may be true for the majority of individuals within a culture, they certainly are not true universally. Likewise, no culture is static. Therefore, culturally sensitive patient teaching requires ongoing work and modification to reflect changes within the patient's culture. There will always be exceptions. Although there is not a standard way to work with patients of different cultures, it does require a comprehensive approach that raises the awareness and sensitivity of health professionals to cultural issues to be incorporated into patient teaching. Health professionals cannot know specific customs, values, and beliefs of every ethnic group. Health professionals should, however, develop an openness to cultural differences and not impose their values on patients from different ethnic backgrounds.

At times, patient teaching involves problem solving and negotiation, identifying barriers that may prevent patients from following through with advice and recommendations given. The same is true with patients from different cultures. Health professionals must be aware of and sensitive to cultural differences, not making assumptions and generalizations based on stereotypes but, rather, attempting to understand the patient as an individual.

COMMUNICATION ISSUES IN CROSS-CULTURAL PATIENT TEACHING

Communicating effectively requires skilled use of various techniques (Berry, 2007). Patient teaching involves interpersonal communication as well as information transfer. Both communication and information transfer are two-way processes. The process of interpersonal communication involves speech and language, body language, personal space and distance, and physical contact, such as touch, all of which are exhibited by both patient and health professional. The process of transferring information is two-dimensional and consists of receiving information from the patient as well as providing the patient with information about his or her condition or treatment with the goal of helping the patient to:

- Understand his or her diagnosis and treatment
- Understand aspects of prevention
- Incorporate the information into daily life
- Make truly informed choices about the extent to which he or she will follow treatment recommendations

Before effective patient teaching can occur, however, health professionals and patients must accurately send and receive both verbal and nonverbal messages. In conducting patient teaching across cultures, it is important to adapt not only the content of the information but also the methods by which the content is conveyed. Communication styles may be different and may be a source of misunderstanding. There should be a concerted effort to make information fit the patient rather than insisting that the patient fit the information. Barriers to effective communication in patient teaching can occur at any time, even when both patient and health professional are from the same culture. When health professionals and patients are from different cultural backgrounds, however, the barriers to effective communication become greater, and a greater opportunity for misunderstanding exists. In addition to such misunderstandings impeding the accurate transfer of information in patient teaching, misunderstandings can also lead to alienation and disintegration of the relationship between patient and health professional.

Language

A significant amount of research has demonstrated the negative impact language barriers can have on health care (Bowen, 2004; Pope, 2004), including miscommunication, reduced comprehension, and nonadherence to treatment (Bowen, 2004). Patients from different cultures may not use the standard language spoken by health professionals or may not speak the language at all. Often, in an attempt to speak the language of the health professional, patients may use simple phrases because of their limited vocabulary in the language. It is at times easy for health professionals to assume, because of a patient's difficulty in using the language, that he or she has limited intelligence. The health professional may begin to think of the patient as a child and begin treating him or her in that way, which only serves to build further barriers to effective patient teaching. In most instances, a patient's inability to use a new language adequately is not a reflection of level of intelligence or education but, rather, merely unfamiliarity and inexperience with the new language.

Even if the language of the health professional is the primary language of the patient, regional differences may exist within the same language. Language variations related to words and expressions may be as important as recognition of differences of values and customs. Subcultures within the same country may also use nonstandard language as the norm, with their own phrases and words to express concepts. Language of the subculture may be a way the patient has found to adapt and function in his or her own world. Although foreign sounding to the health professional, the language of the subculture may be highly developed and structured and quite adequate for conveying ideas. If health professionals cannot relate to patients' language systems, then they probably will have difficulty building rapport.

Likewise, health professionals may, because of their own lack of understanding of the patient's language, attribute inaccurate characteristics or motives to the patient. Misunderstandings that arise from cultural variations in communication may lead to alienation and/or inability to develop trust and rapport, which may result in termination of the patient teaching intervention. Although breakdown in communication can and does occur at times between health professionals and patients from the same culture, the problem can be exacerbated between people from different racial or ethnic backgrounds. Likewise, health professionals from one social class may assume that patients are using the same class rules when communicating and that the words and phrases have the same meaning, whereas this may not be true.

Meanings of language are communicated in many ways. In addition to verbal expression, nonverbal communication is often as meaningful or may be even more meaningful than words expressed. Lack of understanding of the nuances or the importance of nonverbal behaviors in different cultures can also cause misunderstanding and consequently serve as a barrier to effective patient teaching. In addition, the ways words are communicated—such as rate, inflections, loudness, hesitations, and silences—are all used to communicate a variety of different meanings. Gestures, tone, inflections, posture, or eye contact may enhance or negate a message.

For example, people from some cultures may feel uncomfortable with stretches of silence, whereas those from other cultures may give silence specific meaning. Some cultures may use silence as a sign of respect or as a sign of politeness. In other cultures, silence may be used to signify agreement or to emphasize a point. If the health professional is from a culture in which silence is not part of regular communication, a patient teaching interaction in which the patient remains silent may be interpreted as lack of understanding or disinterest on the part of the patient. If the health professional is uncomfortable with silence, he or she may keep talking to fill in the silence or believe that the patient teaching has failed.

Health professionals may expect patients to be inquisitive and open, approaching the patient teaching with a certain degree of sophistication.

Persons not fitting into this framework may be considered resistant or defensive.

Take the case of Ms. Bobnon, an international student who was receiving routine prenatal care from Dr. Tate. At each visit, Dr. Tate attempted to talk with Ms. Bobnon about diet and activity during pregnancy, what to expect at different stages of pregnancy, and how to prepare for the baby. Throughout each visit, Ms. Bobnon remained silent, never asking questions and offering no comment. Dr. Tate became increasingly frustrated and shared with the nurse that he had concern about Ms. Bobnon's ability to care adequately for the baby given that she seemed to have so little interest in the information he had attempted to provide. Dr. Tate did not understand that, whereas in some countries patients are expected to ask questions or state their opinions about their treatment, some cultures may view this as rude and disrespectful, and consequently patients do not ask questions during patient teaching, which was true in Ms. Bobnon's case. Health professionals unaware of such differences may also interpret this reticence of asking questions as a sign of ignorance, a lack of motivation, or an ineffective patient teaching interaction when, in fact, patients may believe they are merely being respectful.

For the most part, health professionals may believe that being frank, open, and direct when conducting patient teaching is most desirable. Many cultures, however, have norms that value indirectness or the use of euphemisms in conversation. People from different cultures may vary in their information orientation. Whereas some cultures may value facts and directness, others may place more importance in having their own questions and concerns answered. In some cultures, indirectness in speech is considered an art. Directness may be considered forceful, or the patient may view the health professional who is direct as being rude and pushy. Such actions may alienate the patient. Under these circumstances, openness and directness, especially if the information is perceived to be a particularly sensitive topic, may be viewed as too blunt or as a source of embarrassment, thus alienating the patient. Take the following example of Mr. Delano.

Mr. Delano, a nurse, had recently begun working in an adolescent health center where most of the patients were of the same ethnic background, a background different from his own. Having worked with adolescents of his own background for a number of years, Mr. Delano prided himself on being able to build rapport quickly and to conduct patient teaching effectively. One program he had been particularly proud of was the acquired immunodeficiency syndrome prevention program he had established at another health clinic. He became increasingly disillusioned and discouraged at the neighborhood health center, however, when it became obvious that not only were the adolescents at this center unreceptive to this information, but they seemed to be avoiding talking with him about other issues as well. Although Mr. Delano interpreted this behavior as the patients' lack of ability to confront the issue, in fact, the patients were offended by what they perceived as Mr. Delano's brashness and insensitivity in being so direct in his discussions.

Volume of speech may also be interpreted differently in other cultures. Speaking in a soft voice may not indicate shyness but rather politeness, and speaking in a loud, brash manner may not indicate anger or hostility but rather interest and enthusiasm. Likewise, the speech patterns or tone of voice of the health professional may be interpreted by the patient as indicating that the health professional is upset, embarrassed, rude, or sarcastic.

Nonverbal Behavior

Nonverbal behavior also has an important impact on interpersonal communication. Culture affects not only verbal language, but also nonverbal use of gestures, touch, and personal space. Nonverbal behavior is culture bound, and consequently the health professional cannot make universal generalizations about different nonverbal behaviors and their meanings. These behaviors operate primarily without the awareness of the individual exhibiting them and often may be a more accurate reflection of feelings than are words. Nonverbal behaviors may be used as a way to exhibit social control, such as getting up and moving to the door as a signal that it is time to end the conversation. Nonverbal behavior is also a way of demonstrating warmth or friendliness. The extent to which these concepts are acceptable to display among strangers or acquaintances, however, varies from culture to culture. For example, in some cultures, a handshake may be a traditional form of greeting, whereas in other cultures, body contact is avoided, but gestures such as bowing are considered polite. In yet other cultures, more intimate forms of greeting, such as hugging, are considered appropriate in most social situations.

Eye contact is another nonverbal behavior that has different meanings in different cultures. In some cultures, eye contact is considered important, demonstrating attention and interest, whereas in other cultures, eye contact may be considered confrontive, aggressive, hostile, or as a sign of disrespect. In patient teaching interactions, eye contact may be interpreted by health professionals as a sign that patients are interested or listening. Aversion of the eyes may be interpreted as a sign of discomfort, guilt, indifference, depression, or disregard. Some cultures, however, assume that merely being there and sitting quietly indicates interest. Styles of communication with the eyes may be different between cultures and may lead to misinterpretations.

Health professionals use patients' nonverbal behavior as cues to discomfort, fatigue, disinterest, embarrassment, or a variety of other factors that can interfere with effective patient teaching. However, when conducting cross-cultural patient teaching, the same rules of interpretation of nonverbal behavior may not be applicable. Being aware of differences in the meaning of nonverbal behavior can help the health professional avoid misinterpretations.

Likewise, health professionals should be aware that their own nonverbal behavior may also be a help or a barrier to effective patient teaching. Individuals from different cultures may be very sensitive to behaviors exhibited by health professionals. In some cultures, greater sensitivity and awareness of the nonverbal behavior of others, especially those in power, may have been learned as a matter of survival. In some instances, the health professional may be unaware that certain nonverbal behaviors are offensive to the patient. In other instances, however, the nonverbal behavior may be the unconscious reflection of the health professional's bias.

Take the case of Dr. Frankel, who had asked Mr. Su, a patient from a cultural background different from her own, to return for blood pressure monitoring due to an elevation of blood pressure on several visits. When Dr. Frankel diagnosed Mr. Su as having hypertension, she took Mr. Su into her office to talk about the condition and its treatment. Rather than sitting beside Mr. Su as she usually did when conducting patient teaching, however, she sat at her desk with Mr. Su placed on the other side. She used less eye contact, and after presenting the information arose from her desk, walked to the door and asked Mr. Su to call her if he had any questions. Although the content of the information was the same as that Dr. Frankel routinely presented, her nonverbal behavior communicated feelings of indifference and disinterest. Attitudes, beliefs, and feelings are deeply ingrained into our total being. No matter how unbiased health professionals believe they have been verbally, if they have not recognized and adequately dealt with their own biases, they may still communicate bias through nonverbal cues.

Use of space as an aspect of culture is an important factor in communication. Reactions and behaviors in interaction with others are, to some extent, a reflection of the spatial dimension to which we are all culturally conditioned. Conversational distance, or the amount of space between two people talking, varies considerably from culture to culture. Some cultures dictate a much closer stance than normally comfortable for people from other cultures. If the patient's conversational distance according to his or her culture is closer than that of the health professional's, and the health professional backs away from the patient, the patient may interpret such behavior as aloofness or the desire not to communicate. On the other hand, the health professional may interpret the close proximity as patients' attempt to become intimate. Personal space may also be interpreted as a sign of dominance and status. The higher the status of the individual, the more space he or she is allowed to occupy.

Even the setting in which patient teaching takes place is important. The placement of furniture where both health professional and patient sit may have implications that could have an impact on the effectiveness of the interaction and can enhance or interfere with the effectiveness of patient teaching.

Body movement may also lead to misunderstanding because the same movement can have contrasting meanings. For instance, whereas in some cultures a raised thumb is given to show approval, in some cultures, the same movement may be considered an insult. In some cultures, nodding the head up and down while the other individual is speaking demonstrates listening and understanding of what is being said. However, not all cultures use this movement. Its absence, therefore, could be interpreted by health professionals as lack of interest or understanding on the part of patients, when in fact it is merely not a behavior commonly used in the patient's culture.

COMMUNICATION STYLE

Communication styles may either enhance or negate the effectiveness of patient teaching. When the communication style of health professionals is different from that of patients from another culture, patient teaching may not be effective, and several problems may arise. The health professional may not seem credible to the patient, and the patient may not incorporate the information or may not attend subsequent sessions. The health professional may terminate patient teaching early as a result of what he or she considers poor motivation or lack of interest on the part of the patient, or the patient and health professional may be unable to establish rapport, which is crucial to effective patient teaching.

It is important for health professionals working with culturally diverse populations to be aware of differences in communication practices and different meanings of nonverbal behavior. Health professionals should guard against possible misinterpretation by patients of actions and/or information and should be aware of how their own nonverbal behaviors may reflect stereotypes or bias about various cultural groups. Health professionals should be able to shift their communication styles and delivery of information to suit the needs of the culturally different patient.

Likewise, it is important to recognize that health professionals cannot understand all variations and nuances of all cultures. When there are personal limits to the extent to which health professionals' communication style can be altered, they may need to seek other alternatives, such as learning more about the specific culture, seeking information from others from the patient's cultural background who can provide insight, or anticipating their own limitations and the impact on the patient. In most instances, however, the health professional can be the most effective by communicating acceptance and understanding of the patient's world view and acknowledging to patients that they are aware that the information they are presenting is from a different cultural perspective. This alone may be enough to bridge the communication gap between patient and health professional.

USE OF AN INTERPRETER

The terms "translation" and "interpretation" are often used synonymously. Translation, however, generally refers to written communication, because translation deals with words. For example, for patient teaching, when preparing brochures for patients with a different language, the health professional may enlist the services of a translator. Interpretation, on the other hand, is a broader concept that usually refers to interpersonal interaction and focuses on spoken interaction in which there are no omissions, additions, editorializing, or distortions (TriAd Research Inc, 2002). Interpretation in patient teaching has greater meaning than just translating words. It is important to also understand the meaning of tones and gestures used in a cultural context (Srivastava, 2007).

When patients and health professionals do not speak the same language, an interpreter, if available, may be used to assist in patient teaching. Use of an interpreter alone, however, does not always ensure that patient teaching will be successful. Just because an individual speaks the same language as the patient does not mean that all communication conveyed between parties will be effective. Whereas information exchange in patient teaching normally takes place between two people, the health professional and the patient, the use of an interpreter adds one more dimension, which can increase the complexity of the interaction.

Interpreters, even though able to communicate in the patient's language, may or may not also be familiar with the patient's culture. Even if the interpreter is familiar with the patient's culture, he or she may consciously or unconsciously insert personal bias into the interpretation from patient to health professional or health professional to patient. In addition, issues of confidentiality may occur if the patient is being given or has asked for information of a particularly sensitive nature.

Although in larger cities professional interpreters may be available, this may not be the case in more rural areas. In instances where a neighbor, family member, or sometimes the patient's child is asked to interpret, health professionals should be aware that the educational and social background of the interpreter is just as important to consider as that of the patient. In order to interpret accurately, the interpreter must understand both the content and the context of the message. The interpreter must also be able to convey information from health professional to patient and from patient to health professional in as unbiased a way as possible. If the interpreter's own values and beliefs are in conflict with the patient's or the health professional's, the information may be slanted toward a particular view of the interpreter rather than given as the information was originally presented.

Patient teaching using an interpreter takes longer. Each message must be verbalized twice. The health professional should attempt to present information with as little technical jargon as possible and attempt to keep explanations simple and unambiguous. The health professional should not forget the patient's presence and should avoid talking only to the interpreter as if the patient were absent. The health professional should face the patient, use direct eye contact, and address the patient in the first person rather than asking the interpreter to convey the information. As the information is provided to the patient by the interpreter, the health professional should be attendant to the patient's response, reactions, and expressions, and if they indicate that the patient is anxious, upset, or has any other negative response, the interpreter should be asked to identify what specifically made the patient respond in that way. At times, it may be important for the health professional to obtain a word-for-word translation of what was said. Obtaining this type of feedback provides the health professional with a chance to clarify or amplify any points that were unclear or misunderstood, as well as provide an opportunity to make sure the message was interpreted accurately.

Although it is helpful in many patient teaching situations to have written materials that can reinforce information the patient has been given verbally, this may be even more important in the case of individuals who speak a different language. If written materials are used, however, it is just as important to make sure the translation is correct in writing as it is to make sure the verbal translation is correct. Having the interpreter back-translate the information can help identify problems or inaccuracies of the original translation so that they may be corrected.

SOCIAL–CULTURAL VARIATIONS IN PATIENT TEACHING

Patient teaching is greatly influenced by the social–cultural framework from which it arises. Identification with the cultural group norm may affect not only patients' health behavior but also the degree to which they adhere to recommendations. As a result, individuals from different cultures may respond quite differently to the same type of information.

Cultural responses to patient teaching on a variety of topics are illustrated by the following examples. For instance, prenatal patient teaching, which is accepted as a routine part of good prenatal care in some cultures, may, in other cultures, be viewed as unnecessary or even a violation of privacy. Some cultures may believe that this type of information is best shared between females in the culture or that such information should be passed from mother to daughter rather than given from a health professional who is a stranger. As another example, patient teaching about tobacco and alcohol use may be viewed differently by patients from different cultures. Although in some cultures, both are taboo, in others, both are used as part of ceremonial ritual. While in some cultures, the use of one or both is considered socially appropriate, in other cultures, the use of one or both may be considered socially irresponsible. Patient response to patient teaching about either will be determined to some extent by the cultural view and tradition from which the patient comes. Diet is also important to ethnic identity, having religious as well as nutritional connotations, including not only what foods are eaten but how they are prepared. Patient teaching about nutrition or diet changes alone may be ineffective, unless the cultural meaning of food and tradition of preparation are understood.

In some cultures, individualization and independence are highly valued. For example, in the United States, patient teaching traditionally emphasizes providing the patient with information about his or her condition and treatment or strategies of prevention of illness, with the goal of empowering them to make informed decisions and be more self-directed in their health and health care. In the United States, patient teaching practice arises out of the belief that patients should be given information from which to make their own decisions and out of the belief that information regarding health and health care will help the individual follow recommendations, which will in turn enhance their well-being (Jennings et al., 2003; Koenig, 2007). Given this philosophy, helping patients to engage in necessary behavior change in accordance with their own goals is the ultimate goal of patient teaching. Although health professionals may emphasize self-determination and self-direction, other cultures may expect the health professional to take an authoritarian approach, valuing the mystique of health professionals and believing they have healing powers.

Information health professionals believe to be necessary for the patient may not be the same information believed by the patient to be necessary. Consequently, patients may not view information the health professional provides to them as important and may not value self-reliance and self-determination in health care and treatment to the same degree as does the health professional. When the views between patient and health professional become too diverse, patients may choose to abandon the setting, and the health professional, seeking help and advice from those whose beliefs and practices more closely resemble his or her own.

Information given may also be in conflict with the patient's traditional beliefs or superstitions regarding cause and/or treatment of illness. Patients in a new culture may be living a dualistic life in which they are attempting to retain traditional values while still trying to live and function in a dominant culture different from their own. This conflict can be the source of considerable stress. Patients may fear retribution if they disagree or allow health professionals to know their true feelings. Consequently, they may take great efforts to hide their true thoughts or their behavior for fear of offending or threatening the health professional. Instead, while appearing to accept the information, they may quietly discount all of it and not follow recommendations. Public appearance of acceptance of information does not necessarily guarantee that the patient will follow the recommendations when in private.

Health professionals may assume that the major goal of patients in healthcare settings is to "get better." In some cultures, however, patients may have a stoic acceptance of poor health with little effort to change. Such patients may accept life, illness, and death as a destiny of nature, not under individual control and not to be interfered with. In other instances, illness may be viewed as a human weakness, and, consequently, admitting illness by receiving treatment or learning more about the illness or treatment may also be viewed in a negative light. Some cultures ascribe a spiritual nature to illness, believing that illness is the will of another who wishes the illness upon them. Such attitudes may be difficult for health professionals to accept unless they understand the cultural context.

SOCIOECONOMIC STATUS AS A CULTURAL VARIABLE

Social and economic status can also contribute to patients' reactions to patient teaching and their ability to follow recommendations. Individuals of lower socioeconomic status or those living in poverty may have yet another layer of values and priorities different from individuals with middle or higher socioeconomic status, even though they may be from the same culture or ethnic group. In some cases, socioeconomic status alone acts as another culture, setting patients with lower socioeconomic status apart from others in their own ethnic culture who are better educated and more financially solvent.

Patients with poor socioeconomic status may have less education and have received poorer health care because of limited access to health care or to good healthcare practices. Consequently, they may view such recommendations as "regular exercise, plenty of rest, and a diet of fresh fruits and vegetables" as a luxury rather than a legitimate recommendation they can follow. Not taking into account patients' economic backgrounds and the role this plays in their current health status is a mistake that can interfere with patient teaching effectiveness.

Lower socioeconomic status often compounds cultural variations. The gap between a health professional who is from a middle-class environment that is predictable and a patient from a lower socioeconomic class environment that is unpredictable may be immense. Individuals from a lower class or socioeconomic background have different access to resources, which may affect the extent to which they are willing or able to follow treatment recommendations. For instance, follow-up visits may be difficult if the patient has no access to transportation. Walking in order to obtain more exercise may be unreasonable if the neighborhood in which the patient lives is unsafe. Other recommendations may involve things the patient cannot afford.

Health professionals may not understand that recommendations that are future oriented, such as issues of prevention, are meaningless to patients who are struggling day to day in the present for basic needs such as food or shelter, factors the health professional may take for granted. Health professionals may view some patients as unable to plan and become frustrated at what they perceive to be lack of motivation. Individuals who are unemployed, underemployed, or for other reasons live in a state of poverty may feel in day-to-day jeopardy and consequently may only be able to concentrate on immediate, short-term goals rather than long-term goals. The health professional may attribute the patient's behaviors and attitudes to cultural differences whereas they are actually due to the adversity of the patient's circumstances. In these instances, patient teaching that focuses on short-term goals and patients' immediate needs will be more effective than patient teaching that focuses on long-term goals.

Because of patients' environments and/or inexperience with being included in their own health care, their expectations may be quite different from those of the health professional. Many patients may expect merely to be given some tangible treatment and may see no reason for additional information. Under these circumstances, providing patients with the amount and type of information they are ready to accept while, at the same time, assuring them that additional information is available if they choose to access it at a later date, will be more efficient than attempting to barrage them with information they are unwilling to hear.

Although poverty and lower educational status impact patient teaching and must be considered, it is just as important to guard against myths and stereotypes about patients from lower socioeconomic backgrounds as it is to refrain from myths and stereotypes about different cultural groups. For example, if a patient with lower socioeconomic status arrives late for an appointment or misses an appointment altogether, the health professional may make the automatic assumption that the patient is irresponsible or unreliable, when in fact the situation occurred because the patient's only means of transportation, the bus, was late or failed to appear.

Rather than making assumptions or basing opinions on stereotypical images, health professionals should attempt to ascertain the reason for the missed appointment. In many instances, for example, the reason for the missed appointment may be related to not owning a car, and thus being dependent on others for their transportation, or owning a car in serious disrepair. Even if public transportation is available, it is at times costly and can be undependable. Patients may also have difficulty arranging child care and may not find it manageable to bring children with them, especially small children. Health professionals must appreciate and be prepared to respond to the needs of the individual, especially if the situation is confounded by economic hardship, discrimination, or other stressors within the environment.

FAMILY ISSUES AND CULTURAL DIVERSITY

The role and influence of family on patients' willingness and ability to carry out treatment recommendations are important in any patient teaching interaction. However, family and specific roles and expectations of family members are not the same across all cultures. Whereas some cultures define the family as the immediate nuclear family, other cultures define family to include not only extended family, but also neighbors, friends, or other people in the community (Chang & Kelly, 2007). Health professionals must define and respect family members' roles, enlist family support for continuing treatment, and increase their confidence in the proposed intervention. It may be important to incorporate the family into patient teaching and to praise the family for its efforts that have helped the patient adhere to medical recommendations.

Cultural beliefs affect family roles and relationships and can have an impact on patient teaching in a number of areas. Child-rearing practices and gender roles are two examples. Discipline—how it is administered and by whom—may have strong cultural overlays that may influence the patient's receptivity to patient teaching about the topic. In addition, gender roles and expectations may make a difference in how, when, and to whom patient teaching is provided and how willing the patient is to follow the recommendations.

In some cultures, men and elders are viewed as having higher status and are regarded as the major decision makers in families, with little input from others. Gender roles, perceptions, and expectations may also be different. Some cultures place major emphasis on the male of the household being independent and the caretaker of his family. If this is the case, it may be difficult if treatment recommendations place the patient in a position where he must be in a dependent role, whether in the hospital or at home. An older patient who does not speak the language of the health professional may feel threatened by having to depend on his or her children to translate information provided. It may be difficult for the patient under these circumstances to maintain dignity and respect in a dependent role that may be required because of the condition. In some cultures, the husband, when he is not the patient, is expected to be given the information and make decisions about the recommendations for his wife. The husband may be resentful if a male presents information directly to his wife or may resent his wife having more knowledge about her condition or treatment than he has. If the husband is the patient, he may feel resentful of having to be dependent on his wife for part of his care.

In some instances, when one family member has become acculturated, strain may be experienced between family members for accepting advice that appears to go beyond the values of the culture. For instance, in cultures where celibacy before marriage is expected, any discussion about contraception prior to marriage may be viewed as offensive.

In some instances, a family member may inherit two different cultural traditions. Reluctance to accept certain treatments should not be viewed as a sign of disinterest or irresponsibility but rather may reflect a conflict between duality of membership in two groups. Even though the patient may have become established in the new culture and is functioning in his or her daily life, the patient's respect for his or her family and cultural traditions may mean that the patient reverts to former cultural practices under some circumstances. This may be true particularly during illness. For instance, in cultures where family is considered integral to the patient's care, the health professional may undermine the patient's cultural concept of extended family by asking to talk with the patient alone without the presence of relatives. Health professionals' persistence in encouraging patients to be self-reliant in their treatment may violate cultural views of appropriate role behaviors and alienate both the patient and his or her family who are viewed as a needed source of support.

ALTERING APPROACHES TO PATIENT TEACHING

To conduct patient teaching effectively with people from different cultures, health professionals must be willing to alter their own behavior, attitudes, and communication styles and to examine their own biases and stereotypes. Patient teaching interventions that are culturally appropriate are patient-centered and are dependent not only on knowledge about different cultures but on cultural sensitivity as well. Health professionals must have the ability to demonstrate tolerance of others' frames of reference and points of view. This does not mean that there must be a blanket acceptance of beliefs or practices that could be harmful. Abusive practices are not acceptable regardless of tradition. When cultural practices are not harmful, they can be incorporated with treatment recommendations. Although there is no cookbook formula for working with patients from different cultures and ethnic backgrounds, there are some general guidelines.

GENERAL GUIDELINES FOR CULTURALLY SENSITIVE PATIENT TEACHING

It is important that the health professional have awareness of cultural differences and how they impact the patient's health and behavior, but it is also important that each patient is assessed individually without making cultural assumptions about a patient's beliefs or health practices. At the same time, it is important that the health professional be aware of his or her own values, prejudices, and stereotypes, and how those may influence the patient teaching interaction.

Health professionals should assess patients' beliefs and maintain openness and flexibility. Questions such as, "What do you think is wrong?" help the health professional assess the patient's perception of the problem. For instance, in some cultures, epilepsy is viewed as spirit possession which has some positive connotations, which in turn may serve as a barrier to the patient's willingness to take antiseizure medication (Galanti, 2008). Assessing the patient's perceptions assists the health professional in dealing with potential barriers to adherence and to alter patient teaching approaches accordingly.

Assessment of the patient's perception of the causes of the condition is also important. For example, if to the question, "What do you think is causing your cold?" the patient responds, "The bad wishes of my neighbor," the health professional, rather than criticizing or discounting the belief, should attempt to learn more about the belief. Health professionals should not discredit patients' cultural beliefs and practices and should treat beliefs, practices, and traditions with respect. The health professional should be aware that regardless of the effectiveness of the recommendations, unless the cause the patient perceives is addressed, the chance that the patient will adhere to the recommendations given by the health professional is slight. Health professionals should attempt to reflect back their interpretation of the patients' perspectives for clarification and to acknowledge they have both heard and respected the patient's point of view by addressing the patient's perceptions in patient teaching.

As much as possible, health professionals should attempt to incorporate the patient's beliefs and practices into the treatment recommendations. If some of the patient's cultural beliefs or practices have the potential for harm, the health professional should consult others who have more insight into the culture so that alternatives may be identified. Depending on the immediacy of the threat and the extent of danger, the health professional may need to obtain more immediate consultation from a supervisor or from other outside agencies. Before this step is taken, however, health professionals must be certain that the perception of harm is accurate and not simply a result of their own bias or lack of understanding of what the belief or practice actually encompasses. For instance, in some cultures, babies are carefully swaddled and kept in the swaddling for hours at a time. Although from a perspective that infants need to have full freedom of movement, the practice may seem appalling; however, if no harm has been shown from this practice, the health professional would hardly be justified in reporting the family for child abuse. The case would be different, of course, if a prenatal patient confided to the health professional that if the baby were not the right gender, it would be drowned at birth.

As with all patients, when working with individuals from a different culture, it is important for health professionals to assess who the patient looks to for social support and advice. Again, rather than attempting to discredit these sources, the health professional should demonstrate understanding of their importance to the patient and include them when appropriate. If, for example, the person of authority and respect is an elder in the group, whether related or not, that person may have more influence on the degree to which the patient is willing to accept and follow treatment recommendations than has the health professional.

In order for patient teaching to be the most effective, the health professional should also assess the individual's concerns about his or her condition and about recommendations. Patients may have concerns that are not immediately apparent to the health professional. For example, the health professional may not understand that the reason the patient is adamantly opposed to taking insulin has nothing to do with fear of injection, but rather with their perception that insulin will cause harm, because a relative, who was diabetic and taking insulin, had to have his or her leg amputated.

Although health professionals, especially if working predominately with one ethnic group, should strive to learn as much as possible about that group, each patient from the culture should be approached as an individual. Health professionals should avoid stereotyping and making assumptions about patients based on the norms of the group without first assessing the individual patient's values and beliefs. Individual variation within cultures exists. Health professionals should also remember that the term "normal" means average. It is a statistical phenomenon that may vary in different cultures. "Normal" is relative.

When communicating with patients from different cultures, health professionals should take into consideration the interaction of class, language, and cultural factors and their impact on verbal and nonverbal behavior. Health professionals should take care not to misinterpret patients' behaviors and to be aware of their own behavior and how patients respond. If, for example, every time the health professional moves close to the patient, the patient moves away, before making the assumption that the patient is unfriendly, the health professional should consider other reasons for the behavior, such as cultural definition of socially appropriate distance. Likewise, the health professional should avoid moving close if he or she observes that the patient's response is one of discomfort.

Health professionals should convey instructions and recommendations in a culturally appropriate manner. Some cultures may consider directives offensive. Other cultures may expect a more direct approach to health advice. Health professionals should be aware of the possible misinterpretation of examples or analogies and should use these with care. Abstract examples may be taken literally. Health professionals should also be aware that some words may not have correlates in all languages or may have a different meaning from the one intended. As much as possible, health professionals should attempt to be clear and concrete in instruction to avoid misunderstanding.

Health professionals should know when to be action-oriented and when to work with patients toward achieving goals at a slower pace. Patients may not care about long-term effects but rather may have different priorities of what is important to them immediately. Helping patients from different cultures through situational problems and dealing with their priorities demonstrates respect, builds greater trust and rapport, and keeps open the possibility of continued discussion and patient teaching.

Above all, health professionals should be genuine. Health professionals should not be afraid to acknowledge unfamiliarity with a culture and should not be afraid to apologize for any faux pas. Statements such as, "I have had little experience with people of your culture, but I would like it if you could help me learn," or "I didn't mean to offend you. Please allow me to try again," convey caring and concern and will be accepted by most people as such. Health professionals should not pretend to know about a culture unless they really do. A brief visit to a country is hardly sufficient for anyone to understand fully the traditions and nuances of that culture. The understanding is most likely superficial and prone to subjective interpretation of the experience. In addition, it negates the differences of different regions of the country, different subcultures, as well as educational and economic variations. Statements such as, "I'm well aware of your customs in Mexico; I spent a week in Tijuana last summer," not only serve to discredit the health professional but may also be offensive.

Conducting patient teaching with patients from another culture can be challenging but also enriching for health professionals. The interaction offers not only the opportunity to help patients but also an opportunity for health professionals to expand their own knowledge of other cultures. Consciously engaging in self-examination and in-depth exploration of personal biases, stereotypes, prejudices, and assumptions about individuals from different cultures or ethnic backgrounds helps the health professional gain increased cultural awareness so he or she is able to engage in culturally sensitive patient teaching with the patient and his or her family, which will increase chances of adherence and positive health outcomes.

REFERENCES

Andrews, M. M., & Boyle, J. S. (2008). *Transcultural concepts in nursing care* (5th ed.). Philadelphia: Wolters Kluwer/Lippincott Williams & Wilkins.

Aziz, V. M. (2009). Cultural aspects of the patient-doctor relationship. *International Psychogeriatrics, 21*(2), 415–417.

Berry, D. (2007). *Health communication theory and practice.* Berkshire, England: Open University Press.

Bowen, S. (2004). *Assessing the responsiveness of health care organizations to culturally diverse groups.* Winnipeg: University of Manitoba, Department of Community Health Sciences.

Cagle, J. G., & Kovacs, P. J. (2009). Education: a complex and empowering social work intervention t the end of life. *Health & Social Work, 34*(1), 17–27.

Campinha-Bacote, J. (2009). A culturally competent model of care for African Americans. *Urologic Nursing, 29*(1), 49–54.

Canino, G., & Guarnaccia, P. (1997). Methodological challenges in the assessment of Hispanic children and adolescents. *Applied Developmental Science, 1*, 124–134.

Chang, M. & Kelly, A. E. (2007). Patient education: Addressing cultural diversity and health literacy issues. *Urologic Nursing, 27*(5), 411–417.

Farahani, M.A., Mohammadi, I., Ahmadi, F., & Maleki, M. (2007). Cultural beliefs and behaviors of clients with coronary artery disease: a necessity in patient education. *SBMU Faculty of Nursing and Midwifery Quarterly, 16*(59), 1.

Galanti, G. (2008). *Caring for patients from different cultures* (4th ed.). Philadelphia: University of Pennsylvania Press.

Giger, J. N., & Davidhizar, R. E. (2004). *Transcultural nursing: Assessment & Intervention* (4th ed.). St. Louis: Mosby.

Jennings, B., Ryndes, T., D'Onofrio, C., & Baily, M. A. (2003). Access to hospice care: Expanding boundaries, overcoming barriers. *Hastings Center Report, 33*, S3–S59.

Kaiser Family Foundation. (2001). *African Americans view of the HIV/AIDS epidemic at 20 years.* Menlo Park, CA: Author.

Kar, S. B., Alcalay, R., & Alex, S. (2001). *Health communication: A multicultural perspective.* London: Sage.

Kingma, M. (2006). *Nurses on the move: Migration and the global health care economy.* Ithaca: Cornell University Press.

Koenig, B. A. (1997). Cultural diversity in decision making. In M. S. Field & C. K. Cassel (Eds.), *Approaching death: Improving care at the end of life* (pp. 363–382). Washington, DC: Institute of Medicine.

Leininger, M. M., & McFarland, M. R. (2006). *Culture care diversity and universality in a world-wide nursing theory* (2nd ed.). Sudbury, MA: Jones and Bartlett.

Leong, F. T. L., Wagner, N. S., & Tara, S. P. (1995). Racial and ethnic variations in help-seeking attitudes. In J. G. Ponterotto, J. M. Casas, L. M. Suzuki, & C. M. Alexander (Eds.), *Handbook of multicultural counseling* (pp. 415–438). Thousand Oaks, CA: Sage.

Lewis, M. (2002). *Multicultural health counseling: Special topics acknowledging diversity.* Boston: Allyn & Bacon.

Pope, C. (2004). *Concept paper: Language access services in nursing.* Washington, DC: US Department of Health & Human Services, Office of Minority Health..

Srivastava, R. (2007). Working with interpreters in healthcare settings. In R. Srivastava. *The healthcare professional's guide to clinical competence* (pp. 125–143). Toronto. Mosby/Elsevier.

TriAd Research, Inc. (2002). *Evaluation of the language and culture facilitation pilot project.* Calgary: Author.

Washam, C. (2009). Study: treatment satisfaction tied to language & culture. *Oncology Times, 31*(3), 19–20.

CHAPTER 8

Communicating Effectively in Patient Teaching: Enhancing Patient Adherence

EXCHANGING INFORMATION

A number of studies have shown that patients want more information about their condition and treatment than health professionals often think (Donovan & Blake, 1992; Luker et al., 1998; Williams, 1993). Effective patient teaching requires more than giving patients information or having them recite facts. To be effective, patient teaching must be based on patients' individual needs and provided in a manner that facilitates their ability to carry out recommendations. This requires a degree of interpersonal skill and sensitivity from the health professional. Health professionals must be able to listen to, observe, and understand what patients are saying before they can give patients information that will be most meaningful to patients and best meet patients' individual needs.

Communication in patient teaching is a two-way process involving interchange between the patient and health professional. It is a complex process that is essential to identifying patients' needs so that patient teaching can be adjusted to best meet those needs and help patients follow recommendations. Although it is vital to communicate information clearly in a way patients are most likely to comprehend and remember, health professionals' skills in patient assessment are just as important. These include the ability to recognize patients' verbal and nonverbal cues, respond accurately and appropriately to those cues, and to provide support and feedback, which are all critical components in patient teaching (Lloyd & Bor, 1996). These skills promote a sense of trust, which, in turn, promotes an open and honest relationship and makes it more likely that health professionals will be able to elicit accurate information from patients, including their concerns, misconceptions, or misunderstandings.

RELATIONSHIP SKILLS: BUILDING RAPPORT

The object of patient teaching is not only to help patients comprehend information but also to help them put the information to use in their daily lives. This is most readily accomplished in the context of the relationship between patient and health professional. The quality of this relationship can have a significant impact on the outcome of treatment and on patients' ability and willingness to carry out recommendations (Roter et al., 1998; Squirer, 1990). Although evidence suggests that one important factor in the relationship may be the professional's ability to communicate information to patients about their condition and treatment, findings also indicate that the health professional's ability to establish rapport with patients is even more important to communication effectiveness (Culos-Reed et al., 2000; Williams, Weinman, & Dale, 1998).

Rapport, although difficult to define, is essential to establishing a good relationship between the patient and health professional. A part of rapport is the health professional's ability to make patients feel cared for and respected as individuals. The degree to which patients feel comfortable with sharing information about themselves, as well as with sharing their feelings and concerns, is determined to a great extent by the health professional's ability to communicate a caring, respectful attitude. Basic aspects of a relationship that facilitate open communication and rapport are acceptance, understanding, empathy, and trust. Although these terms have become platitudes for some, they are essential in building a relationship that can influence the effectiveness of patient teaching.

DEMONSTRATING ACCEPTANCE AND UNDERSTANDING

Acceptance demonstrates respect for people regardless of their circumstances and placement of value on individuals simply because they are human. Acceptance of a person does not mean blind acceptance of all their behavior. For example, showing acceptance of a patient who has emphysema but continues to smoke heavily does not mean condoning the smoking behavior. It does mean continuing to respect and value the patient as a person.

Everyone appreciates being treated in a respectful way. Feeling that one is respected is an integral part of building a relationship. Demonstration of respect facilitates communication and trust and is the first step in building rapport. When patients detect an attitude of indifference or disinterest displayed by health professionals, they are less likely to engage in open communication.

Acceptance of patients is demonstrated by exhibiting a nonjudgmental attitude and accepting patients' views, although they may be different from those of the health professional. An attitude of acceptance establishes open communication and creates an atmosphere that is more conducive to patient receptivity of information and their willingness to follow recommendations. Consider the different impact of each of the following remarks made by health professionals while conducting patient teaching. The patient in the example has liver damage and has been instructed to give up alcohol.

> *Patient*: I don't think I can function without being able to have a drink every now and then. Whenever I'm tense or depressed, alcohol has been the only thing that can help me keep going.
>
> *Health Professional A*: You're just using alcohol as a crutch. It isn't a way to solve problems, and in your case, it'll only make your problems worse.
>
> *Health Professional B*: So coping with some of your feelings is at times difficult for you.

The remark of Health Professional A is judgmental and demonstrates little empathy for the patient's feelings. Such a remark, rather than helping to establish a relationship which would enhance patient teaching, will probably alienate the patient, making the success of further teaching interventions unlikely. The remark of Health Professional B, however, neither judges nor condones. The remark communicates that the health professional recognizes the patient's feelings and accepts them as such. Acceptance is not synonymous with approval; it does, however, establish an atmosphere in which patients can openly share their feelings and concerns. Lack of acceptance may cause patients to withhold information that could be of value to the health professional in developing an effective patient teaching plan. Without a feeling of acceptance, patients may be reluctant to return for further patient teaching.

Health professionals must be able to communicate not only acceptance of patients but also understanding of them, their feelings, and their concerns. Understanding means the ability to grasp patients' perspectives and to interpret the meaning of their words and behavior accurately.

Before acceptance and understanding can be demonstrated, health professionals must first be attentive to what the patient is saying. Flipping through a chart or looking at other material while the patient is trying to describe their situation or express their concerns does little to build rapport. Likewise, even though health professionals may be able to repeat verbatim what the patient has said, such attention is superficial listening at best. Many patient cues may have been missed. Patients who sense a lack of genuine concern may also be reluctant to ask questions or express feelings. Patients want to know that they have been given the health professional's full attention. This means listening to words and ideas as well as being aware of what patients may be expressing through their behavior. Not only the content of what is being said but also the feelings expressed nonverbally must be considered. Giving patients full attention during teaching activities helps demonstrate concern and caring for them as unique individuals and can contribute to the patient's willingness to accept and follow recommendations.

COMMUNICATING EMPATHY

Failure to establish empathy can be a serious barrier to effective patient teaching. Empathy is the ability to view feelings from patients' perspectives and to communicate acceptance and understanding to patients. Health professionals communicate empathy by putting aside their own feelings and values, putting themselves in the patient's shoes, and viewing feelings and attitudes from the patient's perspective. Before beginning patient teaching, it may be helpful for professionals to pause and ask themselves, "How would I feel if I were in the patient's situation? If I were given these recommendations under the circumstances the patient is in, how might I feel? How might this affect my reaction to the recommendations?" Empathy must be an accurate understanding of the patient's perspective. The following example illustrates empathetic and nonempathetic responses.

Mrs. Vicker had just had a mastectomy. In preparation for Mrs. Vicker's discharge from the hospital, the nurse had begun to teach her exercises that had been prescribed to increase her range of motion, as well as how to change her own dressings. During a teaching session, Mrs. Vicker became tearful.

> *Mrs. Vicker*: "I'm so ugly now. I'll never be the same. I'll never be able to function again as I did before, either as a wife or just in general. Sometimes I think it would have been better if I had never consulted the doctor when I found the lump in my breast."
> *Nurse A*: "Don't be silly. The mastectomy saved your life. Lots of women who have had mastectomies lead full, happy lives. There are so many things left for you to enjoy in this world. I think you're just feeling sorry for yourself. You should appreciate what you have."
> *Nurse B*: "I know this isn't easy for you. You're pretty discouraged now, aren't you?"

Nurse A's response not only shows rejection of Mrs. Vicker's feelings but shuts off further expression of concerns that may be important to effective patient teaching. Nurse B's response is empathetic. It demonstrates acceptance and understanding of Mrs. Vicker and encourages her to express her feelings more directly. It is important for health professionals to realize that an empathetic response does not involve giving advice or coming up with solutions. It merely communicates to the patient that the health professional recognizes their feelings and accepts their expression of them.

The creation of a nonjudgmental atmosphere when conducting patient teaching is important in building rapport and, consequently, in conducting effective patient teaching. A positive, noncritical attitude establishes a relationship that increases the probability that patients will be more honest in their responses to health professionals. If patients feel that acceptance is dependent on repeating what they feel the health professional wants to hear, rather than what is actually true, important information that could contribute significantly to the effectiveness of patient teaching may be lost.

Identification of patients' needs and concerns through exploration and discussion is crucial to establishing collaborative goals with the patient. However, before this point can be reached, a relationship built on trust, understanding, acceptance, and honesty must be established.

BUILDING TRUST

Developing trust facilitates rapport as well as establishes credibility. Patients are less likely to follow instructions provided by someone who they do not feel is credible. If a patient feels the health professional is not providing him or her with accurate or appropriate information, does not understand his or her situation, or does not have his or her best interests in mind, the patient will be less likely to accept recommendations, much less follow them.

Part of trust comes from health professionals' ability to communicate genuine concern for patients. Trust also comes from patients' beliefs that health professionals are competent in their skills and that they are approaching patients in a truthful, honest manner. Before patients can trust health professionals' recommendations, they must have some trust and confidence in health professionals themselves.

To some degree, trust is built into the relationship between patient and health professional by virtue of the health professional's expertise and credentials. This is communicated to patients by the health professional's role, title, and academic and/or scientific degrees. Patients already have some expectations about the health professional's knowledge based on the role he or she fills, such as physician, nurse, dietitian, or pharmacist. Although the health professional's title and credentials can be an asset from some vantage points, professional qualifications cannot be relied on solely as a means of guaranteeing successful patient teaching interactions. Maintaining a professional demeanor may be an expected part of professional behavior; however, in order to establish trust, health professionals must also be personable and comfortable with patients and not hide behind learned roles and words.

The manner in which health professionals present information is critical in developing a sense of trust and confidence. If information is presented in an abrupt, matter-of-fact way without demonstrating sensitivity to patients' reactions, patients may be less likely to be convinced that the health professional has any knowledge of or concern for them as individuals. Health professionals who drone on with facts without considering the emotional impact of their statements stand to lose patients' cooperation as well as their trust no matter how well the information is organized.

Health professionals who seem unsure of the information they are presenting also risk losing credibility and trust. Consider the following statement. "I think this is the way Dr. Jacobs wanted you to take your medicine—or maybe it was two times a day rather than three—that's probably right, take it two times a day." The statement does little to instill confidence. The patient may doubt (and rightfully so) the accuracy of the instructions and consequently be reluctant to follow any of the instructions given. Chances are good that the patient will not be eager to seek further advice from the health professional or to seek answers to possible questions. In instances when health professionals do not know the answer or do not have information readily available, they should acknowledge to the patient that they do not know and offer to try to find the answer or the additional information requested.

Effective communication of information includes having a good understanding of the information presented and having confidence that the information presented is accurate. This, of course, necessitates health professionals' willingness to stay abreast of changes in health literature and to review and update their own knowledge base as needed.

Consistency of information provided in patient teaching is also important to developing trust. Health professionals who contradict themselves when presenting information or who contradict information given by other health professionals also may cause the patient to question which information is factual and which recommendations he or she should follow. Consistency of information given by one health professional or by several health professionals working with the same patient is important in building trust. The case of Mrs. Kramer, who had been given diet instructions from both the dietitian and the physician for her diabetes, is an example.

> *Dietitian*: "I note from your chart that you enjoy having a glass of wine before dinner. I've incorporated that into your diet plan by taking away one of the other exchanges, so now you can still enjoy a glass of wine."
> *Mrs. Kramer*: "But Dr. Gephardt said I was to avoid alcohol totally in any form because it could be very harmful to me because of my diabetes."

Mrs. Kramer is put in the position of not knowing who to believe and which instructions are correct. Communication between health professionals conducting patient teaching is crucial to provide consistency. Likewise, the health professional must make sure that information is consistent from one teaching session to another if credibility is to be maintained. The preceding situation might have been avoided had there been better communication between the dietitian and the physician. Neither appeared to have an understanding of what the other would tell the patient. Of course, patients can at times misinterpret information. Under the circumstances, the dietitian should clarify what the patient was actually told by the physician without disrupting the credibility of either of them. The dietitian may respond with a statement such as, "Certainly using alcohol in excess and without appropriate planning can be harmful. Although alcohol in small amounts can be incorporated into the diet plan, all patients are individuals and respond differently. Let me check with your physician and see what is best in your case."

In addition to credibility and consistency, a major variable in developing trust is honesty. Honesty is more than merely being truthful. It conveys a sense of openness between health professional and patient, and promotes confidence that the health professional is being genuine in the interaction with the patient. In the case of Mrs. Squires, newly diagnosed as having diabetes, the nurse had spent several teaching sessions explaining the importance of controlling diabetes with accurate administration of insulin, as well as following the prescribed diet. Consider the effects of each of the following statements made by the nurse.

Mrs. Squires: "It sounds so easy when you talk about it all, but diabetes will still make a big difference in my life. We've always gone to a lot of parties and dinners, and I love sinfully rich desserts. We've lived that kind of life for so long. It's all going to be very difficult. Sometimes I wonder if it's all going to be worth it. I've known people who followed their diet and insulin instructions faithfully and still developed complications. I'll bet you wouldn't think all of this was so easy if you were going to have to do it."

Nurse A: "The people you've mentioned were probably cheating on their diet and insulin all along and you just didn't know. If you value your life and your health, you'll follow the instructions. You'll just have to get your priorities right. If I were you, I wouldn't think twice about following the instructions to the line."

Nurse B: "I know following these instructions won't be easy for you. I, too, would find it very difficult. And you're right, there are no guarantees that following all the instructions will mean you'll remain 100% complication-free. However, we do know that when better control is maintained, the greater are your chances of having fewer complications. Tell me a little more about what you feel will be the most difficult for you."

In her response, Nurse A lost credibility by denying the accuracy of the patient's observations without further exploration and was critical of Mrs. Squires' feelings. The blanket statement that the nurse would have no difficulty deciding what to do conveyed a sense of superiority over Mrs. Squires. This lessens the probability that Mrs. Squires will respond honestly or trust the nurse with her feelings in the future.

Nurse B's response was open and honest not only in acknowledging personal feelings that the task of administering insulin and following a special diet was difficult, but also by showing a willingness to explore Mrs. Squires' feelings further. The nurse demonstrated acceptance of Mrs. Squires' concerns and reinforced her for expressing them. This increased the possibility that Mrs. Squires would feel comfortable expressing concerns in the future. Encouraging Mrs. Squires to be honest in expressing her concerns created the opportunity to provide her with support and to identify alternatives and compromises that may be possible to increase her adherence with the recommendations.

Openness and honesty must always be used with sensitivity and discretion when health professionals provide information. Truth dumping, which consists of the indiscriminate disclosure of facts without regard for a patient's feelings or the impact the information will have, is just as detrimental to the development of trust as being dishonest. Forming a social unit with the patient in which there is mutual caring and respect helps patients come to trust health professionals. This component may be one of the key elements in helping motivate patients to follow health advice.

NONVERBAL COMMUNICATION

Communication is a key component in effective patient teaching. Communication, however, consists of more than verbal exchange. Many messages are also conveyed by body movements, facial expressions, touch, eye contact, and tone of voice. Such nonverbal behaviors communicate the attitudes, beliefs, and emotions of both patient and health professional in subtle ways. Awareness of nonverbal cues can help the health professional to communicate more effectively so that both patient and health professional receive and interpret messages the way they were intended.

Patient Cues

Much information can be gained from the patient's nonverbal cues during a teaching interaction. Cues may indicate the patient's emotional state, a lack of understanding, possible discomfort, or just that further information is needed.

Nonverbal cues help health professionals obtain a more accurate interpretation of patients' statements by linking their behavior to the words they speak. Noting patients' facial expressions as well as their words increases understanding of the meaning of their message. Nonverbal behavior also helps health professionals determine the most appropriate way of responding to a patient at a given time. For example, a different response would be required for a patient who appeared angry than for one who appeared sad.

Nonverbal cues from patients are available to health professionals throughout teaching interactions. How does the patient appear as the health professional enters the room? Is the patient's body posture relaxed or tense? Does the patient appear nervous or at ease? Does the patient's body posture or position change during the teaching session? Does the patient maintain eye contact with the health professional or look around the room or at the floor? Does the person avoid eye contact only when certain issues are discussed? Does the patient's facial expression appear pleasant or worried? Does the patient appear angry or indifferent? What changes occur in the patient's facial expression when various topics are discussed? Does the patient appear attentive or distracted? Does his or her facial expression indicate understanding or confusion; disagreement or acceptance?

For observation of nonverbal behavior to be useful in the teaching interaction, the behavior must be interpreted correctly; however, no communication, verbal or nonverbal, has meaning out of context. For example, if the health professional notes that the patient has begun to fidget during a teaching session, it is difficult to know the meaning of the behavior without gathering further information about it. Fidgeting could mean that the patient is uncomfortable physically or uncomfortable with the content of the information being presented. Fidgeting might also mean that the patient is anxious to end the session because of time constraints.

Nonverbal cues alert health professionals only to the fact that some message is being delivered. In order to interpret the message correctly, the health professional must obtain additional information. Interpreting nonverbal cues without clarification may interfere with the effectiveness of patient teaching. For example, if the health professional observes the patient fidgeting throughout the interaction and interprets the behavior as disinterest when the patient is actually physically uncomfortable, further teaching efforts may be abandoned rather than rescheduled for a time when the patient is more comfortable and, thus, more receptive. Such misinterpretation of cues might communicate to patients that the health professional is insensitive to their needs and thus interfere with building the rapport that is crucial to future teaching interactions.

Noting how closely patients' nonverbal communication parallels their verbal responses can also give health professionals valuable information to facilitate effectiveness in patient teaching. If patients' nonverbal behavior appears to conflict with their verbal responses, health professionals have an indication that further clarification of the message is needed. For example, if a patient states that he or she will have no difficulty following the treatment recommendations but frowns while making the statement, additional information about the response is needed before its meaning and that of the nonverbal behavior can be interpreted correctly. The frown may indicate a lack of understanding of the instructions. It may indicate that the patient disagrees with the treatment prescribed or that the patient will have some difficulty carrying out the recommendations. Without further clarification, the health professional cannot respond in a way that will contribute to the effectiveness of patient teaching, either by giving additional information, negotiating aspects of the recommendations, or helping the patient resolve problems that might interfere with following the instructions. A statement such as, "I notice you were frowning when you said you would have no difficulty following treatment," provides an opportunity for opening additional dialogue and, consequently, clarification of the meaning of the observed behavior.

Observation of nonverbal behavior is, of course, only one part of making communication effective. When nonverbal cues are observed, health professionals need to decide whether behavior should be clarified at the time or merely noted and added to the data already obtained. Whether patients are confronted immediately or observations are noted for future investigation depends on several things. To some extent, timing of the confrontation depends on the relationship between the health professional and the patient. How and when the patient is approached also depends on the health professional's clinical judgment concerning the particular teaching situation. In some instances, it may be better merely to note nonverbal behavior for future reference or so that it can be supplemented with additional observations. In others, failure to clarify the meaning of the nonverbal behavior when it occurs may be a substantial barrier to effective patient teaching.

At times, failure to clarify the meaning of nonverbal behavior is a result of the health professionals' lack of knowledge of how to approach the patient. Clarification of nonverbal behavior should be as nonthreatening and nonaccusing as possible and done in a way that communicates that the health professional is attempting to understand the patient and the meaning of the behavior observed. For example, when a patient is observed to fidget during the teaching interaction, the health professional may say, "You seem to be somewhat uncomfortable. Is there anything I can get for you, or would it be better to stop for today and to continue this teaching at a later time?" At this point, the patient has the option either to deny discomfort or to explain the behavior. If the patient chooses to deny discomfort and offers no explanation for the restlessness, the health professional may note the observation and look for cues that may give additional insight into the behavior. If the patient offers an explanation, such as, "I just can't sit in one spot too long because of my back. Could I just stand up and walk around a little before we go on?" or "My neighbor brought me to the clinic today, and she's been waiting for a long time. I hate to have her wait much longer," the health professional can then take appropriate action based on the additional information received.

Any communication has two frames of reference. In this case, the two frames belong to the patient and the health professional. Continuing the teaching interaction without noting or clarifying nonverbal messages, or interpreting nonverbal behavior without checking for its accuracy, can have an impact on the extent to which patient teaching is effective.

Cues from the Health Professional

It is important for health professionals not only to understand patients and the meaning of patients' nonverbal behavior but also to understand themselves, their usual patterns of communication, and how these factors can influence the teaching interaction. Health professionals need to be aware of unintentional cues and messages they may be conveying to the patient through nonverbal communication.

Nonverbal behaviors of health professionals can be interpreted by patients in a variety of ways. Patients can interpret a hurried approach or poor eye contact as a lack of interest in them as people. Health professionals' projection of approachability may not only have an impact on patients' receptivity to information presented but may also be a factor in patients' willingness to express views honestly or to give the health professional information needed to construct the most effective teaching plan.

The manner in which health professionals present information may also influence the degree to which patients carry out the recommendations (Bultman & Svarstad, 2000; DiMatteo, 2004; DiMatteo, Reiter, & Gambone, 1994; Roter & Hall, 2009). If the health professional fidgets, appears tense or nervous, or seems to lack confidence while presenting information, patients may not take the information seriously or may question its credibility. Presenting information in a disinterested, routine way can also have negative effects. Patients may interpret the manner of presentation to mean that the health professional is not interested in them as individuals or has not considered their special problems and concerns. Patients may therefore not be willing to follow recommendations and may take it upon themselves to modify the instructions as they feel best meets their needs.

Nonverbal cues such as eye contact, a relaxed body posture with no excess gesturing, and a warm and friendly manner communicate that the health professional is accepting of and interested in patients as persons and is considerate of their special needs. Showing attentiveness and a nonhurried approach also indicates a willingness to answer patients' questions. Asking the patient whether he or she has any questions when the health professional's nonverbal behavior contradicts the stated willingness to answer those questions is unlikely to receive an honest response from the patient. Effective patient teaching is dependent on patients' ability to follow the recommendations accurately. If they are unsure of how or why recommendations are to be carried out, the possibility of their following the recommendations accurately is decreased. If, however, patients feel that the health professional demonstrates an openness to questions and a willingness to answer those questions, they will be more willing to ask questions, and it is more likely that doubts, lack of understanding, or misunderstanding can be identified. This type of information exchange affords health professionals an opportunity to correct any problems that may interfere with patients' willingness or ability to carry out the recommendations.

Touch can also be of help in the patient teaching interaction. It can be used to convey acceptance, support, and caring to the patient. Touch can, of course, be overused. If health professionals use touch appropriately and with discretion, it can increase rapport and influence the success of patient teaching. Touching takes many forms—from a simple handshake to a touch of the arm to an arm around the shoulders. How and when touch is used in patient teaching depends on the clinical judgment of health professionals as well as a number of other variables. It stands to reason that using touch to communicate reassurance, support, or acceptance may be less appropriate when explaining why an antibiotic is prescribed for strep throat than it would be when teaching a patient with a terminal illness.

Beginning a teaching session by putting an arm around an individual is obviously not as appropriate as a handshake, especially if this is the first interaction between patient and health professional. In other instances, putting an arm around an individual after the patient has shared a particularly emotional bit of information does more to convey reassurance and acceptance than a handshake.

Other variables to be considered in the use of touch during patient teaching include the age difference between patient and health professional, the gender of each, and cultural differences that may exist between the two. Touch is perceived in different ways by people of different ages, genders, and cultures. From an awareness of variables mentioned in previous chapters, health professionals can increase their skill in determining the degree to which touch should be used in individual teaching encounters. It is important for health professionals to remember that touch, although at times helpful in patient teaching, can also be misinterpreted. Good judgment in the use of touch appropriate to the circumstances can be of great help in enhancing rapport between patient and health professional, thus facilitating the effectiveness of patient teaching.

RESPONDING TO PATIENTS' VERBAL CUES

Throughout the teaching interaction, whether during the initial stages of rapport building and data gathering, information transfer, or evaluation of teaching effectiveness, health professionals' responses to patients' verbal statements can facilitate or hinder the degree to which teaching goals are reached. Knowledge of a variety of available responses can be of value in making the teaching session as productive as possible.

Probing Responses

A probing response is an open-ended statement that is used in an attempt to obtain additional information from the patient. Although such responses may be used most frequently in the initial information-gathering stages of teaching, such responses are helpful whenever health professionals want to obtain additional information. In the initial stages of teaching, when health professionals want to assess patients' understandings or feelings about their conditions, examples of probing statements may be, "Tell me your understanding of your condition," or "I'm wondering if you know anyone else with this condition and, if so, what your impressions have been."

Such statements encourage patients to express their views and are more productive than closed statements requiring a yes or no response, such as, "Do you understand your condition?" or "Do you know anyone else with this condition?" Such closed statements give health professionals very little additional information and may discourage patients from elaborating. Probing statements may be especially valuable in the closing portion of teaching, when health professionals are attempting to evaluate the extent to which patients understand the information given. Closed statements such as, "Do you understand what you're supposed to do?" or "Are the instructions clear?" are likely to elicit an affirmative response regardless of patients' level of understanding. Patients may not wish to reveal that they do not understand and therefore may answer yes regardless of their understanding of the material presented. In some instances, patients may feel that they do understand the material presented and what they are supposed to do when they actually have misinterpreted or misunderstood the advice given. A probing statement such as, "Just so I know that I've been clear in my instructions, could you tell me how you're to take your medicine?" or "Could you briefly summarize for me what we've talked about today?" gives health professionals far more information and provides the opportunity to correct misinformation or misunderstanding before the patient leaves the health facility.

Clarifying Responses

A clarifying statement facilitates correct understanding. Statements of clarification help health professionals make sure they are interpreting patients' verbal statements correctly. Accurate perception of patients' verbal statements is important throughout the teaching interaction. Clarification of patients' statements can help determine, to a great extent, the direction teaching takes. If, for example, after receiving diet instructions, the patient says, "This diet will be almost impossible for me to follow," the health professional may clarify the patient's response with a statement such as, "Do you mean that you will have difficulty because of willpower or because of the lifestyle and schedule you have?"

In assuming that the statement in the preceding example means that the patient has no willpower, the focus of teaching may be misdirected. The actual problem may be that the patient's schedule is such as to render it difficult to have three scheduled meals a day in the amounts specified. If this is the case, the focus of teaching should be directed toward suggestions that could help the patient follow the recommendations.

Reflecting Responses

A reflecting statement facilitates further communication by encouraging patients to elaborate on a statement already made. Reflecting statements can help health professionals gain more understanding of patients' concerns and perspectives, which can in turn facilitate the effectiveness of patient teaching.

For example, Mr. Abernathy was scheduled to be admitted to the hospital for an angiogram as well as other diagnostic procedures. A few days before admission, Mr. Abernathy visited the clinic, at which time the physician explained the procedure to him, and helped him understand what to expect. As the visit with the physician was drawing to a close, Mr. Abernathy said, "I sure hope whoever does this test knows what they're doing. I'd sure hate to end up worse than I am now."

In response to Mr. Abernathy's statement, the physician may have made a reflecting statement, such as, "You're feeling anxious about this test," or "You're nervous about having the test performed." Such a statement would not only facilitate further communication but would also help identify additional information that may indicate the cause for Mr. Abernathy's concern. Was Mr. Abernathy's anxiety partly based on misunderstanding or lack of understanding of what had been said? Had he had previous negative experiences or known others who had negative experiences related to an angiogram? Identifying the patient's concerns and perspectives through reflecting statements helped the physician assess whether Mr. Abernathy needed additional information, clarification of information, or additional reassurance and support.

Statements that close the door on identification of the patient's additional teaching needs produce less than satisfactory results. Such a nonproductive response to Mr. Abernathy's statement might be the following: "Oh, hundreds of patients have this done every week with no problems. The persons doing the test are highly trained and well qualified for the job. It's a highly valuable technique for understanding just what exactly is causing your symptoms. You'll do fine."

It is unlikely that such a statement would elicit further insight into Mr. Abernathy's concerns. While at first glance the statement may appear to give further information and support, it may, in actuality, only indicate to Mr. Abernathy that the physician has little concern for his feelings. In addition, the statement produces a barrier to further communication and, consequently, to identification of further teaching needs. Unless health professionals identify and perceive patients' true concerns, it is difficult to meet patient's needs. Without accurately identifying and addressing patients' fears, concerns, and/or misunderstandings, the health professional takes the chance that the patients will disregard the information, which may produce an end result of nonadherence

Confronting Responses

A confronting response describes an observation of the patient's verbal or nonverbal behavior of which he or she may or may not be aware. Confrontation does not imply that health professionals take on an adversarial role with patients. Rather, it implies that a statement is made that gives honest feedback about what health professionals perceive to be happening with the patient.

Confronting responses should not make inferences about patients' motives for the observed behavior. It merely gives patients an opportunity to elaborate on or deny observations brought to their attention. For example, if at the last minute, a patient has canceled several appointments for patient teaching about hypertension, a statement such as, "I see you've been canceling your appointments at the last minute. Obviously you're having difficulty accepting your condition," may not only be untrue but may actually alienate the patient. A more positive use of confrontation in this situation may be a simple observation of fact, such as, "I see you've canceled several of your appointments."

Confrontation should not take the form of a formulated question such as, "Why are you uncomfortable?" Such a question also assumes that the health professional's interpretation of the observed behavior is correct and can put the patient on the defensive. Confrontation should not communicate hostility but should reflect sympathetic interest. An example of the use of confrontation is illustrated by the following case.

Mrs. James had been scheduled for a hysterectomy. She was seen at the physician's office before admission to the hospital for preoperative teaching and a history and physical examination. The physician began discussing the surgical procedure but noticed that Mrs. James appeared more quiet than usual, her eyes tearing at several points. Several times, the physician asked Mrs. James if she was all right or if anything was bothering her. Each time she responded that nothing was wrong. Toward the end of the teaching session, the physician decided to confront Mrs. James with his observations with the statement, "Although you say nothing is wrong, I see tears in your eyes." Mrs. James began to cry, stating that she feared that she would no longer be perceived as a woman by her husband.

By confronting Mrs. James with his observations, the physician gained information that could then be pursued. The confrontational statement made by the physician consisted of observations, rather than accusations such as, "You aren't telling me the truth. If nothing is wrong, why are you crying?"

If used excessively and inappropriately, confrontation—like other responses—loses its value. Used correctly, however, confrontation can facilitate patient responses that might give the health professional new insights to be used in patient teaching.

INITIATING PATIENT TEACHING

The way people initiate communication can have a significant influence on and set the tone for the rest of the interaction (Berry, 2007). Patient teaching can consist of an informal interaction or it can be part of formal interactions in which patient teaching is the major purpose of the meeting. The way the patient is approached in either of these situations depends on the context, the degree of familiarity the health professional has with the patient, and other specific circumstances.

In situations in which teaching is a routine part of an interaction between patient and health professional, such as during a clinic visit or medical procedure, there is no reason to delimit the teaching portion of the interaction. Patient teaching under these circumstances becomes a normal part of the communication between patient and health professional.

In cases where patient teaching is the only purpose of the interaction, the approach to patient teaching may be different. If the health professional is unfamiliar with the patient, before initiating teaching, the health professional should offer an introduction defining his or her professional role and the purpose of the interaction.

When meeting new patients, health professionals should not make the assumption that patients prefer to be called by their first names. More appropriately, the health professional may give the patient the choice with a statement such as, "Would you prefer I call you Mrs. Smith or Jane?" Such a statement conveys regard for the patient as an individual, helping to build rapport.

When initiating the teaching interaction, health professionals may also put patients at ease through touch, asking how they feel or briefly engaging in some other pleasant form of conversation that communicates a personal interest. The following example illustrates the preceding points. The patient, Mr. Jones, had been referred by a physician to a dietitian, Miss Smith, for special diet instruction.

> *Dietitian*: "Hello, Mr. Jones (smiling and extending hand for handshake). I'm Miss Smith, the dietitian. Dr. Johnson has asked me to talk with you about your diet. (Miss Smith sits down.) Would you rather be called Mr. Jones or Don? (Patient responds.) I see from your chart that you have a little girl who is six. I have a niece her age. They sure have a lot of energy at that age, don't they?"

In the statement, the dietitian has introduced herself and defined her professional role and why she is interacting with the patient. She has also offered a statement that communicates that she knows something about the patient as an individual and that serves to put the patient at ease before moving directly into the teaching to be conducted.

Communication is also enhanced if, when initiating patient teaching, health professionals establish comfort in the environment, such as providing adequate ventilation or a quiet area where there will be minimal distractions. In a physician's office, for example, the physician may say something like, "I wanted to talk with you in a little more detail about your blood pressure, but it's really stuffy in this examining room. Why don't we go to my office where it's a little more comfortable?"

The main thrust of the initial interaction in patient teaching is to gather information that will enable the health professional to individualize the patient teaching approach and to build rapport. Part of this time can also be used to identify patients' current knowledge and/or attitudes about their condition or treatment by encouraging them to express their views or knowledge. This step, whether teaching about acute or chronic disease, is important to efficiency and effectiveness in patient teaching. The following statements are examples of types of approaches health professionals might use to elicit this type of information:

- "From our test results, it appears you have a urinary tract infection. Can you tell me a little bit about what you know about urinary tract infections?"
- "As you know, your diagnosis of emphysema has been confirmed. I want to talk with you about emphysema in more detail, but first would you tell me a little about what you already know about emphysema?"

Both statements give health professionals an opportunity to determine the patient's level of understanding about the condition, avoiding possible redundancy in teaching. Such statements help health professionals discover any misinformation or misperceptions patients may have so that those may be addressed. This approach also helps build rapport by letting patients know that the health professional is concerned about what they think about their condition.

ESTABLISHING GOALS FOR COMMUNICATION IN PATIENT TEACHING

The content of patient teaching depends on the needs and interests of the particular patient, the circumstances under which the teaching is taking place, and the goals to be accomplished. Although major goals in patient teaching are based on reaching collaborative goals with the individual patient, the health professional should also have a well-thought-out plan for patient teaching, which can be adjusted in order to correspond with patient needs.

Depending on the situation, health professionals may become overwhelmed with the amount of information they feel needs to be presented and, in an attempt to cover everything, jump from topic to topic with no clear sense of organization. This type of patient teaching is not only inefficient, but also is ineffective (Bultman & Svarstad, 2000). Although patient needs must be assessed and considered, in order to be efficient and effective in patient teaching, the health professional should also have an organized and predetermined plan with both short- and long-term goals of what he or she hopes to accomplish in the teaching intervention.

When communicating recommendations and determining goals for patient teaching, health professionals should recognize that although some goals can be accomplished in the immediate teaching session, others require days, weeks, or months of teaching before they can be reached. This is especially true when patient teaching involves the development of specific skills or a change of attitude on the part of the patient.

When determining what should be accomplished with patient teaching, it is important that the health professional assess teaching goals realistically. Health professionals may feel that patients should be as well informed as possible in all areas of their health and health care, and overwhelm patients with information and expectations for outcomes. It is important, however, to establish realistic goals and to assess the feasibility of meeting those goals in the context of the individual patient.

For example, it is doubtful that health professionals could expect to be successful in patient teaching if the goal is to eliminate smoking in a 25-year-old patient who smokes two packs of cigarettes a day, has no symptoms, and has no desire to quit smoking. Expecting the patient to be receptive to a long dialogue about hazards of smoking and making recommendations that the patient should cease smoking totally, at this point, is probably an unrealistic goal. Under these circumstances, a more realistic goal might be to assess the patient's reasons for smoking, assess the patient's knowledge about effects of smoking, and to work toward having the patient consider the possibility of cutting down the number of cigarettes smoked each day.

Determining goals for patient teaching does not have to be difficult if health professionals take the time to ask themselves, "What should the patient to be able to do as a result of this instruction?" From this question, the content of patient teaching can also be determined if health professionals ask themselves, "What information does the patient need in order to carry out the instructions?" These two questions will yield different answers for different patients with various illnesses. Different goals and content are obviously required for teaching patients with acute conditions, chronic conditions, or for teaching people about health promotion. In any teaching situation, short- or long-term goals may be established.

For example, when teaching a patient about medication prescribed for a urinary tract infection, short-term goals might be the following:

- The prescription will be filled.
- The patient will take the medication as prescribed.

Once these goals have been identified, the health professional might ask, "What information does the patient need to know to accomplish these goals?" Answers might be:

- The name and type of medication
- The length of time the medication is to be taken
- Why it is important to take the medication as directed
- What the patient should expect from the medication (such as discoloration of urine or potential side effects of the medication)
- Any special action the patient should take (stop the medication and call the physician if rash occurs, etc.)

Unless the patient understands why the medication is important, the patient may not get the prescription filled. Unless the patient understands the importance of taking the medication for its full course, the patient may discontinue it as soon as symptoms subside. He or she may discontinue taking the medication without consulting the physician if side effects occur. By identifying a teaching goal and asking the initial question, "What does the patient need to know in order to reach the goal?" the health professional has identified information the patient should be provided in order to reach the desired outcome.

The same teaching interaction could also identify long-term goals. In the example above, one long-term goal that may be established might be, "The patient will decrease the frequency of reoccurrence of urinary tract infections." To accomplish this goal, the health professional may determine that the patient needs to be aware of ways to prevent urinary tract infection from occurring, such as good hygienic practices or increasing fluid intake.

Short- and long-term goals may also be established for teaching about chronic conditions or health promotion. Because teaching about chronic illness may involve much more complex information, as well as be affected by patient reactions to the condition, short-term goals for each teaching session may be used as building blocks on which the accomplishment of long-term goals can be based. For instance, when teaching patients with diabetes how to inject insulin, short-term goals might be directed toward teaching them to draw up the correct insulin dose and then inject it, while the long-term goal may be to help them independently manage their own insulin injection accurately at home on a daily basis.

Patient teaching for health promotion may also have short- and long-term goals. For example, when teaching a patient about dental hygiene, a short-term goal may be helping the patient learn to brush and floss their teeth appropriately; however, a long-term goal may involve helping the patient avoid caries and gum disease.

In setting goals for patient teaching, health professionals should establish priorities for the sequence of information so that it can be presented in an organized way. When information is necessary to enable patients to function safely and adequately, that information should be covered first. Goals should go from simple to complex, with complex goals being built on those that are less difficult. Goals that are dependent on the accomplishment of prior goals can be included at a later time.

Patient teaching goals should be explicit and measurable. For instance, a goal such as, "For the patient to know about his condition," says little about the specific outcomes to be expected, and it would be difficult to determine the extent to which the goal has been reached. The more explicit health professionals are in determining the behavior patients are to demonstrate as a result of patient teaching, the more efficient and effective teaching will be, because it is directed toward accomplishing that goal.

COMMUNICATING INFORMATION IN PATIENT TEACHING

Although effective patient teaching is greatly dependent on the interpersonal skills of health professionals and their ability to accurately assess patient needs, health professionals' ability to communicate information in a clear, concise manner is also of major importance (Christensen, 2004). Although information alone is insufficient for patient teaching to be effective, patients must have information and be able to understand it before they are able to follow the recommendations. Organizing and presenting the information in a clear way that patients can understand is an important skill in patient teaching.

Approaches to Giving Information

Patient teaching may be done on a formal or informal basis and may be direct or indirect. Varying approaches to patient teaching are appropriate at different times. The approach used is dependent on the circumstances. Informal patient teaching takes place during a regular clinical encounter when the sole purpose of the interaction between patient and health professional is not patient teaching. Although informal patient teaching is done spontaneously rather than at a predetermined time, the need for presentation of information in a clear, organized manner based on the patient's level of need should not be minimized.

Informal patient teaching, for example, may be used when patients' need for information is identified unexpectedly. For example, a preteenager at an office visit for a sore throat may, in passing, ask about menstruation. In this instance, even though unplanned as a teaching intervention, a need for information has been identified and may best be addressed when the need arises, rather than requiring the patient to return at a later time for a formal teaching session.

Informal patient teaching may also be conducted when health professionals observe an additional need for information. For example, the health professional may note, seeing a 2-year-old at an office visit for otitis media, that the child has not had a needed immunization. Although not directly related to the condition or treatment for which the child is being seen, a need for teaching the parents about the importance of immunization is identified. The information need can be addressed informally during the office visit, even though information provided is unrelated to the reason for the visit. Other examples of informal patient teaching may be providing patients with explanations of findings during a physical examination, recommendations for treatment of a condition for which they have sought advice, or any other explanation that is part of their regular clinical encounter.

Formal approaches to patient teaching consist of time set aside for patient teaching of a specific topic. For example, formal approaches to patient teaching may be preoperative instruction, giving patients with chronic disease specific instructions about their condition or care, or giving specific instructions to a hospitalized patient about home care. A formal approach does not mean that health professionals lecture patients or that patients remain passive listeners. Even in formal approaches, patient teaching may take the form of discussion and information exchange between the two parties. As much as possible, patient teaching should remain a two-way process of communication, keeping patients actively involved.

Although presenting information to patients at a time they are ready to receive it and in amounts they are able to comprehend is desirable in most situations, a more direct approach may be necessary in certain situations. If, for example, a child is examined in the emergency room for a head injury, and the decision is made to send the child home for continued observation, a more direct approach to patient teaching may be desirable. Teaching parents signs and symptoms they should be aware of that may indicate complications of the head injury or teaching them what they should do if such symptoms are observed cannot be postponed. Information given to the parents in these circumstances is crucial. The health professional's assurance that the information has been understood is even more critical.

An indirect approach to patient teaching may be used when time is available. In this case, information may be given in an easy, give-and-take method that combines giving information during discussion. This approach assists the health professional to involve patients and identify their feelings and/or concerns. An example of an indirect to patient teaching may be teaching that is provided during prenatal visits over time.

Avoiding Jargon

Health professionals must remember that they have special medical knowledge and a special medical vocabulary, or medical jargon, that the patient may not have. Medical jargon should be avoided. For instance, teaching patients with emphysema about their condition with an explanation such as, "Emphysema means basically that there is dilatation of the alveoli with inherent loss of elasticity," probably will have little meaning to many of them. Time spent giving patients information they cannot understand is not only an inefficient use of time but is also unlikely to reach the anticipated goal of patient teaching. A better explanation might be, "In the lung, there are tiny air sacs in which outside air and air that is inside your body, which is a waste product, are exchanged. In emphysema, these little air sacs become bigger and lose their ability to stretch."

Patient teaching can involve teaching patients medical terms as well. In this case, the lay term may be used with the medical term. While explaining a gastroscopy to a patient, for instance, the health professional may say, "During the procedure, we'll place a hollow tube down your food pipe or esophagus." This technique serves to acquaint patients with the medical terminology while still conveying the content of the message. It also helps health professionals avoid the feeling that by using simpler language they are talking down to patients.

The level of language used when explaining things is determined to some degree by the assessment of patient variables as discussed in preceding chapters. It is also important for health professionals to recognize that patients' ability to form concepts may often be related to their level of language acquisition. The words used and the content, too, may be determined by patients' use of language. Patients with relatively low levels of sophistication may not want or be able to conceptualize the same type of information as those with a greater level of sophistication.

The use of analogies can be helpful in explaining medical terms and concepts to patients. For instance, the heart may be described in terms of a pump, while an aneurysm may be described as of a hose with a weakened area susceptible to different water pressures. Such analogies may help patients conceptualize information in a way that is more meaningful to them.

Health professionals should not make assumptions about patients' level of language and ability to conceptualize without further information gathering. Patients should not automatically be stereotyped to have a particular level of ability to understand without being considered as an individual. Just as it is faulty for health professionals to assume that patients of lower educational levels are unable to understand various explanations, so is it faulty to assume that those with a higher educational level or apparent levels of sophistication necessarily understand medical terminology. An example illustrating this point is the case of Mrs. Lindquist.

Mrs. Lindquist was working on a doctoral degree and had consulted her physician because of excessive uterine bleeding. Upon examination of Mrs. Lindquist, the physician reported that she had a fibroid tumor and that he felt surgery would be necessary. Assuming the patient understood the diagnosis, no further explanation of the condition was given other than routine preoperative teaching. The patient suffered a miserable week until surgery, thinking that any kind of tumor meant cancer.

This type of misunderstanding can be avoided by clarifying medical terms that may be misconstrued. Just as some patients may think that the word tumor is synonymous with the word cancer, numerous other terms may be misunderstood, such as vaginal infection and gonorrhea. When giving explanations, health professionals should clarify each term, saying something such as, "The tumor is benign, which means it isn't cancer," or "You have a vaginal infection, which should not be confused with a venereal disease like gonorrhea." In doing so, health professionals prevent misunderstanding just by spending a few additional seconds of time with the patient.

Clarifying Perceptions

Health professionals should keep in mind that they and their patients may be from significantly different social backgrounds. Differences in social status or background may mean discrepancies in life experiences, values, attitudes, and perceptions. Health professionals and patients may perceive illness differently and may perceive information differently as well. The thought patterns of health professionals may be so different from those of the patient that there may be total unawareness of patients' faulty interpretation of information given. Such is the case of the patient in the following example.

Mr. Castillo was given a prescription for medication for hypertension. He received instructions about hypertension as well as instructions to take his medication once a day. At a follow-up visit, the physician discovered that Mr. Castillo had taken hardly any of the medication. When Mr. Castillo was asked why he had failed to follow the instructions, he stated that he thought he had been following them. He continued that he thought hypertension, although realizing that the term meant high blood pressure, also meant that he would feel extremely tense, which he interpreted to be the cause of his elevated blood pressure. Because he had not felt tense since his last appointment, he had seen no reason to take the medication.

Health professionals should, throughout teaching interactions, periodically check for understanding and interpretation of information presented. Patients should be encouraged to ask questions. Asking simple questions, such as, "Does this make sense to you?" or "Are there points I haven't made clear or that you would like to talk about some more?" give patients the opportunity to clarify any information of which they may be uncertain. Asking patients to summarize information is another means by which their understanding of the information presented can be assessed.

If health professionals keep in mind that the main goal of patient teaching is to communicate information in such a way that patients understand and are able incorporate into their daily lives, the process becomes easier. This means that if slang terms are needed to get a point across, then they should be used. If the patient does not understand the term "urinate," but rather uses the phrase "make water," then using the patient's terminology is the most efficient way to communicate. Health professionals working in an area where slang terminology prevails may save themselves considerable time and create more effective and efficient communication in patient teaching if they take the time to learn some key slang words and phrases and the conceptualizations they denote. It is just as important for the health professional to accurately perceive words that have meaning to the patient as it is for the patient to accurately perceive what is meant by medical terms used.

Being Specific

It is important to be as specific as possible when giving patients instructions. Vague instructions are not likely to be followed as accurately as those that are to the point. Comments such as, "When you go home after surgery, take it easy for a few weeks," can mean different things to different people. To the man who is used to heavy labor, mowing the lawn may seem like taking it easy, even though he uses a push mower.

Several studies illustrate the importance of being specific with instructions. In one study, a diuretic was prescribed for water retention. More than half the patients for whom the medication was prescribed thought that its purpose was to help them retain water rather than eliminate it (Mazzullo, Lasagna, & Griner, 1974). In the same study, an antibiotic was ordered every 6 hours. Only a small number of patients interpreted the instructions to mean every 6 hours around the clock. Patients interpreted the instructions to mean that they should take the pill every 6 hours while they were awake. Consequently, a number of patients for whom the medication was prescribed received only three quarters of the amount of medication prescribed in a day's time.

The more specific health professionals are about recommendations, the more likely patients will be to carry them out accurately. Instead of saying, "Take it easy after surgery," health professionals may specify exactly what is meant by "take it easy." Specific instructions, such as, "Avoid lifting over 10 pounds," or "Avoid going up and down stairs," are more explicit in helping patients know exactly what is meant. With medication, health professionals may specify exact times the medication is to be taken, such as (in the case of every 6 hours) 8 a.m., 2 p.m., 8 p.m., and 2 a.m.; or health professionals may work with the patient in arranging times to suit their individual schedule, such as 6 a.m., 12 noon, 6 p.m., and 12 midnight.

Being specific also means that health professionals emphasize which instructions are most important to follow and elaborate on why recommendations are important. If, for example, a patient is being given two medications—one of which is to be taken as needed but the other to be taken in the treatment of a specific disease—vague instructions about the two medications may be confusing. As a result, the patient may take neither medication accurately. For example, if the physician prescribes an analgesic and an antibiotic for a 3-year-old patient with otitis media, it might be important to give specific instructions to the parents, such as the following.

"I am giving your child a prescription for two medications. One is to help relieve the symptoms, but the other is to treat the cause of the symptoms and fight the infection that is causing them. The first medication is for the symptoms. It's a local anesthetic that will reduce the pain. Fill the ear canal with the drops, and place a cotton plug in the ear canal. Repeat every 2 to 4 hours as necessary to relieve the pain. Usually after 2 days the symptoms will be gone, and you won't need to continue using this medication. The other medication is an antibiotic that will fight the infection. Give your child 1.5 measuring teaspoons by mouth every 8 hours around the clock so the organisms causing the symptoms are killed. You should continue using this medication even though your child may have no further symptoms, otherwise the organism causing the infection may not be killed, and the infection could become full-blown again."

The more specific health professionals can be in giving patients information, the more likely patients will be to have a clear understanding of what they are to do. Consequently, they will more likely be able to carry out recommendations accurately. Being specific takes little extra time if the health professional is aware of the variety of ways in which information may be misinterpreted by the patient. Time spent in making the instructions as specific as possible is time well spent.

HELPING PATIENTS REMEMBER INSTRUCTIONS

It is not enough for patients to understand instructions. They must also be able to remember them. Studies indicate that patient recall of information received during physician visits is generally no more than 50% (Ley, 1972; McGrath, 1999). The reason for such low rates of retention is thought to be linked to large amounts of information given to the patient at one time, the patient's high anxiety, the small amount of medical knowledge held by the patient, and the intellectual level of the patient.

In conducting patient teaching, health professionals should use simple but accurate words and should provide enough information so the patient can put it into perspective. Explanations should be limited in accord with the emotional and intellectual capacity of the patient. Health professionals should be aware that patients may suffer from information overload if they receive too much information at one time. Quantity of information is not always linked with patients' understanding. At times, an abundance of information can fatigue patients and interfere with their remembering.

Specific techniques can be used to help increase patients' ability to recall information. Patients may not remember all the information given, especially if it is complex. Discussion of the information under a topical outline may help patients organize the information in their minds, thus providing a structure that can be more easily remembered. For example, the health professional may say, "I am first going to explain the treatment prescribed for your condition. Then I'll discuss what we expect the treatment to do, and finally I'll discuss how you are to carry out the treatment." If the information is complex, it may be divided into several sessions. For example, "Today I'm going to explain what diabetes is. Tomorrow we'll talk about your diet, and the next day we'll begin to talk about insulin injections." Specific instructions, such as teaching patients to administer their own insulin, may have to be broken down into smaller steps.

When patients are given a large amount of information at one time, they may have difficulty detecting which information is most crucial. Repetition of important instructions facilitates their ability to decipher what is most important as well as helping them to remember the information given. Important instructions may be repeated in a slightly different way, not only to increase retention but to clarify the instructions as well.

Another way to help patients remember instructions is by writing them down or using simple handouts. Although never meant to replace one-to-one communication between the patient and health professional, written instructions may help patients remember instructions after they return home or may clarify instructions they cannot remember clearly. Pictures of simply drawn diagrams can also be used in patient teaching to illustrate points. The phrase, "A picture is worth a thousand words," is important to remember when teaching patients.

In all instances, verbal and written communications should complement each other. Health professionals should remember that the overuse of handouts can be detrimental to effective patient teaching. Although use of handouts alone may appear to be a way to save time, it can also be impersonal. Handouts are of little value if the patient does not understand them or does not read them. Further discussion of the use of handouts and other visual aids in patient teaching appears in Chapter 16.

Helping patients remember instructions should not be a difficult task if the health professional remembers the following:

- Organization of material
- Clarity and specificity of instructions
- Repetition of important points
- Illustration or demonstration of points
- Reinforcement through written instructions.

REFERENCES

Berry, D. (2007). *Health communication: Theory and practice.* Berkshire, England: Open University Press.

Bultman, D. C., & Svarstad, B. L. (2000). Effects of physician communication style on client medication beliefs and adherence with antidepressant treatment. *Social Science and Medicine, 40,* 173–185.

Christensen, A. J. (2004). *Patient adherence to medical treatment regimens: Bridging the gap between behavioral science and biomedicine.* New Haven, CT: Yale University Press.

Culos-Reed, S. N., Rejeski, W. J., McAuley, E., Ockene, J. K., & Roter, D. L. (2000). Predictors of adherence to behaviour change interventions in the elderly. *Controlled Clinical Trials, 21,* 200–205.

Dimatteo, M. R. (2004). Variations in patients' adherence to medical recommendations: A quantitative review of 50 years of research. *Medical Care, 42,* 200–209.

Dimatteo, M. R., Reiter, R. C., & Gambone, J. C. (1994). Enhancing medication adherence through communication and informed collaborative choice. *Health Communication, 5*, 253–266.

Donovan, J. L., & Blake, D. R. (1992). Patient non-compliance: Deviance or reasoned decision-making? *Social Science and Medicine, 34*, 507–513.

Ley, P. (1972). Comprehension, memory and the success of communications with the patient. *Journal of Instructional Health Education, 10*, 23–29.

Lloyd, M., & Bor, R. (1996). *Communication skills for medicine.* Edinburgh: Churchill Livingstone.

Luker, K., Austin, L., Hogg, C. Ferguson, B., & Smith, K. (1997). Nurse-patient relationships: The context of nurse prescribing. *Journal of Advanced Nursing, 28*, 235–242.

Mazzullo, J. M., 3rd, Lasagna, L., & Griner, P. F. (1974). Variations in interpretation of prescription instructions. The need for improved prescribing habits. *Journal of the American Medical Association, 227*(8), 929–931.

McGrath, J. M. (1999). Physicians' prescriptives on communicating prescription drug information. *Qualitative Health Research, 9*(6), 731–745.

Roter, D. L., Hall, J. A., Merisca, R., Nordstrom, B., Cretin, D., & Svarstad, B. (1998). Effectiveness of interventions to improve patient compliance: a meta-analysis. *Medical Care, 36*, 1138–1161.

Roter, D., & Hall, J. A. (2009). Communication and adherence: Moving from prediction to understanding. *Medical Care, 47*(8), 823–825.

Squirer, R. W. (1990). A model of empathic understanding and adherence to treatment regimens in practitioner-patient relationships. *Social Science & Medicine, 30*, 325–339.

Williams, O. A. (1993). Patient knowledge of operative care. *Journal of the Royal Society of Medicine, 86*, 328–331.

Williams, S., Weinman, J., & Dale, J. (1998). Doctor-patient communication and patient satisfaction: a review. *Family Practice, 15*, 480–492.

CHAPTER 9

Building Patient Partnerships: Facilitating Patient Participation in Patient-Centered Teaching

PARTNERSHIP AND COLLABORATION

The concept of partnership between the patient and health professional has been evolving since the 1970s in response to social, cultural, and political changes (Hook, 2006). In 1978, the World Health Organization promoted the concept of partnership when they proposed a social model of health that emphasized patients' right and responsibility to be involved in their own health care (World Health Organization, 1978).

Three characteristics of partnership have been described as follows (Gallant, Beaulieu, & Carnevale, 2002):

- Relationship
- Power sharing
- Negotiation

Partnership is a cornerstone of patient-centered care, which has been defined as behavior that elicits, respects, and incorporates patients' wishes, allows active patient participation, and is related to improved outcomes (Breen et al., 2009; Hartog, 2009). The concept of patient-centered care has expanded to all areas of health care and has been linked to increased patient satisfaction and overall increased quality of care (Wolf et al., 2008), as well as patient adherence (Fuetes et al., 2007; Singleton, 2008).

The concept of patient-centered care when applied to patient teaching consists of patient teaching that is built on a philosophy of partnership and collaboration between the patient and the health professional. Although health professionals may have the knowledge and technical expertise needed to provide the patient with information about his or her condition and treatment, the patient is the expert regarding his or her own body and life experience.

Consequently, the patient's needs, goals, and preferences must be acknowledged and recognized, and incorporated into patient teaching interactions.

Patients are now expected to assume more personal responsibility for health outcomes, and patient participation in health and health care has been promoted as best practices (McKenna & Tooth, 2006; Porche, 2007). Involving patients in their own care empowers them and increases their sense of control and confidence. Effectiveness in patient teaching requires that the health professional think beyond providing information. Effective patient teaching emphasizes a more contextual approach by tailoring the recommendations to the individual and his or her life needs. The notion of involving the patient is important in fostering an atmosphere of cooperation and collaboration between the patient and health professional. Health professionals must be aware of and acknowledge the patient's expressed thoughts and feelings and respectfully come to a mutual agreement about recommendations as well as find strategies to promote the patient's ability to carry out prescribed recommendations (Comstock et al., 2008).

Although part of patient teaching consists of providing patients with information, effective, patient-centered teaching is more encompassing. It refers to helping patients become actively involved in their health and health care, enabling them to make the necessary adjustments in order to improve or maintain health status. Communication is a key component toward reaching this goal, especially when communication is used to engender collaboration and help the patient to make informed choices (DiMatteo, Reiter, & Gambone, 1994; Roter & Hall, 2009).

NEGOTIATION

The term "negotiate" implies conferring with another in order to reach a compromise. In terms of patient teaching, negotiation may be a somewhat foreign term to health professionals who believe that patients who come for help or advice should and will automatically follow the recommendations offered. In such interactions, health professionals and patients are too often at odds, with health professionals making invalid assumptions about the patient's ability or willingness to follow recommendations. Patients, on the other hand, may withhold important information about their inability or unwillingness to follow the recommendations or may never be provided with the opportunity to share their concerns.

The concept of negotiation in patient teaching may be met with varying degrees of acceptance by health professionals. Some may feel that negotiation interferes with what they consider to be the major goal of patient teaching: to offer information that will help patients improve or maintain health. If negotiation is included, some health professionals may fear that patients may not choose what is best for them. Given this point of view, then, it would seem that negotiation could make patient teaching less effective. The problem with this view, of course, is that it assumes health professionals know what is best for patients and their health. This may not be the case.

To make recommendations that patients are unable or unwilling to follow is inefficient and ineffective for both patient and health professional. Conflict exists if health professionals blindly advise patients, expecting them to follow the recommendations without understanding patients' feelings or identifying barriers to patient adherence. Negotiation identifies areas of agreement and disagreement and provides a forum for discussion of solutions. Although some health professionals may find the concept of negotiation alien and not within the framework of health care to which they have grown accustomed, patient teaching can only be as effective as patients' ability and willingness to carry out recommendations. Negotiation is a way to work collaboratively with the patient in order to establish mutually acceptable goals and problem solve to assist patients' ability to reach them.

CHANGE IN PATIENTS' ROLES IN HEALTH CARE

In the past, patients were viewed as passive recipients of health care (Ong et al., 1995). Generally, neither patients nor health professionals expected patients to play any active role in their health care, much less negotiate with the health professional about the recommendations provided. It was expected by both patients and health professionals that health professionals were the ultimate authority by virtue of their expertise and would therefore make the final decision about what was best for patients (Stone, 1979).

Often, information about their health and health care was kept from patients by well-meaning health professionals who rationalized information deprivation with statements such as the following:

- Patients do not have the ability to understand.
- If patients had all the information, they would worry needlessly.
- Patients really do not want to know all the information. That is why they are seeking advice from a health professional.

Some health professionals felt that their professional role would be diminished by sharing too much information with the patient. Other health professionals felt that keeping some mystery in their professional role was in itself therapeutic. Some felt that if patients were given too much information, they would lose respect for the health professional. Still other excuses for failing to give information ranged from, "Patients wouldn't remember anyway," to "Giving the patient information takes too much time."

When patients did challenge the lack of information given to them by health professionals, they were frequently looked upon as "troublesome patients." The "good" patient was thought of as the one who sat passively, offering no criticism and asking few questions. Patients were frequently treated in a paternalistic way, with a benevolent attitude being displayed by health professionals connoting, "What you don't know won't hurt you." When patients did challenge a recommendation or ask a question, they were frequently met with comments such as, "Oh, don't worry about that. I have everything under control," or "I'm not able to disclose that information. You'll have to ask your physician."

As patients became more sophisticated about health and health-related topics through the media, Internet, and other sources, faith in health professionals as the final authority diminished. The advent of self-help and patient information groups increased patients' desires for increased involvement in their care. Media publicity also decreased patients' view of health professionals as omnipotent guardians of their health; in some instances, it increased distrust of health professionals themselves.

At the same time, studies conducted in patient adherence indicated that many formerly held beliefs about patients and about giving patients information about their condition and treatment were in error. Health professionals began to realize that if information was conveyed properly, patients could understand explanations and that, through various strategies, their recall of information could be increased. Contrary to previously held beliefs, patients did want more information about their condition and treatment (Beisecker & Beisecker, 1990; Donovan & Blake, 1992; Luker et al., 1997; Williams, 1993); rather than having more problems as a result of knowing what to expect, patients who were better informed had fewer problems (Stewart, 1995). Also in contrast to earlier beliefs, patients—instead of losing respect for the health professional as a result of having more information—were more satisfied with the care they received if adequate information was given (Dansky, Colbert, & Irwin, 1996).

Patient teaching, if conducted efficiently, can save health professionals time by decreasing unnecessary phone calls and return visits. Withholding information can increase patients' anxiety rather than decrease it. Patients frequently misinterpret a lack of information as meaning that the truth is so negative that it cannot be shared with them. In addition, patients are much more anxious if they do not know what to expect, even if by being informed they know they can expect pain or discomfort.

Although increased information has many positive results, information alone is not associated with patient adherence (Blessing-Moore, 1996). Although health professionals now tend to agree that patients should be informed, it has also become increasingly evident that health professionals—if they are to affect positive outcomes in patient adherence—must take another step. Patients need to feel that they are not only recipients of information, but they also play an active part in their own health. Even though patients now receive more information, they still are often not actively engaged in the teaching process. It becomes increasingly obvious that effective patient teaching is a shared responsibility between patient and health professional.

MODELS OF PROFESSIONAL RELATIONSHIPS AND NEGOTIATION

Szasz and Hollender (1956) described three types of relationships that embrace models of interaction in the physician–patient relationship. These conceptual models are:

- Activity–passivity
- Guidance–cooperation
- Mutual participation

Although described more than a half a century ago, examples of these relationships can still be found in interactions between health professionals and patients today. These conceptual models can also be applied to interactions between patients and health professionals. The success of patient teaching may be determined to a great extent by the model of interaction health professionals use when conducting patient teaching.

Perhaps the oldest of the three models and the one most used in the past was the activity–passivity model. In this model, health professionals took an active role, assuming full responsibility for determining goals. Patients assumed a passive role, being recipients of care and having little input in the treatment or care being received. This model, if applied to patient teaching, might be reflected in the one-sided communication of information given by the health professional to the patient in which there is little or no consideration for the patient's feelings or ability to follow the advice given. The teaching method would probably resemble a lecture approach, and the patient would have little opportunity to respond to the information presented. Although this model is the least desirable for effective patient teaching, under special circumstances it may be necessary: In the case of an emergency, for example, when the patient or family must be given instructions quickly, and there is little opportunity or necessity for negotiation. Use of this model under less stressful circumstances is likely to achieve less than the desired results.

The second model, that of guidance–cooperation, is probably more familiar to health professionals. In this model, although patients are more active than in the previous model, most of the responsibility for goal setting still belongs to the health professional. This model implies that by virtue of health professionals' training, they possess special knowledge and expertise that patients seek for their perceived needs. The model assumes that because patients are seeking help, they are also willing to cooperate with health professionals. Using this model, it may be assumed that the major goal of patient teaching is to help patients gain information so they will be able to follow recommendations given by health professionals. Because patients are in the position of seeking help, it may be assumed by health professionals that they are also willing to "cooperate" and "comply" with the recommendations given. Carried to a further extreme, the model may be one in which the major goal of patient teaching is to enforce patient adherence by attempting to shape or mold patients' behavior according to goals of the health professional rather than those of the patient.

The guidance–cooperation model places health professionals in a paternalistic role. Patients are expected to comply with the recommendations. There is little opportunity for patient input or disagreement with the recommendations. Even though characteristics of patients may be taken into consideration when determining the manner in which instructions are given, and even though patients may be encouraged to be actively involved in the teaching process by asking questions or offering feedback about their level of comprehension, the possibility that health professionals might actually negotiate the recommendations with patients is not recognized. This model removes the patient from the decision-making process and from assuming responsibility for participating in goal setting. Although this model may, at first glance, seem more efficient, it probably results in less effective patient teaching by lessening the mutual participation between patient and health professional in the teaching relationship.

The last of the three models, the mutual participation model, might also be called the model of negotiation. This model assumes both patient and health professional to be equal members of the interaction. Patients and health professionals work together, sharing information and reaching a mutual agreement about treatment goals. In patient teaching, patients become active participants in the process, forming a partnership with health professionals in decision making. The patient's own experiences provide clues for the most effective plan. Health professionals essentially are facilitators as well as educators, helping patients to help themselves. Such an approach does not mean that health professionals abandon what is medically sound advice, nor does it mean that persuasion in patient teaching in this model has no place. It does mean that health professionals base patient teaching on the situation of the individual patient and work with the patient to problem solve to best meet his or her needs.

Each model of interaction between patient and health professional may be appropriate at different times. It would obviously be inappropriate to engage in a mutual participation model with a small child or under emergency circumstances, just as it would be inappropriate to engage in an activity–passivity model when discussing elective cosmetic surgery with a patient. The health professional's judgment and awareness of the use of different models in various teaching situations are critical. In most teaching situations, however, respecting the patients' needs and rights, working with patients in defining goals, and problem solving with them to establish a plan for reaching those goals will most likely result in effective patient teaching.

In the first two models, agreement between patient and health professional is taken for granted. Both models assume that patients do not know enough to dispute the word of health professionals. In both the first two models, it is assumed that health professionals know what is right and best for patients and that the major goal of patient teaching is to influence patients so that they accept the health professional's views or plans, with little alteration.

The model of mutual participation is characterized by high degrees of empathy and recognition of patients' individual needs. In this model, health professionals do not profess to know what is best for patients or all the variables patients must face in order to follow recommendations. The model is based on negotiation—two-way communication of information and equality between patients and health professionals. Although health professionals and patients have different levels of knowledge (i.e., medical knowledge of health professionals and knowledge of patients of their own psychosocial needs), it is a combination of both that best enable the patients to follow the recommendations. If patients have no knowledge of what they are to do, recommendations cannot be followed. On the other hand, if health professionals have no knowledge of the problems and barriers patients experience in following recommendations, it is unlikely that the recommendations will be followed.

Even when a point of disagreement is reached, it is far better for health professionals to recognize areas of dissension and seek alterations that may still be within the framework of a therapeutic outcome than to be unaware of alterations in treatment the patient may establish independently. Focusing on points on which patients and health professionals do agree and continuing to search for alternatives and solutions in areas where they disagree can enhance patient satisfaction as well as adherence.

SHARED RESPONSIBILITY IN PATIENT TEACHING

The mutual participation model, if used in patient teaching—although assigning the patient more responsibility in the patient–professional interaction—does not lessen the responsibility of health professionals; it merely alters the focus of the responsibility.

Patients' personal responsibility is the central theme of negotiation. The responsibility of health professionals, however, is to identify concerns, values, or problems that may interfere with patients' success in following recommendations. To do this, health professionals must build an atmosphere of trust in which patients feel comfortable.

Health professionals have the responsibility not only to communicate instructions in a way patients can understand but also to assess whether patients can follow recommendations. In patient teaching, therefore, health professionals must address issues relevant to the patients' situations that may be a barrier to carrying out recommendations. The mark of success in patient teaching is not the patients' ability to regurgitate information but their ability to incorporate instructions into their daily lives, away from the direct supervision of health professionals. During patient teaching interactions, health professionals should identify patients' feelings about the information and recommendations provided and assess problems or limitations they may have in carrying out instructions. Only in this way can health professionals help patients discover alternatives and solutions that may increase the likelihood that they will be able to follow through with the plan. This is best accomplished when patients have had a part in formulating the plan.

Passive patients who have little to do with formulating the plan for treatment are also likely to feel less responsibility and commitment for carrying it out. If, as in the activity–passivity model, health professionals accept full responsibility for decisions about the recommendations patients are to follow, patients may also delegate full responsibility to the health professional for treatment failure, rather than examining the possibility that their own actions or lack of action contributed to the problem. In assigning major responsibility for positive treatment outcomes to health professionals, rather than accepting their role in carrying out recommendations, patients may place unrealistic demands and expectations on health professionals. If the patient's expectations are not met, the result may be anger and hostility directed toward health professional. The point can be illustrated with the case of Mr. Morris.

At 32 years of age, Mr. Morris was obese and hypertensive. His physician, concerned about the elevated blood pressure, talked with him about hypertension. The physician used an active–passive model of interaction, being directive and parental in giving instructions. The physician's statement was, "I want to get your blood pressure down. In order to do this, I'm ordering this medication and a low-salt/low-calorie diet. The diet I'm prescribing will help you lose weight as well as help lower your blood pressure. I'm referring you to the dietitian for further explanation of the diet. I'll monitor how effective my plan for lowering your blood pressure has been by having you return for follow-up visits."

After several follow-up visits, it was noted that Mr. Morris had not lost weight, nor was his blood pressure any lower. Upon leaving the physician's office, Mr. Morris, exasperated, made the following remark to a friend: "I've been spending all this money going to that doctor for my blood pressure, and still it's no better and I haven't lost an ounce. I don't think she knows what she's talking about. She just wants my money. I'm not going back if she can't seem to help me."

Mr. Morris did not accept responsibility for his role in contributing to the treatment failure. Even though he was placed on a low-salt/low-calorie diet, he frequently ate snack foods filled with salt and calories. Likewise, he sometimes forgot to take his medication and had neglected to have the prescription filled immediately because of its expense. Because the physician had accepted most of the responsibility for Mr. Morris's treatment, Mr. Morris placed most of the blame for treatment failure on her, expecting her to "heal" him. Had the physician taken a less dominant role, including Mr. Morris as an active participant in his own health care, the outcome might have been quite different.

Motivating patients to accept responsibility for their health and treatment begins by engaging them as active participants in the patient teaching interaction from the start. Whereas some patients may find it difficult to assume responsibility for their actions, health professionals may work toward this goal. With Mr. Morris, more active participation could have been solicited with a statement from the physician such as, "We're going to have to work together to get your blood pressure down. There are two things we need to do in order for that to happen. One is to work on helping you to reduce your weight and to decrease your salt intake, and the other is to have you take a medication to reduce your blood pressure. We'll talk together about how we can best work that out for you. I can prescribe these things, but obviously most of it will have to be up to you to follow the instructions at home. Let's talk about any problems you feel you may have in doing these things."

Such an approach assigns a portion of the responsibility to Mr. Morris and communicates to him that the physician believes that he is a responsible adult and expects him to take an active role in his health care and treatment.

Through patient teaching, health professionals not only communicate information but provide help and support to patients so that they may come to terms with problems and feelings they have in carrying out the recommendations. Health professionals can provide assistance by exploring patients' feelings and concerns and by working with them to find solutions. If patients say they are unable to follow the recommendations, health professionals may focus on alternatives that can assist them. In the case of Mr. Morris, the dietitian and/or the physician might have reached some compromises on the diet, or perhaps a less expensive medication for hypertension could have been prescribed. As it stood, Mr. Morris felt little commitment for carrying out the recommendations and, consequently, did not do so.

Just as it is important for health professionals to include patients in the patient teaching process and to help them assume shared responsibility for outcomes, it is also important that the health professional realize overemphasizing patient responsibility can have undesirable effects. If patients are made to feel that they have sole responsibility and control of their health, they may become overwhelmed and defeated, thus abandoning the treatment recommendations. Placing the responsibility solely on the patient also precludes involvement of the health professional in identifying potential problems that may be overcome with problem solving. If this view is held too strongly by the health professional, little will be done to help the patient overcome barriers in the way of following recommendations. In other instances, patients may come to feel that if they have sole responsibility for their health, the health professional has no expertise of value to them and consequently they may neglect recommendations. The end result, in any of these instances is patient nonadherence.

In the previous example, an overwhelming amount of the burden would have been placed on Mr. Morris had he been told, "Whether you have a stroke or not because of your blood pressure is up to you." Such a statement would most likely decrease rapport between the physician and Mr. Morris. Another nonproductive attitude by the physician might be expressed as, "I gave the advice and he didn't follow it, so there's nothing I can do." This approach leaves Mr. Morris with no alternatives. This type of statement also damages the relationship between Mr. Morris and the physician, which may be crucial in working out solutions so he can follow the recommendations. A more productive statement might be, "Despite the diet and medication we talked about last time, there still is no weight loss. Can we try to figure out why? Can we talk about any problems you might have been having in following the recommendations?"

Health professionals who are committed to effective patient teaching must also accept some of the responsibility for its outcome. Health professionals, of course, have the responsibility to communicate the information necessary to help patients to understand the recommendations and why they are important. Just as important, however, is the health professional's responsibility to determine any obstacles or barriers that could hinder successful communication or prevent patients from following recommendations. This means that health professionals must also be aware of patients' limitations in accepting health advice or in following the recommendations.

THE BOUNDARIES OF PATIENT TEACHING

Just as patients' perspectives on illness might differ from the perspective of health professionals, so there may be differences in the way recommendations are perceived. Although health professionals may not perceive recommendations as being difficult or unreasonable to carry out, patients may view them in quite a different light.

As mentioned in previous chapters, patients' beliefs, values, and social influences may have significant impact on the extent to which they follow any given recommendations. To conduct patient teaching without considering the impact the recommendations have on patients' lives is to discount their point of view. Values held by health professionals may not be the same as those held by patients. Recommendations that seem simple to health professionals may be overwhelming to patients when trying to implement them. Patient teaching outcomes held as ideal by health professionals may not be the outcomes that patients value.

It is not surprising that the degree to which patients are willing to follow recommendations is related somewhat to their perceptions of the cost associated with following instructions. Although cost in terms of financial considerations may certainly be an issue, cost may be measured in a variety of other ways as well. To patients, cost may also be measured in terms of pain and discomfort, lack of function, risk, or perceived loss of self-esteem. Cost is, of course, evaluated subjectively by patients and assessed in terms of their own lives and the impact that following or not following recommendations will have on them. This concept has relevance whether it is used in teaching patients about acute illness, chronic disease, or preventive practices. Not only must patients believe that treatment will be effective; they must also believe that the treatment or change in lifestyle will be worth the cost.

Mr. Ueda's case illustrates this point. Mr. Ueda was a 58-year-old pharmacist who owned and operated two pharmacies in the small city in which he lived. He had had angina for several years; he continued his work at full pace as much as possible until the condition became so incapacitating that bypass surgery was recommended. Mr. Ueda had an uneventful postoperative course and, before leaving the hospital, received a series of patient teaching sessions concerning recommendations for him upon returning home.

One of the recommendations given Mr. Ueda was that he cut down on his hours of work and, preferably, that he relinquish some of his responsibility at both pharmacies, taking on more of a supervisory role. Reasons for a slower pace were provided, and Mr. Ueda appeared to understand the possible consequences of not cutting down his workload. Only a week after his discharge from the hospital, however, the physician received a worried call from Mr. Ueda's wife, stating that he had returned to nearly a full workload at both pharmacies. Obviously upset, she asked that at Mr. Ueda's next visit, the physician make a special effort to "talk some sense into him" so that he would be encouraged to follow recommendations. At the next visit, the physician began to talk with Mr. Ueda about his obvious nonadherence. Mr. Ueda replied that he had spent much time and effort developing the pharmacies and took much pride in being actively involved in their management. Although he fully understood what the additional strain of maintaining his current level of activity might mean, he was also aware of the personal loss he would experience if he would cut back on his involvement. Although he was willing to follow the other recommendations given, the personal cost of decreasing his involvement with the pharmacies was, to him, not worth the benefits that the physician and Mr. Ueda's wife believed the decreased workload would bring. Mr. Ueda stated, "What would extra years of life mean to me if I were miserable sitting at home? If as a result of my work I have a shorter life, at least the time I have had will be well spent. I can only hope that if I die early as a result, that it will happen at work where I have invested so much of myself."

The physician, realizing that additional lecturing or informing Mr. Ueda of the reasons why the recommendations should be followed would be to no avail, began to think of ways that alterations could be reached. The physician negotiated with Mr. Ueda, arranging some rest periods during the day as well as talking with him about the possibility of working 6 days with shorter hours instead of 10 hours for 5 days. Through this process of negotiation, the physician and Mr. Ueda were able to reach a satisfactory plan that more closely approximated the goals of both. Without such negotiation, the additional time and effort spent in patient teaching would have been less than effective. The value that the physician and Mr. Ueda's wife placed on the possibility of longer life as a result of decreased activity was not shared by Mr. Ueda. Negotiating recommendations within the framework of Mr. Ueda's values increased the likelihood that Mr. Ueda would more closely adhere to the new recommendations.

WHEN NEGOTIATION FAILS

It appears that effective patient teaching is most likely the result of mutual participation, respect, and shared decision making between patients and health professionals. Patients' personalities, values, attitudes, and life situations are all key components of the process. Likewise, the personalities, attitudes, and values, as well as the skills, of health professionals in communicating health advice also affect the success of patient teaching.

The concept of negotiation is not to assure patients that they receive only what they want in terms of treatment recommendations. It is rather a process by which both patient and health professional engage in discussion to determine goals that can be acceptable to both and to establish what each is willing to compromise to reach the mutually established goals. Health professionals seek to offer advice they feel is professionally appropriate, whereas patients seek to reach goals that are consistent with their own expectations and priorities. Compromises in patient teaching are acceptable as long as both patient and health professional are able to maintain their own particular standards.

Although the concept of negotiation would seem the ideal solution in ensuring that patient teaching goals are reached, the reality of all human encounters is that conflict is bound to occur at some point. Obviously, the nature of the condition for which patient teaching is being conducted is also a major factor in the degree to which negotiated goals can be established. For instance, patients with insulin-dependent diabetes who object to injecting themselves with insulin may have few alternatives that can be negotiated. In addition, time or circumstances will usually preclude negotiation in emergency situations.

There are times, however, when patients and health professionals may be unable to reach an acceptable compromise even when negotiation of alternatives would be possible. Sometimes, even the best attempts to understand the patient's perspective may result in stalemate. What happens when there appears to be a stalemate between the patient and health professional? Several courses of action can be taken.

One course of action may be coercion, in which either the patient or the health professional or both attempt to coerce the other into accepting their point of view. Coercion may be used to punish the other with the threat of rejection. The health professional may try to coerce the patient with a statement such as, "Miss Lorig, if you won't make a commitment to losing weight as we discussed, then it's useless to go on with these teaching sessions, and I won't see you anymore."

The patient's use of coercion of the health professional may also be an attempt to punish by rejection with such a statement as, "I really don't see why I can't be given more Valium for my symptoms. The relaxation exercises you've talked with me about will never work. If you won't see that I get more Valium, then I'll just go to someone else who will."

Coercion by health professionals alienates patients. If punishment in the form of rejection is also used, then health professionals lose the opportunity not only to supply future patient teaching but also to provide support in other aspects of the treatment recommendations that patients may be willing to follow.

A more productive means of handling the problem may be for the health professional to accept the fact that the patient is not following the recommendations as recommended. The health professional can then work with the patient in areas of the recommendations in which he or she is cooperating. The health professional can monitor the patient's progress and remain available to answer questions, offering alternatives when and if the patient is ready to accept them.

Such an approach does not mean that health professionals show approval of patients' nonadherent behavior. Health professionals may still be honest with patients about views of why the recommendations should be followed. By demonstrating acceptance of the patient as a person despite the nonadherence, however, and by keeping channels of communication open, the possibility for further patient teaching and negotiation is also kept open. As an example, take the case of Mr. Lepig, who refused to have a screening colonoscopy, a procedure strongly recommended by his physician. The physician stated, "Mr. Lepig, you know I disagree with your decision not to have a colonoscopy and I hope at some point you may reconsider, but I accept your decision and, if in the future you change your mind, I will be happy to arrange it for you. In the meantime, please know that I'm here to answer any questions you may have and to continue to work with you on other goals on which we do agree."

Rather than berating Mr. Lepig for his choice, or merely avoiding the issue of disagreement, the physician attempted to be honest with Mr. Lepig while, at the same time, leaving open the opportunity for future interactions.

When patients demonstrate coercion and attempt rejection of the health professional as a way to get what they want, especially when the request goes against the health professional's judgments and standards, such demands need not necessarily be met. The health professional may explain why the demands cannot be met and continue to demonstrate a willingness to work with the patient despite areas of disagreement. Health professionals obviously cannot control patients' behavior or whether or not they will return. Health professionals can, however, continue to show respect and acceptance of patients as individuals with differing opinions. This approach may increase the probability that additional patient teaching can be accomplished in the future.

Another unproductive course of action that may be adopted by either patient or health professional when negotiation fails to reach a compromise is to ignore the problem. Patients, realizing that a stalemate has been reached, may merely resign themselves to agreeing outwardly with the health professional when in actuality they disagree with the recommendations and have little intention of following them. The health professional, uncomfortable with a situation in which there is conflict, may pretend that the conflict is resolved and discontinue further discussion. In additional encounters between patient and health professional, the charade may be maintained. The patient may not admit to not following advice. The health professional, to avoid further confrontation, may avoid asking the extent to which the patient is following the recommendations.

Avoidance of confrontation over conflicts in negotiation does not appear to be the most effective solution to the problem. When disagreements are reached and cannot be resolved, it is more effective for both patient and health professional to be open and honest about areas of disagreement, focusing on areas in which agreement can be reached. In doing so, health professionals are able to obtain an accurate picture of patients and their progress. Patients then have the option of returning to the health professional at a later time for advice and information without losing face.

The case of Mr. Perkins illustrates productive outcomes of the appropriate handling of occasions when negotiation between patient and health professional fails. Mr. Perkins had arteriosclerosis and subsequently was diagnosed as having an aortic aneurysm, which was repaired. The nurse practitioner working with Mr. Perkins's family doctor visited him while he still was in the hospital to begin discharge planning and to conduct patient teaching. Mr. Perkins had been a heavy smoker for many years, a behavior that was definitely contraindicated because of the arteriosclerosis and the surgery he had experienced.

In addition to other instructions for discharge, the nurse discussed techniques that might be helpful to Mr. Perkins in stopping smoking. The nurse's approach was open and warm, and feedback from Mr. Perkins regarding his perceptions and feelings about the recommendations were frequently elicited by the nurse. With regard to the instructions to quit smoking, Mr. Perkins said, "I've been smoking for over 30 years. That isn't a habit that would be easy to break even if I wanted to."

The nurse responded with various attempts at negotiation—ranging from having Mr. Perkins cut down on the number of cigarettes smoked to, at the very least, switching to cigarettes that contained less tar and nicotine. Mr. Perkins, out of exasperation, finally said, "I enjoy smoking. I like the cigarettes I've smoked for 30 years, and I don't intend to stop."

The nurse, recognizing the futility of continuing to negotiate further, stated the following, "Mr. Perkins, you know from our discussion why the advice to stop smoking is crucial. I can't, however, force you to stop and I can't tell you that it's okay if you don't. I'll continue to help you with other aspects of your treatment, though, and if you do change your mind about smoking, please contact me and we'll go over ways that that might be accomplished."

The nurse's attitude toward Mr. Perkins was one of cooperation and respect for his decision while still communicating that his choice was not within the standards of what was thought to be therapeutically best. At subsequent visits to the physician's office, the nurse continued to ask Mr. Perkins about his smoking as well as other aspects of his recommendations, offering him support and encouragement for following the other instructions while still leaving open the option to work with him to stop smoking.

Although Mr. Perkins may never stop smoking, because of the nurse's attitude many other goals for patient teaching were accomplished. Failure at negotiation does not mean that nothing more is to be accomplished. It means the health professional remains alert and aware of other issues in which positive outcomes might be affected for the patient.

FACILITATING PATIENT DECISION MAKING

A variety of factors determine how patients make decisions about the extent to which they follow recommendations. Recommendations may invoke conflict when patients are attempting to decide which recommendations they are willing or able to follow. Following recommendations may mean that the patient accepts some short-term losses or inconvenience in order to reach the long-term goals that adherence proposes to attain. In some instances, the short-term effects of following the treatment may not seem worth the effort taken to reach the long-term goals. Such might be the case of patients following recommendations for preventive health practices. The time and effort spent in exercising, dieting, or quitting smoking may not have immediate results that are reinforcing enough to motivate patients to continue, especially when the long-term goals seem nebulous at best. In terms of treatment recommendations for various conditions, the "cure" may seem worse than the treatment itself, causing patients to discontinue treatment despite their knowledge of the consequences. This may be true in the instance of medications that have side effects or treatments that involve discomfort; it may also be true when treatment interferes with patients' other priorities. Such was the case of Mrs. O'Fallin.

Mrs. O'Fallin was pregnant with her fourth child and had suffered kidney damage in the past. She continued to have recurrent urinary tract infections, which were watched closely by the physician and treated aggressively to prevent the infection from affecting her kidneys. She had returned to her physician for a prenatal visit after having been seen by the physician for a urinary tract infection a week previously. At that time, she had been given a prescription for antibiotics along with instructions on how to take the medication and why taking the medication as directed was crucial. At the prenatal visit, the physician was shocked to learn that Mrs. O'Fallin had not had the prescription filled despite knowing the risk involved if recommendations were not followed.

Mrs. O'Fallin's explanation of how she reached her decision seemed to her quite simple. Her husband was temporarily laid off from his job. Their youngest child had been quite ill and required medication. Money was not available to fill both the prescriptions for Mrs. O'Fallin and their child. Mrs. O'Fallin, therefore, chose to risk her own health rather than risking the health of her child. The physician saw the situation in quite a different light. From the physician's standpoint, Mrs. O'Fallin's health was crucial to her unborn child as well as to the continuing care of her other children. Mrs. O'Fallin's decision not to follow recommendations was, however, based on her beliefs and priorities despite knowledge and explanation of the risk involved.

In making decisions about the extent to which instructions will be followed, patients can react in a variety of ways depending on how they balance the consequences of following or not following instructions.

- Patients may totally ignore the information given and continue in their current pattern of action or inaction despite the consequences to their health and well-being. Such might be the case with persons with diabetes who continue to fail to follow dietary restrictions or take their oral medications regularly, despite the clear explanation given of the potential consequences of not doing so.
- Patients may totally adopt the recommendations given without question, being complacent and passive in the process. In this situation, patients place the decision of what is best solely in the hands of the health professional who is providing them with recommendations, basing their strict adherence to the recommendations on the faith that the health professional's advice is sound.
- Patients may appear to have decided to follow instructions but actually choose to follow only selected aspects of the recommendations, procrastinating about the rest or blaming others for their inability to follow all of them. Excuses such as, "My wife forgot to remind me to take my medication on vacation," or "I was waiting until I tie up a few loose ends at work to begin the treatment," may be examples of this process of decision making.
- Instructions given may seem so threatening or so impossible that patients, discounting the instructions, frantically search for what they consider easier solutions to their problems. Such may be the case of patients who, after receiving instructions, elect to seek more "natural" means in the form of health foods and other folk remedies instead.
- Patients weigh the pros and cons of the instructions given, ask questions, seek additional information, and make a decision of whether or not to follow the instructions based on their investigation and assimilation of the information available. An example of this type of decision-making pattern may be determined by patients who, before deciding whether or not to have elective surgery, research the risks versus the gains, seek a second opinion, and base their decision on facts gathered.

The last pattern of decision making, except in emergencies when there is no time to gather additional facts, probably leads to the best decisions. Although health professionals cannot coerce patients into this form of decision making, they can do various things to facilitate the process.

First, when involved in patient teaching, health professionals should be realistic in relaying the consequences of following or not following the instructions. Reasons for following instructions should be based on facts regarding the probability that the outcome adherence will be positive, rather than making promises based on personal bias or conjecture. Such statements as, "If you'd quit smoking, you'll live to be a hundred," are unrealistic in terms of the outcomes patients can expect if they follow instructions. A better statement, based on fact, may be, "There is considerable evidence supporting the view that smoking is linked to a variety of diseases and that, as a whole, persons who smoke less tend to have increased longevity." The second statement, based on fact, is more likely to be taken seriously by the patient than one that appears to have no supporting evidence.

When following or not following instructions seems critical to a patient's well-being, health professionals may be tempted to use threat and fear arousal in an attempt to motivate the patient to make the decision to adhere. Studies indicate, however, that as the degree of fear is increased, adherence to recommendations decreases (Leventhal, 1971). If the consequences of not following recommendations are blown out of proportion or are based more on emotions than fact, patients may be less apt to take recommendations seriously. If, for example, the health professional says, "If you don't take your medication for your hypertension as directed, you're going to have a stroke and die," the patient only has to know of one other individual who has not adhered with the same recommendations and has had no serious consequences to discount the credibility of the statement.

Fear arousal can also raise patients' anxiety levels to a degree that they deny that the threat exists to protect themselves from increased anxiety. Under these circumstances, patients may react to the preceding statement by ignoring the health advice totally rather than admitting the seriousness of their condition.

Before patients can be motivated to action or before they can make an adequate decision about the extent to which they will follow recommendations, they must be given a realistic view of the consequences of following or not following the recommendations. A statement by the health professional, such as, "Just take these medications for your hypertension as directed," will do little to help patients in decision making. By receiving information based on fact, however, patients are better able to weigh the risks and benefits of following the instructions realistically and make a more rational decision on how closely they will adhere to them. Consider a statement such as, "Hypertension, if uncontrolled by medication, could lead to stroke. The purpose of the medication that has been prescribed is to help you to keep your blood pressure at a safe level." The statement communicates the seriousness of the condition and the importance of following the recommendations without being unnecessarily alarmist in the warning.

The second way health professionals can help patients in decision making is by helping increase their awareness of their use of excuses and rationalizations and how these are interfering with following recommendations. In confronting patients with their excuses or rationalizations, health professionals should not actively accuse patients of making excuses but rather refute the excuses or rationalization with factual information.

As an example, a patient may say, "If I have a Papanicolaou smear and they find cancer, there is nothing they can do, anyway." Rather than telling the patient she is wrong or that she is being unreasonable, it is more productive for the health professional to counter with facts, such as the cure rate for cervical cancer when it is detected early.

Rather than attacking patients' use of excuses or rationalizations, health professionals should raise patients' awareness and assist patients in acknowledging their tendency to rationalize. This technique helps patients explore excuses they are making so that more effective decision making may result.

Another way health professionals can help patients to make decisions about following recommendations is to prepare them realistically for what they might expect from following or not following the recommendations. The information should address both positive and negative effects that may result if recommendations are followed. Health professionals frequently refrain from sharing possible side effects of treatment or medication for fear that patients will be less likely to follow recommendations or that patients' knowledge of potential side effects will increase their chances of developing them. Withholding such information often has effects opposite those intended. Patients who have not been forewarned about what to expect may be more likely to discontinue treatment if negative effects are experienced. If patients know what to anticipate, are reassured, and are told what to do if negative side effects occur, however, the likelihood that they will continue treatment is increased.

There is also little evidence to support the belief that patients who are informed about possible side effects are more likely to develop them. Realistic expectations can help patients cope more effectively with negative effects of following recommendations as well as help them experience a more active sense of control.

Patients' verbal commitment to following negotiated recommendations can be helpful in increasing the effectiveness of patient teaching. Many people feel uncomfortable going back on their word, especially when the commitment made to a particular action is made verbally in the presence of a respected and esteemed person. Such might be the case of a patient making a commitment to follow instructions in the presence of the health professional who has provided them.

Such a commitment may be obtained by the health professional, with a statement such as, "Now that we've reached an agreement and appear to have worked out most of the problems that there seemed to be with regard to the instructions, tell me what exactly you are going to do when you go home."

Commitment may also be more formalized in terms of establishing a contract between patient and health professional that outlines specifically what is expected.

Facilitation of decision making is helpful to health professionals in effective negotiation in patient teaching. Although patients have final control over whether or not instructions will be followed, guiding patients in effective decision making is an important aspect in patient teaching.

PATIENT CONTRACTING AS A TOOL IN PATIENT TEACHING

Contracts consist of written or verbal agreements between the patient and health professional that clearly outline terms and expectations and can be used to increase patient adherence (Bosch-Capblanch et al., 2007). Patient contracting in patient teaching is one method that can be used to help patients follow recommendations and to help them reach mutually accepted goals that have been decided on through negotiation. Negotiation was previously described as discussing or bargaining to reach an agreement. Contracting is an active process in which patients and health professionals work together to establish specific measurable goals. Whereas negotiation establishes a general framework for the partnership, contracting specifies the particulars. Responsibility to reach the goal is shared rather than being one-sided. Both patient and health professional clearly know and agree on what can be realistically expected from each other.

The process of contracting is based on a theory of learning. It specifies that behavior is increased when there are positive consequences that closely follow performance of that behavior. Through contracting, patient teaching goals are made in measurable and observable terms. Through specific identification of what the patient is to do, the patient knows what to expect, the health professional is able to facilitate the meeting of specific goals by reinforcing behavior that contributes to meeting the goals, and there is an observable process through which patient progress can be monitored.

Contracting focuses on increasing patients' skills in carrying out recommendations, emphasizing patients' strengths rather than weaknesses. If certain instructions seem unmanageable or overwhelming, rather than dwelling on patients' inability to carry out recommendations or on the mammoth nature of the task, emphasis is placed on small parts of the task that the patient can accomplish. Breaking recommendations into small, attainable steps makes the plan more realistic for the patient to follow. Through feedback and monitoring of progress, health professionals are able to reinforce patients at each level of attainment, as well as noting problems patients may have with various aspects of the recommendations. If problems occur at different points, the contract can be negotiated, and additional strategies that might help the patient attain the goal can be used. Rather than emphasizing patients' failures to adhere to recommendations, contracting emphasizes what has been accomplished and continually searches for additional methods to help patients follow the recommendations that have been decided on.

Just as with other approaches to effective patient teaching, contracting must be based on patient needs in order to be effective. This means that assessment of the patient and the current situation is essential if contracting is to be optimal. Identifying and exploring background information regarding the patient's current lifestyle and activities enables health professionals to be aware of patient strengths that can be used to facilitate following instructions. In addition, health professionals are able to identify potential barriers that may need to be altered if the goals are to be reached. Gathering this type of background information helps the health professional assist the patient to build a framework from which they can make their own decisions. After mutual goals have been established, health professionals are then able to supply information patients want and need to reach the goals.

HELPING PATIENTS IDENTIFY GOALS

Recommendations that appear simple to implement to the health professional may seem overwhelming to the patient. Recommendations may seem unrealistic to patients, and thus many of them may be abandoned. The goal of health professionals may be to help patients carry out all the recommendations at once, without realizing that such an ambitious goal may actually sabotage the possibility of carrying out any of them. Patients, discouraged at what appears to be impossible goals, may selectively choose recommendations to follow or may give up the treatment recommendations completely. A more realistic approach may be to identify with patients' short-term goals and strategies that can help them eventually reach the long-term goals. The case of Mr. Gunter is an example.

Mr. Gunter had rheumatoid arthritis. The physician had talked with him about the importance of energy conservation in treating the condition and specified the importance of alternating periods of work, activity, therapeutic exercise, and rest in order to avoid fatigue. The physician had asked that the nurse conduct more in-depth patient teaching with Mr. Gunter about his condition and treatment.

The nurse spent considerable time talking with Mr. Gunter about energy conservation, in addition to other aspects of treatment. The nurse began by helping Mr. Gunter establish some goals and priorities. The first step was to obtain background information concerning his daily activities and to help him to decide which of those activities were the most critical to him.

At first, Mr. Gunter became frustrated at establishing any priorities of activity. He stated, "I can't change my job, and I don't want to be the only inactive one when I'm home with my family. All my activity is important. I just don't see how I'm ever going to be able to get these rest periods in." In talking with Mr. Gunter, the nurse discussed the possibility that everyone engages in a certain amount of activity because it is expected rather than actually examining whether or not the task is worth doing. In helping Mr. Gunter establish some priorities about activity, the nurse asked him to ask himself the following questions about his activities: "Does this task really need to be done? Why does it have to be done? What would happen if it were eliminated? What makes it so hard to think of giving up this task? Is this something that has to be done by me or could someone else help to do it?"

In establishing priorities, the nurse was careful to help Mr. Gunter not exclude tasks for his own enjoyment. Having energy left over to enjoy activities with his family because of rest periods established during the day became rewarding in itself and reinforced Mr. Gunter to continue the recommendations. By working with Mr. Gunter to establish how these rest periods could be accomplished at work, the physician's recommendations for energy conservation were broken down into small, manageable steps with strategies that allowed Mr. Gunter to reach the established goals.

At several points during the establishment of priorities, Mr. Gunter appeared reluctant to make the commitment to rest at specified periods. The nurse continued negotiating and continued further exploration of Mr. Gunter's resistance by saying, "We don't seem to be able to agree on time throughout the day when you could rest. What do you think might make it easier for you to rest?" The statement prompted Mr. Gunter to relay his concerns about what fellow workers would think about his taking frequent rest periods. The nurse and Mr. Gunter were then able to talk about potential problems and to establish strategies for coping with them.

Goals in patient teaching may be numerous. Health professionals may not have the time or opportunity to address all the issues of complicated recommendations at one time. It might be important to remember, however, that accomplishing short-term goals is a step toward accomplishing long-term goals. Those teaching situations in which there will not be ongoing contact with the patient are better geared toward establishment of short-term, prioritized goals that can be reached. In cases where there will be ongoing, continued contact with the patient over time, such as in a clinic setting, short-term goals can be building blocks toward the end goal.

Recommendations that require complex lifestyle changes may be more difficult for patients to accomplish than those requiring only simple, short-term changes. For example, following strict, long-term diet recommendations will probably be more difficult for patients to accomplish than taking one pill a day for 1 week. If health professionals are unaware of the differences in the level of difficulty and expect patients to have complete success with each of the recommendations, both patient and health professional may become disillusioned and disappointed if the patient fails. Establishing less complicated, short-term goals with which patients will have a better chance of success can enhance motivation as well as create additional opportunities for patient teaching. For instance, if a goal is to have a patient stop smoking cigarettes completely, a more realistic goal and point of negotiation might be to establish a maximum number of cigarettes he or she will smoke during the day rather than setting the goal of complete cessation too quickly—a goal that will probably be met with failure. Although both health professional and patient may agree on an ultimate end, the goal is more easily reached if it is tackled in small steps.

MAKING GOALS OBSERVABLE

One of the difficulties in determining the effectiveness of patient teaching is often establishing what outcomes are expected and how those outcomes may actually be measured. Joint establishment of goals between patient and health professional is important, but making the goals specific is just as crucial. Contracting helps establish outcomes that are less vague, more observable, and consequently more easily measured by patient and health professional.

For example, in the previous case, one of the goals that Mr. Gunter and the nurse agreed on was that he would lie down in the lounge at work during coffee breaks in the morning and afternoon, as well as for 30 minutes during his lunch hour. Mr. Gunter was asked to keep a record of how often the goal was reached. Upon returning to the clinic, the nurse noted that Mr. Gunter frequently missed lying down during the lunch break. The nurse helped Mr. Gunter examine factors that interfered with his accomplishing that part of the recommendations. The main problem appeared to be that another employee frequently rested in the lounge, leaving no space available for Mr. Gunter during his lunch hour. Rest periods during the coffee breaks appeared to present no problem.

The nurse discussed the possibility of staggering lunch times or of finding another place to rest, but neither of these approaches was feasible. The nurse was able to negotiate with Mr. Gunter, however, that on days when he was unable to rest at noon, he would lie down for 30 minutes upon returning home. At subsequent visits, it was found that this solution tended to be more satisfactory for Mr. Gunter, thus increasing his amount of rest time during the day. If the goal for teaching outcomes had only been based on Mr. Gunter's knowledge of the importance of rest, or had the goal only been that he have frequent rest periods during the day, neither patient nor health professional would have been able to determine efficiently the extent to which the instructions facilitated the outcome, nor would barriers that impeded reaching the goals have been identified and overcome.

Unless goals are clearly specified, health professionals cannot assume that terms mean the same thing to the patient as they do to them. In Mr. Gunter's case, instructions such as, "Take frequent rest periods throughout the day," may have meant sitting down once or twice during the day, whereas the nurse's concept of the recommendations was something quite different.

If the patient has difficulty attaining a goal, he or she may be encouraged to keep a diary in which the patient records events that occur in relation to following instructions. In this way, the patient and health professional may be able to examine more closely the factors that interfere with the patient's progress and therefore discuss alternatives that would help the patient to attain the goal.

An example is the case of Mr. Henry, who was given dietary instructions in which specific recommendations were, "Avoid caffeinated beverages such as coffee, tea, and cola drinks." By keeping a diary of his activities during the day and the extent to which instructions were followed, Mr. Henry discovered that the major time for nonadherence occurred in the morning shortly after arriving at work. In more fully investigating the circumstances, he discovered that every morning when walking past the lounge to his office, he smelled the aroma of coffee that was served there. The aroma was sufficient stimulus for him to be tempted to have a cup of coffee. By identifying specific situations contributing to his nonadherence, Mr. Henry and the health professional were able to establish ways in which the problem could be dealt with. As one solution, Mr. Henry agreed to try walking to his office another way to avoid walking past the coffee room.

By making instructions specific and observable, goals can be counted, measured, and recorded. By keeping a diary, situations that may interfere with adherence can be described. Contracting can be used to establish a procedure in which both health professionals and patients know what the expectations are and to provide a mechanism for continual evaluation and feedback that can be useful in modifying instructions as need indicates.

REINFORCING PATIENT BEHAVIOR

A reinforcer is anything that is a positive consequence of behavior and increases the likelihood that the behavior will occur. In the case of patient teaching, it may seem that the behavior that maintains or enhances patients' health or sense of well-being should in and of itself be positive enough in consequence to ensure that they will follow recommendations given. It is obvious, though, that this is not the case. Not all patients place the same value on health itself. Likewise, some treatments, although having positive consequences on long-term health, may cause short-term discomfort and inconvenience, which decrease patient motivation to follow the recommendations before the long-term reinforcement is reached.

Contracting uses reinforcement as a way to increase the likelihood that patients will follow instructions to reach agreed-upon goals. Because all persons do not come from the same environment or background, what is reinforcing for one individual may not be reinforcing for another. A significant part of successful contracting is to identify factors that can be used as reinforcement to help patients reach their goals. It is important that health professionals be aware of their own value judgments so as not to impose on patients those things health professionals consider reinforcing. To work effectively, reinforcers have to be meaningful to patients. The issue is not to identify acceptable reinforcers but to find effective reinforcers unique to the individual that will help him or her reach a specified goal.

Reinforcers for patients may change over time as people's circumstances change. Health professionals using contracting in patient teaching therefore must be aware of the changes that occur and the consequences those changes have on patient behavior. Reinforcers may involve praise and recognition, attention, or, in some instances, more tangible factors. The health professional and patient together may discuss what potential reinforcers are available. Some reinforcers may be a natural part of patients' daily lives. These can be used and capitalized on. For instance, a patient who is trying to lose weight and is praised by her husband every time another pound is lost probably has a more powerful reinforcer in her immediate environment than any number of tangible reinforcers the patient and health professional could come up with. In this instance, the contract between patient and health professional would consist of a specified number of pounds to be lost by the patient, perhaps weekly. Although the health professional might continue to reinforce the patient through praise for progress at each visit, the health professional, also aware of the potency of the husband's praise, might reinforce him as well for his positive contribution to the patient's success. Just as a spouse, friends, or other individuals in the patient's life can be positive reinforcers, they also have the potential to sabotage the patient's success. Health professionals who are aware of the importance of social reinforcers can consider these variables and include them as factors in the patient teaching plan.

In other situations, praise of the patient by the health professional may be reinforcing. In some instances, helping patients to determine ways they can reinforce their own behavior may be important. In the case of the patient on a diet, a reinforcer might be to buy a new article of clothing every time a specified number of pounds has been lost.

Reinforcement is most effective if applied in a consistent, systematic way. If, for example, the health professional praises a patient at one visit for losing weight but then neglects to give him or her praise on subsequent visits, the effect of the initial reinforcement may be lost. It is also important for health professionals to recognize that removing unpleasant factors associated with certain behavior may also be reinforcing and therefore increase the likelihood that the patient will follow directions. If, for example, a patient experiences negative side effects from antihypertensive medication and an alternative medication is not feasible, the professional may be able to tell the patient that with sufficient weight loss, the medication could be discontinued. The potential of having the medication removed may in itself be reinforcing and increase the likelihood of the patient's losing weight.

Nearly anything can be a reinforcer. When negotiating a contract, it is important for the health professional to remember that, to be effective, reinforcers must be important to the patient. Reinforcers must also be accessible and consistently applied if they are to increase patients' ability to follow instructions. The best way to find reinforcers is to talk to and listen to the patient. Because the reinforcer must be important to the patient, the unilateral selection of reinforcers by health professionals is of little value.

HELPING PATIENTS TO DECREASE BEHAVIOR

Although many instructions in patient teaching focus on helping patients do something, such as follow a diet or take their medication at regular intervals, sometimes instructions are directed toward helping them decrease behavior, such as smoking. It is important for health professionals to remember that it is easier to increase a behavior than to change a behavior that has become a daily part of the patient's lifestyle.

To decrease behavior through contracting, it is again important that patients and health professionals establish baseline records of the frequency with which the behavior is being performed. Situations that surround the behavior when it occurs should also be identified. For many such activities, the behavior patients want to decrease may be so much a part of their daily routine that they are unaware that it is occurring. They may also be unaware of what stimulates the behavior to occur.

In smoking, for example, patients may note through record keeping that every time they have a cup of coffee, they also smoke a cigarette. They may find that even though they frequently do not drink the coffee, merely getting it is the stimulus to smoke a cigarette. One way to help the patient cut down on smoking, then, may be for the patient to avoid having coffee. By avoiding getting the coffee, the stimulus for a cigarette is decreased. Although in most cases, asking the patient to make two major changes in lifestyle at one time may make the likelihood of success more difficult, in this case the behaviors are linked so closely, one serving as a cue for the other, that change of one necessitates change in the other. Without such record keeping, the patient may have been totally unaware of the correlation between the two behaviors or the frequency of having a cigarette. In recording the baseline data, it is also important that patients be aware of events that may be reinforcing them to continue the behavior. In the same example, although the coffee served as the stimulus to smoke, the reinforcer might be that a coworker, when seeing the patient light a cigarette, would come over to join him. Thus, a pleasant social encounter resulted from the patient lighting a cigarette. Removing the coffee as a cue for cigarette smoking as well as removing the pleasant consequences of smoking may help decrease the smoking behavior of the patient. Further help may be offered by helping the patient to find ways of having the same pleasant social interaction without smoking.

Obviously, the more complex the behavior the patient is trying to decrease, the more complicated are events surrounding the behavior; consequently, they are more difficult for the patient to record. To obtain a more complete pattern of behavior, it may be helpful to include family members in recording behaviors. Family members may observe circumstances surrounding the behavior of which the patient may be totally unaware. Including the family in contracting can help members understand how to provide reinforcers for the patient's success at decreasing behavior. Working with family members can also help them to realize what they may be doing unknowingly that makes it more difficult for the patient to decrease behavior.

An example of including family to assist patients to reach their goals may be illustrated by the same example of smoking used previously. If a family member consistently offered the patient coffee at home without realizing that the gesture offered a cue to smoke, one step in helping the patient to decrease smoking would be to help that family member understand how he or she was contributing to the patient's behavior. On the other hand, if the family member joined the patient on seeing him or her light a cigarette, the attention may serve as a reinforcer for smoking. The family member then may be encouraged to seek other situations in which to give the patient time and attention, thus avoiding reinforcing the patient when smoking. It is important for the health professional to know that including the family in contracting should also be a patient's decision. A secret coalition between health professional and family is not the optimal way to help patients reach their goals or to build an atmosphere of mutual trust and respect.

One of the major difficulties in decreasing behavior is, of course, identifying all the reinforcers that encourage various behaviors to continue. In many instances, if reinforcers are identified, they may not all be controlled. Many reinforcers are subtle. It is important for health professionals to recognize that a variety of techniques may be needed to decrease behavior effectively. By keeping records, the patient and health professional can keep track of the degree to which behavior is decreased. If behavior is not decreased as a result of using the current techniques, this is a clue that another strategy should be tried.

HELPING PATIENTS REMEMBER WITH CONTRACTING

Contracting helps patients and health professionals identify problems the patient may be having in following the instructions given in patient teaching. Although there may be many variables attached to patients' inability to follow instructions, one factor may simply be that they have difficulty remembering what they are supposed to do. Health professionals can help patients find ways to help them remember what they are to do by providing cues for the desired behavior.

For example, there may be many reasons for patients not to keep a follow-up appointment. If the health professional finds that a major reason for the patient's consistent failure to keep appointments is the inability to remember the time, a series of strategies may be implemented. Examples of such strategies may be making a phone call to the patient the day before the appointment as a reminder, having the patient write the appointment on a calendar immediately upon returning home, or asking a family member to remind the patient of the appointment. No matter what technique is chosen, the strategy is designed to provide cues to the patient that will initiate the desired behavior.

The same strategy may be used to help patients remember to take medication or to follow a variety of other instructions; if, for example, the patient is to take a medication before meals but has difficulty remembering to take the medication before lunch at work, the health professional may help the patient to identify reminder cues. Cues might consist of attaching a reminder note to the money to be used to buy lunch or placing a cue elsewhere in the patient's environment to stimulate the desired action of taking the medication.

Family or friends can also help patients to remember what they are supposed to do. Both patient and significant others must, however, express a willingness and interest in having this type of involvement. Before enlisting the help of family or friends, it is important for the health professional to be aware of the relationship between the significant others and the patient. Health professionals should avoid placing patients in a situation in which reminders become nagging rather than a positive stimulus to carry out the desired behavior. Health professionals must also recognize that although enlisting the help of family or friends can be beneficial, under other circumstances, it could foster a dependent relationship in which patients assume increasingly less responsibility for their own care. A careful evaluation of the patient's family circumstances is critical if the desired outcome is to be reached.

CONSIDERATIONS IN THE USE OF CONTRACTING

A variety of issues should be considered when using contracting to increase patient adherence. There are definite advantages to contracting. First, it is a positive approach that focuses on future actions that can be taken rather than dwelling on past failures or difficulties the patient had in following recommendations. Second, in contracting, problems or instructions are translated into specific behavior, which prevents inaccurate perceptions of what is to be done. Both health professionals and patients have the same perceptions of goals and behaviors. Expectations are clearly outlined. Because goals and behaviors are explicit, there is a system for monitoring the extent to which the desired behaviors are reached. There is also a means for identification of specific problems that may interfere with carrying out the instructions. Contracting requires health professionals to focus on patients' environments and ways in which the environment influences their ability to carry out instructions. The patient and health professional work together to determine goals and strategies as to how those goals can be reached.

Despite its many advantages in patient teaching, contracting also has some pitfalls. For contracting to work effectively, health professionals should have ongoing contact with patients during which progress may be monitored and problems, if they arise, identified and dealt with. In many healthcare settings, this is not feasible. Health professionals may have only one contact with the patient, limiting the extent to which ongoing monitoring, reinforcement, and negotiating can be conducted. This, however, does not eliminate the possibility of ongoing follow-up.

Health professionals frequently neglect to recognize that contracting, like other forms of patient teaching, is a highly complex process involving detailed assessment of the patient and the environment. The process requires a commitment by the health professional to work with patients in reaching their goals. The application of contracting in a haphazard way can be more detrimental than helpful and can be perceived by patients as a cold and technical way of approaching their problem. To be effective, the health professional must work closely and consistently with the patient in establishing goals and reinforcing and monitoring their attainment.

Contracting may also be viewed by some as dealing so specifically with observable behavior that the feelings and emotions of the patient are ignored. To be effective, contracting must consider these aspects and how they are reflected in the patient behavior observed. Contracting must be specific to the individual and his or her particular circumstances rather than a series of the same strategies applied to all individuals in the same condition. The plan must remain flexible and must accommodate individual patient needs.

Contracting is not a means to coerce patients into adherence with recommendations. It is a technique by which health professionals work with patients to find ways that may help them follow instructions most effectively. Ideally, contracting gradually enhances the patient's own self-control and self-regulation, consequently increasing each person's responsibility for personal health.

Contracting alone may not be sufficient to reach all goals of patient teaching. It is a tool that can be used for some patients in a variety of teaching situations. Not all patients may be comfortable with this approach, nor will all health professionals be willing to adopt it. Constraints on both patient and health professional must be considered. If applied appropriately, with good judgment, and in the right circumstances, contracting and continued negotiation can be one means to increase the effectiveness of patient teaching.

REFERENCES

Beisecker, A., & Beisecker, T. (1990). Patient information-seeking behaviors when communicating with doctors. *Medical Care, 28,* 19–28.

Blessing-Moore, J. (1996). Does asthma education change behavior? To know is not to do. *Chest, 109,* 9–19.

Bosch-Capblanch, X., Abba, K., Prictor, M., & Garner, P. (2007). Contracts between patients and healthcare practitioners for improving patients' adherence to treatment, prevention and health promotion activities. *Cochrane Database System of Systematic Reviews,* (2), CD004808.

Breen, G. M., Wan, T. T., Zhang, N. J., Marathe, S. S., Seblega, B. K., & Pack, S. C. (2009). Improving doctor-patient communication: examining innovative modalities vis-à-vis effective patient-centric care management technology. *Journal of Medical Systems, 33*(2), 155–162.

Comstrock, D. L., Hammer, T. R., Strentzsch, J., Cannon, K., Parsons, J., & Salazar, G. (2008). Relational-cultural theory: A framework for bridging relational, multicultural, and social justice competencies. *Journal of Counseling & Development, 86,* 279–287.

Dansky, K. H., Colbert, C. J., & Irwin, P. (1996). Developing and using a patient satisfaction survey: a case study. *College Health, 45,* 83–88.

DiMatteo, M. R. Reiter, R. C., & Gambone, J. C. (1994). Enhancing medication adherence through communication and informed collaborative choice. *Health Communication, 5,* 253–266.

Donovan, J. L., & Blake, D. R. (1992). Patient non-compliance: Deviance or reasoned decision-making? *Social Science and Medicine, 34,* 507–513.

Fuertes, J. N., Mislowack, A., Bennett, J., Paul, L., Gilbert, T. C., Fontan, G., et al. (2007). The physician-patient working alliance. *Patient Education & Counseling, 66*(1), 29–36.

Gallant, M. H., Beaulieu, M. C. & Carnevale, F. (2002). Partnership: Analysis of the concept within the nurse-client relationship. *Journal of Advanced Nursing, 40*(2), 149–157.

Hartog, C. S. (2009). Elements of effective communication-Rediscoveries from homeopathy. *Patient Education and Counseling, 77*(2), 172–178.

Hook, M. (2006). Partnering with patients- a concept ready for action. *Journal of Advanced Nursing, 56*(2), 133–143.

Leventhal, H. (1971). Fear appeals and persuasion: the differentiation of a motivational construct. *American Journal of Public Health, 61*(6), 1208–1224.

Luker, K., Austin, L., Hogg, C., Ferguson, B., & Smith, K. (1997). Nurse-patient relationships: the context of nurse prescribing. *Journal of Advanced Nursing, 28*, 235–242.

McKenna, K., & Tooth, L. (2006). *Client education: A partnership approach for health practitioners.* San Diego, CA: Plural Publishing.

Ong, L. M., d eHaes, J. C., Hoos, A. M., & Lammes, E. B. (1995). Doctor-patient communication: A review of the literature. *Social Science Medicine, 40*, 903–918.

Porche, R. A. (2007). *The Joint Commission guide to patient and family education* (2nd ed.). Oakbrook Terrace, IL: The Joint Commission.

Roter, D., & Hall, J. A. (2009). Communication and adherence: Moving from prediction to understanding. *Medical Care, 47*(8), 823–825.

Singleton, T. (2008). How to improve patient adherence. *Podiatry Management, 27*(8), 145–146.

Stewart, M. A. (1995). Effective physician-patient communication and health outcomes: A review. *Canadian Medical Association Journal, 152*, 1423–1433.

Stone, G. C. (1979). Patient compliance and the role of the expert. *Journal of Social Issues, 35*(1), 34–59.

Szasz, T. S., & Hollender, M. H. (1956). A contribution to the philosophy of medicine: The basic models of the doctor–patient relationship. *Archives of Internal Medicine, 97*, 585–592.

Williams, O. A. (1993). Patient knowledge of operative care. *Journal of the Royal Society of Medicine, 86*, 328–331.

Wolf, D. M., Lehman, L., Quinlin, R., Zullo, T., & Hoffman, L. (2008). Effect of patient-centered care on patient satisfaction and quality of care. *Journal of Nursing Care Quality, 23*(4), 316–321.

World Health Organization. (1978). *Primary health care, report of the International Conference on Primary Health Care, Alma-Ata, USSR, 6–12 September 1978.* Geneva: World Health Organization.

CHAPTER 10

Health Literacy in Patient Education and Patient Adherence

LITERACY

In a world of technological advances and increasing college attendance, it is difficult to believe that a significant number of individuals are unable to read or write or lack the ability to handle numerical information, skills needed to function effectively in society. Although literacy originally was defined as the ability to read and write, the definition has been broadened to include skills such as comprehension, problem solving, and reasoning. Educational attainment is not always an indication of an individual's literacy. Surprisingly, the National Adult Literacy Survey conducted in 1992 found that many individuals with low literacy skills are high school graduates and, in some instances, college graduates (Kirsch, 1993). Unfortunately, a higher educational level may not mean that an individual has attained a level of literacy competence.

Individuals with low literacy skills are indistinguishable from others. Low literacy is not limited to individuals with low intelligence, low educational levels, or low socioeconomic status. Individuals of all socioeconomic and educational levels may experience the problem and cannot be identified through appearance or casual conversation.

Approximately one quarter of the US population has rudimentary literacy skills and is unable to understand written materials that require only basic reading proficiency (Mayer & Vallaire, 2007; National Work Group on Literacy and Health, 1998). Literacy, however, extends to more than reading. It is a complex concept, including a constellation of skills that, in addition to reading, impacts the individual's vocabulary development (Doak, Doak, & Root, 1996) and, consequently, their ability to think, organize, interpret, and analyze information (Lasater & Mehler, 1998).

In the United States, literacy is described as, "an individual's ability to read, write, and speak English, and compute and solve problems at levels of proficiency necessary to function on the job and in society, to achieve one's goals, and develop one's knowledge and potential" (Irwin, 1991).

In 1992, the US Department of Education surveyed 26,000 adults through the National Adult Literacy Survey to assess literacy in the United States population. Researchers, recognizing that literacy is comprised of a broad variety of skills, designed the 1992 National Adult Literacy Survey to assess literacy on three scales (Kirsch, 1993):

- Prose—referring to the knowledge and skills needed to locate and use information
- Document—referring to the ability to locate and use information contained within graphs, tables, insurance forms, etc.
- Quantitative—the ability to apply math skills to everyday life, such as in balancing a checkbook

Results of the survey indicated that about one fourth of the adult population in the United States are unable to understand written information that requires only basic levels of reading ability (Weiss & Coyne, 1997). Reasons for low literacy are numerous. Some individuals may have never learned to read as a result of inadequate education. In some instances, low literacy may be related to cognitive impairment associated with conditions such as traumatic brain injury, stroke, meningitis, or dementia. In other instances, affective disorders, such as depression, learning disorders, conditions such as attention deficit hyperactivity disorder, anxiety, or stress may contribute to low literacy (Mayer & Vallaire, 2007). Some individuals, as a result of inadequate educational opportunities, may have limited vocabulary development that interferes with their ability to read, comprehend, conceptualize, synthesize, or adequately formulate questions (Doak et al., 1996). In other instances, individuals from different countries may experience low literacy because they do not understand the language, even though they are highly literate in their own language.

Individuals may experience low literacy in different ways. Some individuals may be unable to read words while others can read words but are unable to attach meaning to what is written. Even though individuals possess adequate reading skills, they may still be unable to grasp the meaning of words or to comprehend the concepts the words are meant to convey. Others may be unable to conceptualize information in a way that enables them to apply it in their daily lives. In other instances, individuals may have difficulty with language fluency or vocabulary, rather than comprehension.

In addition to interfering with the individual's ability to read signs, directions, or other written material, low literacy can have an impact on the person's ability to work and to enjoy many leisure activities that are taken for granted, such as reading a newspaper, a book, or a magazine, or reading to children or grandchildren.

MYTHS ABOUT LOW LITERACY

Many myths and stereotypes surround beliefs about low literacy. Just as myths and stereotypes interfere with adequate appraisal in social situations, so can they become a barrier to the health professional finding the best way to help patients learn. Because of preconceived views of low literacy, health professionals may not even assess this important factor in interacting with patients.

The stereotypical view often held about people with low literacy skills is that they are from a lower socioeconomic level, use poor grammar, and are uneducated. Although there are correlations between literacy and economic status, minority and immigrant status, and educational level, most individuals with low literacy in the United States are Caucasian and native born (Mayer & Vallaire, 2007). Low literacy is found in many types of individuals and is not limited to a specific group or educational or socioeconomic stratum (Lasater and Mehler, 1998).

Another misconception about low literacy held by health professionals, at least until recently, is that while low literacy exists in many parts of the world, it does not exist in the United States, where education for children is mandated by law. As more research is conducted, this too has been demonstrated to be a myth. Results from the 1993 National Adult Literacy Survey revealed the magnitude of the problem in this country (National Center for Education Statistics, 1993). Almost half of the US adult population has deficiencies in reading or computational skills (American Medical Association, 1999).

A common belief among health professionals is that patients unable to read will let their health professionals know. This most often is not the case (Weiss & Coyne, 1997; Williams et al., 1995). If patients are unwilling to admit that they do not understand everything the health professional has said because they fear that the health professional will see them as stupid, then admitting that they are unable to understand or read the written word may be even more difficult. There is considerable social stigma attached to the inability to read, particularly in a situation where the health professional may be viewed as educationally elite. Patients may go to great extremes to hide their low literacy. Such statements as, "I can't read this now, I forgot my glasses," or "I'd like to take this home to read it more thoroughly when I have the time and am not so preoccupied," can easily be overlooked as possible cues for further assessment of level of literacy.

Perhaps an even more destructive view by health professionals of low literacy is that it is directly related to intelligence. This is also a myth with no basis in fact (Doak et al., 1996). Although some individuals with low literacy skills may have additional problems related to cognitive function, in many instances, individuals may have high intellectual skills in certain areas but are nonfunctional in reading, and may show exceptional capacity to compensate for their reading difficulties.

HEALTH LITERACY

Low literacy affects all areas of individuals' lives, including health. Literacy when applied relative to health is called *health literacy*. Studies have consistently shown low literacy to be linked with decreased health status, higher use of health services, and increased health costs (Baker et al., 1998; Baker et al., 2002; Baker et al., 2004; Braveman et al., 1988; Davis & Wolf, 2004; DeWalt et al., 2004; Paasche-Orlow et al., 2005; Weiss et al., 1992). Low health literacy has also been linked to poor adherence with recommendations (Bernhardt & Cameron, 2003).

An individual's health literacy may be lower than their general literacy (American Medical Association, 1999). Although the terms literacy and health literacy are often used interchangeably, and although there is some overlap between the two concepts, there are also some important distinctions. Whereas literacy refers to the individual's ability to read, write, and understand written and verbal language in their native tongue, the concept of health literacy is much broader. Health literacy includes a wide range of skills that patients develop over time to seek, comprehend, evaluate, and use health information and concepts to make informed decisions, assess health risks, and increase quality of life (Zarcadoolas, Pleasant, & Greer, 2006). The World Health Organization (1998) has described health literacy as, "the cognitive and social skills which determine the motivation and ability of individuals to gain access to, understand and use information in ways which promote and maintain good health." Health literacy has also been defined as, "the degree to which individuals have the capacity to obtain, process, and understand basic health information and services needed to make appropriate health decisions" (Institute of Medicine, 2004; US Department of Health and Human Services, 2000).

In both definitions, it is evident that health literacy means more than having knowledge or being able to read pamphlets and make appointments. Low health literacy affects the individual's ability to comprehend recommendations regarding his or her condition or care, and his or her ability to learn about preventive practices and health promotion. In addition, it may affect access to care if the individual is unable to locate resources from lists or directories, or if the individual is unable to fill out forms or applications. Finally, it may hinder the individual's ability to comprehend his or her rights, or understand informed consent, making the individual more vulnerable to undergoing procedures or engaging in activities he or she may not understand and may not want. Definitions of health literacy imply the possession of personal skills and confidence that empowers individuals to use health information effectively in order to take action to improve their personal health. Although individuals with low general literacy often also have low health literacy, people can have high literacy but low health literacy, or low general literacy but demonstrate relatively high health literacy. For example, an individual with a Doctor of Philosophy degree in English Literature may not understand that taking multiple over-the-counter drugs could interfere with the effectiveness of his prescribed medication, while a woman with a general educational development degree may be able to manage the care of her child with cystic fibrosis very well.

People who possess skills and abilities to successfully maneuver and function in the healthcare setting in order to promote, attain, or maintain their health are said to have *functional health literacy*. Functional health literacy has been defined as the ability to read, understand, and act on health information in everyday life (Rudd, Kirsch, & Yamamoto, 2004). Functional health literacy encompasses more than a single skill or ability. It includes a combination of skills, such as reading and writing, but also includes the ability to clearly and accurately express physical, psychological, or emotional states to the health professional despite power differential between the patient and the health professional; the ability to ask questions about their health, health care, or recommendations; motivation to receive health information; the capacity to understand information; and independence from a third party to interpret or translate information to them for understanding health information (Schwartzberg, VanGeest, & Wang, 2005). Given the amount of health information currently available on the Internet, functional health literacy skills may also include ability to use a computer and navigate the Internet (Berry, 2007).

Cognitive abilities that have been associated with functional health literacy include verbal fluency, the ability to understand word meanings, the ability to separate key concepts from less relevant points, and to be able to understand and interpret numbers (Doak et al., 1998). Individuals who have low functional health literacy skills would be unable to read a medication label, understand directions of how to take their prescriptions correctly, understand information about their condition, understand discharge instructions, or to decipher recommendations that are more important than others. In addition, individuals with low verbal language skills may be less able to describe their symptoms accurately, which could have an impact on the ability to accurately arrive at a diagnosis of a health condition. Results from the most recent survey of literacy skill among adults were used to develop the Health Literacy Scale, which describes different levels of health literacy (National Assessment of Adult Literacy, 2003):

1. Proficient—ability to perform complex activities such as searching a document to define medical terms or other information
2. Intermediate—capable of conducting moderately challenging tasks such as finding an age range for a particular vaccination from a childhood vaccination chart
3. Basic—ability to complete simple tasks such as giving two precautions which should be followed if taking a particular medication, based on information in a clearly written pamphlet
4. Below basic—demonstrates lowest level of performance such as identifying what is permissible to eat or drink before having a medical test based on set of short instructions
5. Not literate in English

Health literacy tasks, as defined by the National Assessment of Adult Literacy (2003), include:

• Clinical—involving the patient's ability to fill out forms, understand recommendations, and understand how to take medication
• Prevention—ability to follow guidelines for age appropriate health services; engage in self-care and management
• Navigation of the healthcare system such as understanding rights and responsibilities, informed consent, and insurance issues

Health literacy has been found to have significant negative effects on patients' health, leading to poor adherence, participation in unhealthy practices, and adverse health outcomes (Bernhardt & Cameron, 2003; Davis & Wolf, 2004; Wolf, Gazmararian, & Baker, 2005), including potentially harmful or life-threatening mistakes (Bastable, 2006; Nielson-Bohlman, Panzer, & Kindig, 2004; Osborne, 2005). Individuals with low health literacy will have difficulty reading patient education brochures, discharge instructions, informed consent documents, directions regarding how to take their medications, package inserts, which contain essential information about a medication and its use and side effects, or explanations on a food exchange list.

The impact of low literacy on the individual's health and health care has only recently been realized. Patients' ability to understand health information is a prerequisite to patient adherence (Lasater & Mehler, 1998; Mayeaux et al., 1996). Patients need to be able to read and understand instructions, prescriptions, informed consent, and other written documents to optimize their potential for following recommendations through their own informed choice. Too often, however, patients are given written materials, including informed consent forms, without consideration of whether or not they can read and/or comprehend the material.

Ability or inability to read and understand health information also can affect the degree to which patients follow preventive health practices. With the increasing amount of health information available in magazines and newspapers, as well as brochures, pamphlets, books, and other written materials designed to help individuals be better informed about health and health care, it is easy to assume that everyone has the opportunity to be well informed. For those unable to read these materials, however, this is not the case.

Take the example of Mrs. Peterson, a concerned mother who wanted to do the best for her children but had not had them immunized. A single parent with no family, Mrs. Peterson had decided to move to a large city several hundred miles from her home. Before moving, she asked a friend who previously had lived in the city for the name of a clinic where she could receive health care for her children. Several months after moving to the city, Mrs. Peterson brought her children to the clinic recommended by her friend for a routine checkup. The nurses at the clinic discussed the importance of childhood immunizations with Mrs. Peterson, and she seemed genuinely interested and concerned. They also told her of the availability of free immunizations at the local Health Department and advised her that she could call there for further information. When Mrs. Peterson returned to the clinic a few months later, the nurses discovered that she still had not obtained the immunizations for her children. They were shocked at what they perceived as Mrs. Peterson's lack of motivation to obtain the immunizations despite their encouragement to do so.

"I know Mrs. Peterson is having financial difficulty," one nurse exclaimed, "but it's not as if she has to pay for the immunizations. The announcement of their cost-free availability at the health department is posted all over the clinic waiting room and every examining room. She couldn't have helped but see them. Besides, we also included the notice along with the financial statement for her last visit, and she came in personally to pay that bill, so I know she saw the notice. I become so angry when parents are irresponsible."

The nurse's assumption, of course, was that Mrs. Peterson was able to read the notices. What the nurse did not know was that Mrs. Peterson was unable to read. Although she had asked several of her neighbors about the Health Department, its location, and the days immunizations may be available, they had said they were unsure. They suggested that she look up the number in the telephone book and call the Health Department directly. Not knowing her neighbors, she was embarrassed to tell them that she could not look up the number because she could not read. She was equally embarrassed to admit this to the nurses at the clinic, fearing that they may consider her unfit to care for her children. Obviously, she was also unable to read the announcements that had been posted.

Mrs. Peterson's example is only one of many similar situations that occur only too frequently in healthcare facilities. The extent of low literacy in the general population is unknown. It is estimated that nearly 20% of the adult population in America has reading skills below the fifth-grade level (Davidhizar & Brownson, 1999). Many more individuals are only marginally competent (Doak et al., 1996). This means many of the patient education materials available for patients about prevention or explanation of disease or illness and directions regarding treatment recommendations are all of little benefit for this group.

Health professionals should, of course, always take the time to thoroughly explain aspects of illness and prescribed treatment to patients and should never depend on patient education materials alone. When information is complex, however, written patient education materials are used as supplemental material that patients can take home to read, review, and synthesize at their leisure. For those unable to read, however, these materials are of little benefit. Health professionals should take the time to assess the degree to which patients can read and comprehend materials they are given.

Low literacy is often not identified in everyday life. People may go to great lengths to hide their inability to read or to understand the written word. In healthcare settings, unless the problem is identified and adequately compensated for by the health professional, it can have potentially serious consequences. Take, for example, Mr. Kelly, who had been diagnosed as having diabetes. He had collapsed at work, was admitted to the hospital, and at that time had received his diagnosis. During his hospital stay, as well as a few weeks after his discharge, he received patient teaching about diabetes and its management from the diabetes education team. He appeared to comprehend the information they presented and took home all the material they provided for review and more thorough study, as suggested. Two months after his hospital discharge, he was admitted to the hospital emergency department in a diabetic coma. During the course of his hospitalization, a member of the diabetic education team approached Mr. Kelly to assess his understanding of the recommendations and to provide any additional instruction that might be needed. The following dialogue ensued.

Diabetic educator: "Did the materials I gave you before provide enough information?"
Mr. Kelly: "Oh yes! There were pages and pages. There's a lot of information there."

Diabetic educator: "I was wondering what we might be able to do to help you to avoid going into a coma again. Do you have any idea of how this might have happened?"

Mr. Kelly: "Well everything you told me when we talked before was so clear. I understood everything, really, but then after I got home I couldn't remember exactly what you said about everything so I did the best I could, but I guess that wasn't enough."

Diabetic educator: "We give people the materials you took home for that reason. Didn't they help?"

Mr. Kelly: "I know they would have if I could have read them. The pictures are all real helpful, but you see, I never learned to read."

No one had thought to check Mr. Kelly's ability to read, understand, and use the materials he was given. As a result, the use of materials as a backup was futile.

Use of patient education materials as a substitute for direct information given by the health professional is always an ineffective way to teach patients. When patients have low literacy skills, the patient education materials are even less effective. The key to effective patient teaching is to provide information to patients in a way that will best increase their understanding. Before that can be done, health professionals must be able to assess patients' strengths and weaknesses. Assessing patients' literacy skills is no exception.

IDENTIFICATION OF PATIENTS WITH LOW LITERACY

Recognizing that low literacy is a potential problem is the first step to identifying patients with low health literacy. Although the health professional should be aware of prevalence of low health literacy in some groups, they should avoid preconceived ideas about the type of patients who may experience health literacy and should not assume that they can recognize patients with low literacy skills. Even patients with higher literacy levels may face difficulties when they are confronted with terms that are unfamiliar or when they are under physical or emotional stress (Merriman, Ades, & Seffrin, 2002; Schillinger et al., 2006).

It is difficult to identify patients with low health literacy skills. Self-reported educational levels are not always an accurate reflection of the patient's ability to read or comprehend. Because of social stigma attached to low literacy, patients are often not forthcoming about their inability to read or understand information. Many people attempt to hide their inability. Because they are often ashamed and anxious, they attempt to guard their secret and not inform health professionals of their inability to read or understand explanations or recommendations.

Unless the problem is identified and adequately addressed, however, patient teaching will have little impact. Health professionals should be observant for cues that may suggest low health literacy and assess the reading ability and understanding level of patients before conducting patient teaching. For instance, if the patient consistently "forgets" his or her glasses or consistently asks to take materials home to read rather than reading forms or patient education materials at the time of the interaction, the health professional may suspect that literacy is a problem. Likewise, if the patient consistently asks to have a family member or friend with them when forms need to be completed or when written patient education materials are provided, there may be a problem with literacy.

Even when the health professional suspects that patients may have difficulty reading or understanding, they may feel uncomfortable or not know how to address the issue with the patient. As a result, the problem goes unresolved, and the patient does not receive the assistance needed to fully incorporate information provided in the patient teaching interaction.

Direct questioning of patients about their reading ability has been shown to be highly ineffective. Patients go to great lengths to hide their reading difficulties, or when they do admit having difficulty reading, they often underreport the extent (Parikh et al., 1996). Merely asking patients whether they are able to understand the material is insufficient because most patients with limited literacy skills will probably attempt to hide this deficiency (Weiss and Coyne, 1997).

Establishing a trusting, accepting, and shame-free environment in which the patient feels comfortable with the health professional is the first step in identifying difficulties with literacy. As in most areas of assessment of patients' strengths and weaknesses, the best method of assessment of degree of literacy involves observing, being alert to cues, and conducting sensitive and timely direct questioning. The task is made easier in an atmosphere of genuine concern, trust, and conveyance of a sincere desire to help. Take the example of Mr. Hahn. Mr. Hahn had been a patient of Dr. Marshall for almost a year after being referred to her for treatment of ulcerative colitis.

Dr. Marshall had taken considerable time teaching Mr. Hahn about his condition and treatment and had given him a number of books and patient education materials to increase his understanding. Mr. Hahn always gratefully took the materials and, when returning the books Dr. Marshall had lent him, always made a point of telling her how much he appreciated her lending the books to him. Dr. Marshall never questioned Mr. Hahn's ability to read until one day at a visit. She gave Mr. Hahn information on a new treatment alternative, saying,

"I'm still tied up with another patient, but I'd like you to read this while you're waiting so we can discuss it today before you leave."

Upon returning later to discuss the material with Mr. Hahn, Dr. Marshall said, "Well, Mr. Hahn, what do you think?" "I'm not interested," Mr. Hahn replied. "Really? I'm surprised," Dr. Marshall said with astonishment. "What were your major objections?" Mr. Hahn refused to give any specifics saying only that he would take the material home to think about it.

The next day, Dr. Marshall received an enthusiastic call from Mr. Hahn saying that he would like an appointment with her as soon as possible to discuss beginning the new treatment. When he returned to Dr. Marshall's office, she asked Mr. Hahn why he had suddenly changed his mind. Mr. Hahn shrugged, dismissing the question; however, when Dr. Marshall gave Mr. Hahn the questionnaire that was required to be filled out by all patients beginning the new treatment protocol, Mr. Hahn threw it down saying, "I don't know why I have to do this."

Dr. Marshall proceeded to talk with Mr. Hahn and finally said, "Mr. Hahn, you know a lot of people in our country have difficulty reading. I wondered if maybe that applies to you. If it does, please let me help." Mr. Hahn began to cry, telling Dr. Marshall of the complex ways he had learned to cover up his disability. Dr. Marshall made the appropriate referrals, and Mr. Hahn not only began the new treatment but learned to read as well.

Patients' low literacy can have profound effects on their health and health care. Given that the purpose of patient teaching is to communicate information to patients that they can use to promote their own health and well-being, it is important that health professionals spend time assessing patient literacy skills, make appropriate alterations when necessary, and, in some instances, as in the case of Mr. Hahn, make referrals as necessary.

SCREENING FOR HEALTH LITERACY

Screening for health literacy can contribute to the effectiveness of patient teaching; however, there are currently no standardized quick methods that comprehensively assess patients' health literacy levels. Several instruments have been developed that can be used to assess patients' ability to read health-related materials, although most instruments have been used more for research purposes than clinical application (Davis & Wolf, 2004). One instrument, the Rapid Estimate of Adult Literacy in Medicine (REALM), is a screening tool designed to identify patients with limited reading skills and estimating patient reading levels so that the health professional can tailor information to the patient's level of competence (Davis et al., 1991) The REALM is a medical word recognition and pronunciation test and was designed to be used with patients in healthcare settings. It is designed to assess adult patients' ability to read common medical words and can be administered in about 3 to 5 minutes. It consists of a list of 66 medical terms arranged in order of difficulty starting with one-syllable words and moving to words containing more syllables and higher pronunciation difficulty. The patient is asked to read down the list aloud. The patient's score consists of the number of words pronounced correctly, with possible range of score being 0–66. Scores are then categorized into grade equivalency with 0–18 correct responses corresponding to third grade or below, 19–44 correct responses to fourth to sixth grade, 45–60 correct responses to seventh to eighth grade, and 61–66 correct responses to ninth grade or above. A shorter version of the REALM, which can be administered in 1–2 minutes by individuals with minimal training, has also been developed (Davis et al., 1993).

Another instrument, the Test of Functional Health Literacy in Adults (TOFHLA), measures the functional literacy of patients and was developed using actual healthcare materials such as informed consent forms, appointment slips, instructions for diagnostic tests, and prescription labels (Parker et al., 1995). The test consists of 50 items that measure the individual's ability to read and comprehend written health materials and 17 numerical ability items that measure the individual's ability to read and understand numbers. It takes approximately 22 minutes to administer. For the reading portion of the test, individuals are presented with passages that are missing every fifth to seventh word. They are then asked to choose the word that would be most appropriate based on grammar and the context of the sentence from a list of four words. Each correct response is scored as 1. Each correct response in the numerical section is also scored as 1. The scores of the reading comprehension section are scaled and then added to the numerical score after it has been converted. The total score is then placed within one to three categories: inadequate functional health literacy, marginal functional health literacy, or adequate functional health literacy. A Spanish version of the TOFHLA and a short-form version that requires approximately 12 minutes to administer are also available.

A third instrument, the Wide-Range Achievement Test (WRAT), originally developed in 1941 (Jastak & Wilkinson, 1993), is a nationally standardized achievement test that measures basic skills necessary for learning, communication, conceptualizing, reading, spelling, and performing mathematical calculations. It is currently in its fourth edition. There are two levels of testing: one level for children from grades K–12 and the other extending to age 94. Administration time varies with the age and ability of the individual; however, general administration time for children under the age of 7 is between 15–25 minutes and 30–45 minutes for older children and adults. Items are scored as a 1 for every correct answer. The total score is then converted to standard scores and compared to the scores of others who have taken the test. Since the WRAT is an achievement test, it only measures basic academic skills and does not measure fundamental skills as they may be applied to healthcare situations.

As with any type of testing, results must be considered within the context of the individual. Scores may either overestimate or underestimate the individual's skills or abilities and does not take into account compensatory procedures individuals may have developed.

ASSESSING READABILITY OF MATERIALS

Patients read at different levels. Therefore, it is important that written patient education materials given to a patient match the patient's reading ability. Materials that are appropriate for someone reading at the 10th-grade level may not be appropriate for someone reading at the 5th-grade level or below. Both vocabulary and sentence structure influence readability of materials. To know which level may be best for a particular patient, the health professional should have some understanding of how to assess readability of materials to be used for patient teaching.

Although there is no universally accepted way to assess the degree of difficulty of reading materials, there are a number of different formulas and tools that can be used. The range of rating may vary with the procedure used, but these formulas can provide at least cursory information related to readability. Perhaps one of the simplest and easiest formulas to use is the Simple Measure of Gobbledygook (SMOG) formula. The SMOG formula is one of a number of formulas used to establish readability. It is quick, easy to use, and predicts grade level difficulty within 1.5 grades 68% of the time. The procedure for using the SMOG is as follows (Doak et al., 1996):

1. Choose 10 consecutive sentences near the beginning of the material to be reviewed.
2. Choose 10 consecutive sentences from the middle and 10 consecutive sentences from the end of the material.
3. In these 30 sentences, count the number of words containing three or more syllables, including repetitions.
4. Consider hyphenated words as one word. Proper nouns are also counted. Numerals and abbreviations should be counted as they would if the words were written out. For instance, the numeral 25 consists of three syllables, 20 consists of two syllables, and 5 has one syllable. The abbreviation Dec. for December consists of three syllables. When sentences are divided by a colon, each portion of the sentence is considered a separate sentence.
5. Compare the total number of words containing three or more syllables with the SMOG Conversion Table (Table 10-1).

Table 10-1   SMOG Conversion Table

Word Count	Grade Level	Word Count	Grade Level
0–2	4	73–90	12
3–6	5	91–110	13
7–12	6	111–132	14
13–20	7	133–156	15
21–30	8	157–182	16
31–42	9	183–210	17
43–56	10	211–240	18
57–72	11		

The SMOG formula is only one of a number of tools available to measure readability. The SMOG is generally most useful when used for shorter materials. There are also a variety of computer software programs available to measure readability. It is important, however, that health professionals remember that although patients' ability to read written material is important, even more important is their ability to comprehend the content and concepts contained within.

Other tools that can be used to asses readability of materials include the Fry Readability formula and the Suitability of Assessment of Materials (SAM) (Doak et al., 1996). The Fry Readability formula applies from grades 1 through 17 and assesses samples of text throughout the document rather than testing the readability of every word and sentence. The procedure for using the Fry Formula consists of the following (London, 1999):

1. Select three 100-word passages from the material.
2. Count the number of sentences in each 100-word passage.
3. Count the total number of syllables in each 100-word passage.
4. Calculate the average number of sentences and average number of syllables from the three passages and divide the totals by three.
5. Plot the totals on the Fry Graph for Estimating Readability to estimate readability grade level.

The SAM was originally developed for use with print materials and illustrations, but has also been applied to video and audiotaped instructions. Use of the SAM can pinpoint deficiencies in patient education materials, helping health professionals determine the suitability of the material for a certain patient population or enabling the health professional to correct the deficiencies before the materials are used. Materials are evaluated based on the criteria determined for each of the SAM factors, i.e. factors that affect readability, such as the relative difficulty of decoding words and understanding meaning. After scores for each factor are obtained, they are totaled and then converted to percentages which are then categorized as superior, adequate, or not suitable as patient education material.

TEACHING PATIENTS WITH LOW LITERACY SKILLS

A number of factors have been found to exacerbate communication difficulties for individuals with low health literacy (Fang et al., 2006; Sudore et al., 2007). Several of these issues can impact patient teaching effectiveness when the health professional is working with a patient with low literacy skills.

First, health professionals may be unaware that patients have difficulty understanding verbal or written communication. There is often little information about health literacy that is provided to health professionals either during their professional education or as a part of continuing education activities; consequently, the possibility that patients have difficulty with comprehension or reading is frequently not considered during routine clinical interactions. In addition, even when a patient's health literacy needs are identified, the health professional may be uncomfortable confronting the issue or may be unaware of how to meet the patient's health literacy needs.

A second barrier includes the health professional's perception of time constraints. In many healthcare settings, high patient volume and limited resources may create a sense that there is too little time to assess the patient's health literacy or take steps to modify patient teaching to accommodate low health literacy. A third barrier consists of different culture or language between patient and health professional, and a fourth barrier consists of the health professional's reliance on only one mode of communication, either verbal or written, in order to communicate patient information. Health professionals may rely too heavily on written materials as a means of communicating health information to patients (Sudore et al., 2009; Schillinger et al., 2004).

Many of these barriers can be overcome through awareness of the potential of health literacy problems, careful planning, and team involvement. Patients with low health literacy are capable of learning and understanding information if the problem is identified and sufficient time is taken to present the information that meets the patient's needs (Doak et al., 1996; National Work Group on Literacy and Health, 1998).

While some people have never learned to read, others may be able to read but are unable to fully comprehend what is written. In the latter instance, the person may be able to read the words but unable to grasp their meaning. How health professionals alter patient teaching depends on the specific situation at hand.

Verbal Communication

Much information about the patient's condition or treatment recommendations is communicated to them verbally. During patient teaching, organization of information and presentation of information in a logical sequence is especially important. Health professionals should be sensitive to the patient's need to remember the material without benefit of written materials for review. Health professionals should attempt to avoid proceeding too rapidly and should present the most important information first, repeating it throughout the interaction. As much as possible, focus should be on what patients are expected to do rather than overloading them with peripheral information. It may be beneficial to present smaller amounts of information over several sessions rather than presenting the patient with all the information in one setting. Information should be presented in logical segments using terms with which the patient is familiar. Jargon should be avoided. Analogies should be simple with familiar themes. When patient teaching involves a task, such as reading a thermometer or giving an injection, demonstrations may help patients achieve understanding. Likewise, having the patient perform a repeat demonstration enables the health professional to check the patient's understanding of the procedure he or she is to perform.

In all instances, the health professional should review and restate information presented, but when patients have low literacy skills, reviewing information is essential. The patient's understanding of the information should be verified by having the patient confirm his or her understanding in his or her own words. Because of the patient's potential sensitivity to the problem of low literacy, health professionals should take care that the patient is not treated in a condescending manner. The patient's understanding of information can be obtained with a simple statement such as, "Just so I can be sure I have been clear in my explanation, could you briefly summarize the information we've just discussed?" "How are you to take your medication?" or "What foods are you to avoid?" etc.

The patient's response to the previous statement gives the health professional the opportunity to identify any misunderstanding and then to fill in or correct any information that was missed or misunderstood. Interaction and feedback from the patient should be encouraged frequently. When the patient has not understood or has misunderstood information, the health professional should attempt to present the information in a slightly different way, using the patient's frame of reference as much as possible.

Patients with low literacy skills are capable of learning and understanding explanations and recommendations if health professionals take time to present information in a way that best meets patients' needs. Although these interventions may at first seem time consuming, the results in terms of increased effectiveness in patient teaching of patients with low literacy skills can be worth the extra effort.

If the patient's literacy problem involves fluency and vocabulary, the health professional should be especially cautious not to use jargon and should make sure that the words used are actually conveying the intended message. For example, Ms. Wayne, the patient educator at the outpatient health facility, had been asked to give a presentation on cancer to a group of senior citizens. She said, "Any change in color of your stool is an important sign that you should report to your doctor." One man participating in the group raised his hand and asked, "I haven't talked with my doctor yet, but I am remodeling my bathroom. Is one color better than the other?" Terms that are common to health professionals are not always familiar to patients. Health professionals should, as much as possible, use whatever terms best convey the message to the patient.

Written Communication

Although a number of written patient education materials are available, patients with low literacy skills may not have the skills necessary to utilize the materials. Some patients are able to read simple material but are not able to read more complex information. A brief pamphlet or instruction sheet outlining information may be easier for patients to assimilate than material that contains comprehensive explanations. Health professionals should assess written materials for readability in all instances and match the reading level with patients' needs.

Organization of material is also important. Material should contain only essential information—that which is most important for the patient to know. For instance, although it may be helpful for a patient with diabetes to know the exact mechanism of the disease, it may be most important for them to know signs of diabetic coma and insulin shock and steps to take if either of them should occur. Those items most important for the patient to know should be listed first. The use of headings also helps patients to focus on key concepts of the message contained within the handout and presents patients with the opportunity to retrieve specific information easily for review. Underlining or highlighting in color may help draw patients' attention to important points they are to remember. Material should be arranged in logical, sequential steps of presentation.

Health professionals can select a number of commercially prepared patient education materials that are written at a level compatible with patients' ability. In some instances, it may be more practical for health professionals to develop their own materials. If this is the case, health professionals should remember to avoid jargon, use simple terms with few syllables, and use short sentences. The use of words should be consistent and the material contained within the pamphlet should be directly related to what the health professional wants the patient to be able to do after receiving the information. Low literacy materials used for patient teaching should be written with large print for ease of reading.

In some instances, patients with limited literacy skills may need more time to read or to absorb material. Providing patient education materials to the patient before the teaching session so they may become familiar with the hand-outs may be helpful. In other instances, it may be helpful for the health professional to read the material aloud while the patient follows along.

Visual presentation of concepts can add to patients' ability to comprehend and remember material presented. The adage "a picture is worth a thousand words" is particularly true for patients with low literacy skills. Handouts with graphic representations to illustrate points should be used as much as possible. If pictures are used to convey concepts, the health professional should ensure that the visual aids are not demeaning to the patient or that they do not treat the patient in a childlike manner. Visual aids are meant to enhance the patients' ability to learn, not to create an emotional barrier because of embarrassment.

Audiovisual aids can be used to supplement patient teaching. Patients might be encouraged to return to review audiovisual aids as often as they like, or if practical, audiovisual materials may be loaned to the patient so they are able to review the material at home.

HELPING PATIENTS BECOME ACTIVATED

Although much of the focus of health literacy is on reading ability and under-standing health information, health literacy extends to a much broader context. In addition to reading and understanding, patients must be able to navigate the health system, become their own advocates, and take an active and responsi-ble role in their own health and health care. Today's healthcare system can be daunting and complicated even for individuals who are highly skilled (Nielson-Bohlman et al., 2004). For individuals with low literacy and low health literacy, the situation may seem overwhelming. Many individuals with low health literacy may find the healthcare setting complex and intimidating, and may lack confi-dence and skills required to become fully active in their own care. Consequently, the role of the health professional in patient teaching goes beyond providing the patient with information, but includes helping the patient gain the skills and abili-ties required to be an active participant in his or her health care.

Helping patients become "activated in their health" means helping them develop the ability to manage their own health and health care (Hibbard, 2006).

As with many other issues in patient teaching, behavior change, attitude, and skills develop in stages over time. There are stages to becoming fully competent in managing health (Hibbard et al., 2005):

Stage 1: The patient does not yet believe he or she has an active and important role in his or her health.

Stage 2: The patient believes he or she should be active participants in his or her health; however, the patient lacks the confidence and knowledge to take action.

Stage 3: The patient begins to take action.

Stage 4: The patient maintains behavior over time.

Numerous research studies have demonstrated that health literacy is a strong predictor of overall health status. Health professionals are in a critical position to identify patients with low health literacy and help them become active participants in their health. A relationship between the health professional and patient that is based on trust, respect, understanding, and sensitivity constitutes a strong bond that impacts not only on the effectiveness of patient teaching, but has the potential to improve the patient's overall quality of life through helping him or her obtain the skills and abilities needed to improve his or her health.

REFERENCES

American Medical Association, (1999). Health literacy: report of the council on scientific affairs. *Journal of the American Medical Association, 281*(6), 552–557.

Baker, D. W., Gazmararian, J. A., Williams, M. V., Scott, T., Parker, R. M., Green, D., Ren, J., & Peel, J. (2002). Functional health literacy and the risk of hospital admission among Medicare managed care enrollees. *American Journal of Public Health, 92*(8), 1278–1283.

Baker, D. W., Gazmararian, J. A., Williams, M. V., Scott, T., Parker, R. M., Green, D., Ren, J., & Peel, J. (2004). Health literacy and use of outpatient physician services by Medicare managed care enrollees. *Journal of General Internal Medicine, 19*(3), 215–220.

Baker, D. W., Parker, R. M., Williams, M. V., & Clark, W. S. (1998). Health literacy and the risk of hospital admission. *Journal of General Internal Medicine, 13*(12), 791–798.

Bastable, S. B. (2006). *Essentials of patient education.* Sudbury, MA: Jones and Bartlett.

Bernhardt, J. M., & Cameron, K. A. (2003). Accessing, understanding, and applying health communication messages: the challenge of health literacy. In T. L. Thompson, A. M. Dorsey, K. I. Miller, & R. Parrott (Eds.). *Handbook of health communication* (pp 583–605). Mahwah, NJ: Lawrence Erlbaum Associates.

Berry, D. (2007). *Health communication: Theory and practice.* Berkshire, England: Open University Press/McGraw-Hill.

Braveman, P., Oliva, G., Miller, M. G., Schaaf, V. M., & Reiter, R. (1988). Women without health insurance: Links between access, poverty, ethnicity, and health. *Western Journal of Medicine, 149,* 708–711.

Davidhizar, R. E., & Brownson, K. (1999). Literacy, cultural diversity, and client education. *Health Care Manager,* 18, 11.

Davis, T. C., Crouch, M. A., Long, S. W., Jackson, R. H., Bates, P., George, R. B., et al. (1991). Rapid assessment of literacy levels of adult primary care patients. *Family Medicine, 23*(6), 433–435.

Davis, T. C., Long, S. W., Jackson, R. H., Mayeaux, E. J., George, R. B., Murphy, P. W., et al. (1993). Rapid estimate of adult literacy in medicine: a shortened screening instrument. *Family Medicine, 25*(6), 391–395.

Davis, T., & Wolf, M. (2004). Health literacy: Implications for family medicine. *Family Medicine, 36,* 595–598.

DeWalt, D. A., Berkman, N. D., Sheridan, S., Lohr, K. N. & Pignone, M. P. (2004). Literacy and health outcomes: A systematic review of the literature. *Journal of General Internal Medicine, 19,* 1228–1239.

Doak, C. C., Doak, L. G., Friedell, G. H., & Meade, C. D. (1998). Improving comprehension for cancer patients with low literacy skills: Strategies for clinicians. *CA-A Cancer Journal for Clinicians, 48,* 151–162.

Doak, C. C., Doak, L. G., & Root, J. (1996). *Teaching patients with low literacy skills* (2nd ed.). Philadelphia: Lippincott Williams & Wilkins.

Fang, M., Machtinger, E. L., Wang, F., & Schillinger, D. (2006). Health literacy and anticoagulation-related outcomes among patients taking warfarin. *Journal of General Internal Medicine, 21*(8), 841–846.

Hibbard, J. (2006). Panel 3: Toward an informed and engaged public: Both health literacy and patient activation contribute to consumer's ability to manage the truth. In Office of the Surgeon General. *Proceedings of the Surgeon General's Workshop on Improving Health Literacy.* (pp. 32–33). Bethesda, MD: National Institutes of Health.

Hibbard, J. H., Mahoney, E. R., Stockard, J., & Tusler, M. (2005). Development and testing of a short form of the patient activation measure. *Health Services Research, 40,* 1918–1930.

Institute of Medicine. (2004). *Health literacy: A prescription to end confusion.* Washington DC: Institute of Medicine, Board of Neuroscience and Behavioral Health, Committee on Health Literacy.

Irwin, P. (1991). National Literacy Act of 1991: Major provisions of P.L. 102-73. CRS report for congress. Washington, DC. Library of Congress, Congressional Research Service

Jastak, S., & Wilkinson, G. S. (1993). *Wide-range achievement test. Review 3.* Wilmington, DE: Jastak Associates.

Kirsch, I. S. (1993). *Adult literacy in America: A first look at the results of the National Adult Literacy Survey.* Washington DC: National Center or Education Statistics. Retrieved July 24, 2009, from http://eric.ed.gov/ERICWebPortal/contentdelivery/servlet/ERICServlet?accno=ED358375

Lasater, L., & Mehler, P. S. (1998). The illiterate patient: Screening and management. *Hospital Practice,* April 15, 163–170.

London, F. (1999). *No time to teach: A nurse's guide to patient and family education.* Philadelphia: Lippincott Williams & Wilkins.

Mayeaux, E. J., Murphy, P. W., Arnold, C., Jackson, R. H., & Sentell, T. (1996). Improving patient education for patients with low literacy skills. *American Family Physician, 53*(1), 205–211.

Mayer, G. G., & Vallaire, M. (2007). *Health literacy in primary care: A clinician's guide*. New York: Springer.

Merriman, B., Ades, T., & Seffrin, J. R. (2002). Health literacy in the information age: Communicating cancer information to patients and families. *CA Cancer Journal for Clinicians, 52*, 130–133.

National Assessment of Adult Literacy. (2003). Washington, DC: US Department of Education, National Center for Education Statistics. Retrieved December 2nd, 2009 from http://nces.ed.gov/NAAL/health_dev.asp

National Center for Education Statistics. 1993. *Adult literacy in America: a first look at the results of the National Adult Literacy Survey* (2nd ed.). Washington, DC: US Department of Education.

National Work Group on Literacy and Health. (1998). Communicating with patients who have limited literacy skills: Report of the National Work Group on Literacy and Health. *Journal of Family Practice, 46*, 168–176.

Nielson-Bohlman, L., Panzer, A. M., & Kindig, D. A. (2004). *Health literacy: A prescription to end confusion*. Washington, DC: National Academics Press.

Osborne, H. (2005). *Health literacy from A to Z: Practical ways to communicate your health message*. Sudbury, MA: Jones and Bartlett.

Paasche-Orlow, M. K., Riekert, K. A., Bilderback., A., Chanmugam, A., Hill, P., Rand, C. S., et al. (2005). Tailored education may reduce health literacy disparities I asthma self-management. *American Journal of Respiratory and Critical Care Medicine, 172*, 980–986.

Parikh, N. S., Parker, R. M., Nurss, J. R., Baker, D. W., & Williams, M. V. (1996). Shame and health literacy: the unspoken connection. *Patient Education and Counseling, 27*, 33–39.

Parker, R. M., Baker, D. W., Williams, M. V., & Nurss, J. R. (1995). The test of functional health literacy in adults: a new instrument for measuring patients' literacy skills. *Journal of General Internal Medicine, 10*(10), 537–541.

Rudd, R., Kirsch, I. S., Yamamoto, K. (2004). *Literacy and health in America*. Princeton, NJ: Center for Global Assessment, Policy Information Center, Research and Development, Educational Testing Services.

Schillinger, D., Bindman, A., Stewart, A., Wang, F., & Piette, J. (2004). Health literacy and the quality of physician-patient interpersonal communication. *Patient Education and Counseling, 3*, 315–323.

Schillinger, D., Machtinger, E., Wang, F., Rodriguez, M., & Bindman, A. (2006). The importance of establishing regimen concordance in preventing medication errors in anticoagulant care. *Journal of Health Communication, 11*(6), 555–567.

Schwartzberg, J. G., Van Geest, J. B., & Wang, C. C. (Eds.). (2005). *Understanding health literacy: Implications for medicine and public health*. Chicago, IL: AMA Press.

Sudore, R. L., Landefeld, C. S., Barnes, D. E., Lindquist, K., Williams, B. A., Brody, R., & Schillinger, D. (2007). An advance directive redesigned to meet the literacy level of most adults: A randomized trial. *Patient Education and Counseling, 69*(1–3), 165–195.

Sudore, R. L., Landefeld, C. S., Perez-Stable, E. J., Bibbins-Domingo, K., Williams, B. A., & Schillingr, D. (2009). Unraveling the relationship between literacy, language proficiency and patient-physician communication. *Patient Education and Counseling, 75*(3), 398–402.

US Department of Health and Human Services. (2000). *Healthy People 2010* (2nd ed.). Washington, DC: U.S. Government Printing Office. Retrieved July 20, 2009, from http://www.healthypeople.gov/Document/HTML/Volume1/11healthcom.htm#_Toc490471359

Weiss, B. D., & Coyne, C. (1997). Communicating with patients who cannot read. *New England Journal of Medicine, 4*, 272–273.

Weiss, B. D., Hart, G., McGee, D. L., & D'Estelle, S. (1992). Health status of illiterate adults: Relation between literacy and health status among persons with low literacy skills. *Journal of the American Board of Family Practice, 5*, 257–264.

Williams, M. V., Parker, R. M., Baker, D. W., Parikh, N. S., Pitkin, K., Coates, W. C., & Nurss, J. R. (1995). Inadequate functional health literacy among patients at two public hospitals. *Journal of the American Medical Association, 274*, 1677–1682.

Wolf, M. S., Gazmararian, J. A., & Baker, D. W. (2005). Health literacy and functional health status among older adults. *Archives of Internal Medicine, 165*(17), 1946NPH–1952.

World Health Organization. (1998). *Health promotion glossary*. Geneva, WHO. Retrieved July 23, 2009, from www.who.int/hpr/NPH/docs/hp_glossary_en.pdf.

Zarcadoolas, C., Pleasant, A. F., & Grer, D. S. (2006). *Advancing health literacy: A framework for understanding and action*. San Francisco, CA: Jossey-Bass.

CHAPTER 11

Patient Teaching and Complementary and Alternative Medicine

COMPLEMENTARY, ALTERNATIVE, AND INTEGRATIVE MEDICINE

Complementary and alternative practices have roots in vastly different cultures and are based on multiple healing traditions from around the world, some of which were in use long before the existence of Western medicine (Guerrera, 2007). *Complementary medicine* consists of using both nontraditional therapies and traditional therapies, whereas *alternative medicine* utilizes nontraditional therapies in place of conventional practices (National Center for Complementary and Alternative Medicine [NCCAM] 2000).

Today, the term "complementary or alternative medicine" (CAM) is usually used to described diverse products or practices that are outside of mainstream Western medical practice for promoting health and preventing or treating disease (Gevitz, 1988; Harpham, 2001; O'Connor, 1995). The National Library of Medicine defines CAM treatments as, "medical products and practices that are not part of standard care" (National Library of Medicine, 2005).

CAM encompasses a wide range of products and practices, and often incorporates a broad spectrum of beliefs (Zollman & Vickers, 2000). Complementary medicine and alternative medicine are sometimes described separately. Complementary medicine may be thought of as an approach used together with conventional Western medicine practices, while alternative medicine is sometimes thought of as therapies that replace conventional therapy. For example, a physician prescribing biofeedback in addition to conventional medications to treat symptoms of chronic headaches would be using a complementary approach, whereas if the physician used only herbal preparations to treat chronic headaches, rather than conventional means, he or she would be using an alternative approach.

The term *integrative medicine* is not synonymous with CAM but rather is a philosophy of practice that focuses on healing and health rather than disease, emphasizing the relationship between the patient and the health professional (Rakel, 2007). Integrative medicine combines conventional therapies with complementary and alternative therapies for which there is evidence of effectiveness and safety (NCCAM, 2000).

Despite the differences in origin of various complementary and alternative practices, a common philosophy shared by most is that healing comes from within a person (Hufford, 1997; Josefek, 2000). The basic tenet of CAM is the relationship of health and healing to the harmony of the mind, body, and spirit (Rakel, 2007). In this context, complementary and alternative methods of treatment stress that the body possesses an intrinsic healing capacity. Rather than using external influences used in conventional medicine, such as drugs or surgery, CAM seeks to enhance the body's ability to fight disease and promote healing from within. Complementary and alternative therapies focus on the patient as a whole, are highly individualized, and are based on the compatibility of the method with the individual patient. CAM practices range from use of chiropractors, naturopaths, massage therapists, spiritual healers, or folk healers to the self-administered use of herbal remedies, megavitamin therapy, or special diets. Below is a listing of categories of CAM procedures as outlined by the National Institutes of Health's National Center for Complementary and Alternative Medicine (NCCAM) (1994).

- Alternative medical systems such as homeopathic or naturopathic medicine
- Mind/body or behavioral interventions such as yoga or meditation
- Biologically based therapies such as herbs or dietary supplements
- Manipulative and body-based methods such as chiropractic manipulation or massage
- Energy therapies including biofield therapies such as Reiki and therapeutic touch or bioelectromagnetic-based therapies such as pulsed fields or alternating current or direct current fields

GROWTH OF COMPLEMENTARY AND ALTERNATIVE MEDICINE USE

Complementary or alternative therapies were once viewed by conventional health professionals as countercultural. A common belief was that CAM practices were not dominant in general, although CAM was used by a fringe of the general patient population. A study by Eisenberg and colleagues (1993) changed this view. Their study indicated that patients' use of complementary and alternative therapies was much higher than previously believed. In a follow-up study, Eisenberg and colleagues (1998) found that 42% of adults were found to have used at least one alternative therapy during the previous year, with a significantly higher proportion of patients who saw an alternative medicine practitioner in 1997 than in 1990. There are some indications that the rate of use of CAM is actually greater than most studies indicate (Lazar & O'Connor, 1997). As a generally increasing pattern of CAM use has been seen across a range of conditions, recognition of its impact on conventional, mainstream health care has generated significant interest from the conventional healthcare community.

Use of complementary and alternative therapies remains prevalent (Owen et al., 2001). Expenditures for alternative forms of treatment have been estimated at more than $21 billion in 1997, an increase of 45% from 1990 to 1997 (Eisenberg et al., 1998). Growth of the use of alternative methods by patients stimulated the formation of the National Institutes of Health's (NIH) Office of Alternative Medicine (OAM), which was established in 1993 to evaluate the safety and efficacy of alternative and complementary methods. The OAM was replaced by the NCCAM under the 1999 Omnibus Appropriations Bill, enacted by Congress (Josefek, 2000). The NCCAM has now grown to be an autonomous center within NIH with the ability to fund projects directly (Dokken & Sydnor-Greenberg, 2000). One of the goals of NCCAM is to "integrate CAM practices into conventional medicine" (NCCAM, 2000).

WHO USES COMPLEMENTARY AND ALTERNATIVE MEDICINE: MYTHS AND MISCONCEPTIONS

Preconceived ideas existed about types of patients most likely to use complementary or alternative methods of health care. It was assumed that patients using these methods were often poorly educated, naive, gullible, or from a lower socioeconomic status (Herbert, 1997; Thompson, 1990). A number of studies have shown these beliefs to be faulty (Astin, 1998; Cassileth et al., 1984; Eisenberg et al., 1993; Feldman, 1990). Patients more likely to use complementary or alternative therapies have been found to be women, Caucasian, between the ages of 35 and 49, highly educated, and affluent (Eisenberg, 2005).

The assumption that use of CAM was more common in immigrants has also been dispelled. The assumption was that CAM usage was especially common in those groups who were recent immigrants and who might cling to traditional folk health practices of their culture, especially if they had limited financial resources or limited access to mainstream health care (Pachter, 1993). Although CAM use is prevalent in this group, use appears to be more prevalent in immigrants who are better educated and in a higher socioeconomic status, not just in groups with limited financial means or limited healthcare access (Miller, 1990).

A common belief held by many health professionals was that patients using conventional care would not use CAM. The converse thought was that patients who used CAM would use those methods alone for health maintenance or treatment of disease, rather than using conventional medical approaches. Research has found both of these beliefs to be false. Patients have been found to use complementary and alternative therapies even though they also use healthcare resources (Eisenberg et al., 1998; Elder, Gillcrist, & Minz, 1997; Spigelblatt, Laine-Ammara, & Pless, 1994) and often seek health advice from conventional health providers as well as advice from alternative health providers at the same time (Applewhite, 1995; Eisenberg et al., 1998; Spigelblatt et al., 1994). In addition, patients have been found to often use both conventional and alternative therapies simultaneously for the same condition (Eisenberg et al., 1993).

The once-held view that patients with serious or terminal conditions were more likely to use CAM out of desperation to reverse the disease process has also been found to be inaccurate. Although use of complementary and alternative therapies is common among patients with chronic or end-stage conditions, many of these patients appear to use complementary or alternative methods for general health maintenance rather than as a desperate attempt to cure the disease (Anderson et al., 1993; Cassileth et al., 1984).

Health professionals are often unaware of the number of patients using CAM and the number of complementary and alternative therapies available to patients. Even if health professionals are aware of CAM use for some medical conditions, there may be lack of awareness that patients may also use CAM for purposes unrelated to their medical condition, such as for general health maintenance. There may be the assumption that complementary or alternative methods used by patients are limited to one type. Types and numbers of complementary or alternative methods used by patients appear to vary widely. According to one study, 73 different types of alternative methods were found to be used by patients in a middle- to upper-middle-class community in the United States (McGuire, 1988). When the extent of CAM use by patients in mainstream health care is considered, the importance of exploration of use of complementary and alternative methods by patients as well as an understanding of how these practices impact patient care is obvious.

PATIENT DISCLOSURE ABOUT COMPLEMENTARY AND ALTERNATIVE MEDICINE USE

Despite widespread use of complementary or alternative methods, studies have shown that most patients do not consult nor inform health professionals about their complementary or alternative practices (Eisenberg et al, 1998; Planta, Gundersen, & Petitt, 2000). Eisenberg (1997) found that nearly 60–70% of patients who use CAM practices did not discuss their practices with their physician. Although patients frequently express interest in discussing complementary or alternative methods with health professionals and prefer that health professionals take a more active role in using complementary or alternative strategies, they frequently are reluctant to ask questions or bring up the subject (Visser, Peters, & Rasker, 1992).

Lack of disclosure of CAM practices can be attributed to a variety of reasons. Patients may not approach the subject with health professionals for fear of having their question dismissed or the use of complementary or alternative methods ridiculed or censured. They may be concerned that by admitting to use of or interest in alternative methods they will be categorized as "crocks" or considered to be outside the normal realms of society. Patients may fear that the health professional will view them as ungrateful or disloyal if they were to disclose their use of unconventional therapies. In some instances, they may not disclose use because they believe health professionals lack adequate knowledge about CAM and consequently would be unable to answer questions or provide guidance even if the subject were approached (Crigger, 2000).

In other cases, patients may not believe that CAM therapies are relevant to conventional medical care. Patients may not consider alternative methods as an integrated part of their health care or may be unaware of potential interactions between some alternative and conventional therapies. They may believe that CAM therapies are harmless and, consequently, insignificant to address with their conventional health professional. They may view conventional health professionals and complementary or alternative practitioners as separate entities, therefore reserving discussion of CAM practices for CAM practitioners.

Of course, another major reason patients do not discuss alternative therapies with health professionals may be because they are not asked. Despite increasing evidence that many more patients use complementary and alternative methods than once thought, many health professionals do not routinely ask patients whether they use CAM or include questions about use of complementary or alternative methods as part of routine health history. Studies have indicated that patients do not necessarily try to hide their use of complementary or alternative methods from health professionals. They have indicated willingness to disclose their use of CAM if the health professional asks (Planta et al., 2000). Including discussion about CAM in routine patient encounters would seem to be a means of facilitating communication and rapport between patient and health professional as well as contributing to general patient care.

ATTITUDES OF HEALTH PROFESSIONALS TOWARD COMPLEMENTARY AND ALTERNATIVE MEDICINE

Attitudes about complementary and alternative approaches to health care vary among health professionals (Berman et al., 1995; Ernst, Resch, & White, 1995)

Whereas some health professionals believe that some forms of complementary or alternative therapy may be effective (Astin, 1998; Zollman & Vickers, 1999), a number of other health professionals are skeptical or at times hostile to their use (Crigger, 2000). Some health professionals may still view CAM as "outside the mainstream" of conventional health care and therefore consider it to be inappropriate. Others may object to complementary or alternative practices because many of these methods are unproven and lack scientific evidence of effectiveness. Although concern about proven effectiveness may be valid, it should be noted that some widely used conventional therapies have not been proven, have later been shown to be ineffective in treatment of disease, or in some instances have been found to be harmful (Panush, 2000). Likewise, some complimentary and alternative therapies have been shown to be effective in treatment of some conditions and symptoms (Williams et al., 2000).

Some health professionals may avoid discussion of CAM with patients because they lack adequate knowledge of these practices. Most health professionals have had little or no training about complementary or alternative practices (Eisenberg et al., 1993; Morgan et al., 1998). Only recently has training about CAM been included into the curriculum of some professional schools (Rampes et al., 1997). Consequently, health professionals may have limited knowledge about CAM, use of specific therapies, and the potential benefits as well as risks of each. Because of inadequate information, health professionals may have negative views of CAM and the use of recognized CAM practices.

Whether health professionals advocate or criticize use of complementary or alternative methods to treat disease or to promote health, the data indicate that patients are using them. To work more effectively with patients, it is important for health professionals to put misconceptions aside and learn how to talk with patients about alternative practices. Being aware of the extent of use of complementary and alternative methods by patients who are also using conventional healthcare resources is a first step. Learning how to approach patients about alternative method use requires an open and non-judgmental attitude on the part of health professionals. Holding negative and dismissive attitudes toward alternative methods or attempting to coerce patients to abandon their use will not prevent use of these methods but rather tend to discourage patients from being forthcoming about complementary or alternative method use. Open and nonjudgmental questioning of patients may help increase health professionals' knowledge of patient use of CAM and help health professionals and patients work together toward better health (Elder et al., 1997). Coming to understand patient motivations for use of alternative methods is of utmost importance in beginning to establish a dialogue with patients about alternative methods.

PATIENT MOTIVATION FOR USING COMPLEMENTARY AND ALTERNATIVE MEDICINE

Each patient brings individual beliefs, expectations, and fears to their experience with health and illness. Patients' decisions to use complementary or alternative practices for treatment of disease or health promotion, either exclusively or in conjunction with conventional health care, are complex. No one theory accounts for the increasing trend toward patient use of CAM for prevention, treatment, or cure of disease. Each patient has a unique notion of perceived vulnerability to disease, a personal family history which may contribute to health or disease, an acquired knowledge base from family, friends, or the media from which beliefs about health and disease are patterned, as well as their own subjective experience with symptoms or disease.

Although patients may, at times, make decisions to use CAM out of emotion rather than logic, health professionals should recognize that patients' decisions to use complementary or alternative methods are often based on their own unique method of problem solving and rational decision making. If patients had success with an alternative method once, they reason that it will work again. They may not have taken into account the fact that their condition may have had self-limiting symptoms or that success with the alternative method the first time was coincidence. Take, for example, the following case.

Mrs. Schneider's 10-year-old daughter, Pamela, had been diagnosed with leukemia. Pamela underwent chemotherapy, but she experienced severe side effects from the treatment. Mrs. Schneider, distraught by her daughter's diagnosis as well as the side effects of the chemotherapy, was persuaded by her neighbor to try "metabolic therapy" for Pamela instead. Mrs. Schneider, anxious to have her daughter avoid the severe side effects that had been experienced with previous chemotherapy but also anxious to prevent further progression of the disease, took her neighbor's advice and began giving Pamela large doses of vitamins as well as other dietary supplements, rather than having her undergo additional chemotherapy. After a year, there was no evidence of progression of Pamela's disease even though she had not undergone additional chemotherapy. Mrs. Schneider was convinced that the vitamins and dietary supplements were responsible. She did not, however, consider that the initial chemotherapy may have been responsible and that Pamela would have gone into remission regardless of the vitamins and dietary supplements.

Patients may base their decision to use CAM from observations of the perceived success that others have experienced with the treatment. For example, Mr. Lindquist had become increasingly unable to engage in many activities he enjoyed, including hiking, because of osteoarthritis of his right knee. He consulted his physician, who recommended knee replacement. As much as Mr. Lindquist enjoyed hiking, he feared surgery more. He discussed his concerns about surgery and his frustration at the thought of having to give up hiking with a close friend. His friend told Mr. Lindquist that several years earlier he had been faced with the same type of situation, and rather than having surgery, he had opted to try an herbal remedy. The friend assured Mr. Lindquist that within a month of taking Pau d'arco, a South American Indian folk medicine, his knee problems vanished and he was able to continue all the activities he had enjoyed previously. Mr. Lindquist, delighted to receive from a trusted friend such a positive endorsement of a remedy that would help him avoid surgery but still enable him to continue his activities, chose to abandon the idea of surgery in favor of herbal remedy. He was unaware that his friend had actually only had a knee sprain rather than osteoarthritis.

In some instances, patients choose complementary or alternative methods because they have found traditional treatments to be ineffective in producing the desired outcome (Jensen, 1990; Lazar & O'Connor, 1997). When all conventional methods of treatment have been exhausted with no desired effect, patients may turn to complementary or alternative means. Take, for example, Mr. Gunther. He had experienced recurring shoulder pain, possibly the result of repetitive motion injury related to his job. Dr. Phelps prescribed medication to reduce inflammation and gave Mr. Gunther a referral to physical therapy for consultation. Mr. Gunther took the medication as prescribed, attended the physical therapy consultation, and performed exercises as recommended daily. During Mr. Gunther's routine physical exam several months later, Dr. Phelps asked him about his shoulder. Mr. Gunther disclosed that he had abandoned the prescribed medication as well as the prescribed exercise. He stated that he was now regularly going to see a chiropractor. When Dr. Phelps questioned Mr. Gunther about his reasons for abandoning the prescribed medical treatment he replied, "Well, I did everything that medical personnel told me to do and I still didn't get better, so I went to the chiropractor. I'm continuing to go to him because he's the only one who has been able to help me feel better."

Patients' choice to use alternative therapies may at times be the result of unrealistic expectations for control of symptoms or cure of disease. Health professionals may have neglected to give patients adequate information regarding the length of time after treatment in which patients could expect symptoms to subside, or they may have failed to specify that the purpose of treatment was to control symptoms rather than cure the disease. For example, Ms. Minjeta was seen by her physician because of symptoms of frequency and burning on urination. She consulted her physician, who, after confirming with urine culture that she had a urinary tract infection, prescribed an antibiotic. After 2 days of treatment, however, Ms. Minjeta stopped taking the antibiotic and began self-treatment with St. John's wort. When she confided in her neighbor, Mrs. Jones, who was a nurse, that she had abandoned the physician-prescribed treatment in favor of an herbal remedy, Mrs. Jones questioned her as to why. Ms. Minjeta responded, "I took the medicine for 2 days and I didn't get better so I stopped taking it. Why bother taking medicine when it doesn't work."

In many instances, conventional treatments still have little to offer with regard to curing disease and often are ineffective in controlling symptoms, particularly when chronic pain is associated (Lazar & O'Connor, 1997). In choosing complementary or alternative treatments, patients may still be seeking the same effect (e.g., relief of symptoms) or cure they sought but did not receive with standard approaches. For example, Ms. Philbeck had been diagnosed with multiple sclerosis. Ms. Ellis, the nurse practitioner who had been following Ms. Philbeck's case, became concerned after several follow-up appointments were missed. She called Ms. Philbeck who told her plainly that she would no longer be seeking health care at the clinic. Instead, she was seeing a spiritual healer and using crystals, as well as a number of other mineral substances because, in her words, "I want my condition to be cured. So-called modern medicine is still in the stone age regarding treatment of multiple sclerosis. When I keep coming to you I keep having exacerbations of my disease. Since I've been seeing the spiritual healer, I've been in remission and I have every reason to believe that I'll be cured."

In other instances, patients may choose alternative methods because they have experienced adverse effects from traditional methods (Cassileth et al., 1984). Mr. Adams was placed on an antihypertensive medication by his physician. After a month, however, he stopped taking the medication and switched to herbal preparations. He confided in a friend that he had stopped taking the prescribed medication because of the side effects he experienced. He stated that he chose the herbal preparation so he would have a smaller chance of side effects.

Patients may find traditional methods to be too complicated or technological (Furnham & Forey, 1994) and turn to complementary or alternative methods, which they perceive to be simpler or easier to understand. Likewise, in a time in which there is growing distrust of the healthcare industry, and in which patients desire more autonomy or control over their health matters, they may feel that conventional approaches to health care are too authoritarian (Riesmann, 1994). Patients may feel they have more control over their health care, feeling a greater sense of autonomy and empowerment, when they use CAM (Kaptchuk & Eisenberg, 1998). Health care under conventional practice may be viewed as too fragmented, so that patients seek complementary or alternative methods that they believe to hold a more holistic philosophy of health. Patients may believe that conventional health care treats the symptoms but not the underlying cause of the disease. They may feel that conventional methods do not address spiritual factors in health and may believe that complementary or alternative methods are more congruent with their own health beliefs.

Concerns about toxicity or complications from use of conventional methods may also be a reason patients choose complementary or alternative methods, which they perceive to be more natural. They may feel that complementary or alternative therapies put them at less risk than methods used in conventional care, which they may consider to be mechanistic or synthetic.

The meaning individual patients attribute to pain and disease can affect their ability or inability to cope with their symptoms or disease. CAM may be more consistent with the beliefs some patients have about health or illness (Vincent & Furnham, 1996) or may be more consistent with the patient's religious perspectives (Fuller, 1989). For example, some religious teachings propose that illness is caused by false beliefs. In this instance, followers of those teachings may believe that healing is possible only through prayer and by replacing bad thoughts with good ones.

Complementary or alternative methods are not always used as a replacement for conventional therapies. At times, complementary or alternative methods are used in conjunction with conventional therapies prescribed to achieve therapeutic goals. For instance, patients may use prescribed anti-inflammatory agents for arthritis while also using meditation. They may take antihypertensive drugs for control of hypertension as well as engage in relaxation techniques to help lower blood pressure.

Some patients may believe that conventional therapies are too expensive and consequently seek complementary or alternative therapies because they believe them to be less expensive (Murray & Rubel, 1992). Complementary and alternative methods are not, however, always cheaper. Because many third-party payers do not include CAM as appropriate for reimbursement, many patients are forced to pay out-of-pocket for complementary or alternative therapies.

Some patients may feel especially vulnerable to disease. They may interpret various body sensations as abnormal and, related to their perceived vulnerability, develop excess concerns about their symptoms. For example, Mrs. Jorgenson had been experiencing pain in her abdomen. After having a medical workup that was negative, she began taking ginseng stating, "The doctor says nothing is wrong but both my mother and grandmother died of stomach cancer. I'm taking ginseng just in case."

Cultural variations may determine the extent to which alternative methods are used as well as the methods chosen (Hufford, 1988; O'Connor, 1995). Traditional beliefs of various cultures regarding wellness, sickness, and treatment may be very different from conventional healthcare treatments. The beliefs, traditions, and customs handed down through many generations may play a principal role in the establishment of individual health practices. Consequently, when the patient chooses complementary or alternative methods in response to health and disease, it may be because complementary or alternative methods are more in keeping with the patient's values and beliefs.

To many patients, even those not influenced by a particular cultural group, their own beliefs and values may be viewed as in conflict with the approaches of conventional health care. As a result, a dual healthcare system may exist, leading to confusion and unsatisfactory results. By exploring and understanding patients' values, beliefs, goals, and differing philosophies of health care, both conventional and CAM practices may be successfully integrated in a way that complement each other and achieve satisfactory results for both. To achieve this result, however, communication about patients' beliefs, values, goals, and use of complementary or alternative health practices must first be addressed.

IMPORTANCE OF DISCUSSING COMPLEMENTARY AND ALTERNATIVE MEDICINE

Given the prevalence of use of complementary and alternative methods, patients should be asked routinely about their use of such therapies. However, many health professionals fail to approach the subject with patients. Omission of the subject may be in part because health professionals are unfamiliar with CAM and, consequently, are reluctant to bring up the issue for fear of appearing to be uninformed. To best assist patients make informed choices and use complementary or alternative therapies appropriately, health professionals need to be knowledgeable about them. Health professionals should attempt to familiarize themselves with the philosophy, historical development, underlying concepts, and basic principles of various complementary and alternative practices, as well as attempt to understand more common CAM therapies in depth. In addition to gaining information about CAM practices in general, health professionals should also attempt to understand patients' assumptions and expectations of the CAM methods they may be utilizing. To do this, of course, the subject must first be approached with patients.

There are many reasons why health professionals should be informed of the extent and type of complementary or alternative practices patients use. For instance, some alternative methods have demonstrated beneficial effects, such as pain control by acupuncture (Richardson & Vincent, 1986). Research has also shown that using the patient's own physical and mental resources for health and healing can have direct effects on the immune, endocrine, and nervous systems (Cohen, Tyrrel, & Smith, 1991; Goleman & Gurin, 1993). Once knowledgeable about CAM methods, health professionals can help patients identify therapies that may be most beneficial for their particular condition.

In some instances, CAM methods may be used before more conventional treatments, which may carry greater risks. Not all complementary or alternative methods are devoid of risk, however. In addition to potential adverse effects of some complementary and alternative therapies themselves, when used in combination with conventional therapies, adverse interactions can occur. By being aware of patient use of complementary or alternative methods, health professionals can coordinate efforts so that adverse interactions of methods can be prevented, as well as identify precautions that may need to be taken if alternative and conventional methods are being used simultaneously.

Awareness of patient use of CAM therapies can also help health professionals assist patients in assessing whether the positives of CAM use outweigh the negatives. For instance, although a number of insurers and managed care organizations in the United States now offer alternative method programs and benefits (Pelletier, Astin, & Haskell, 1997), for many patients, use of complementary and alternative methods constitute a large out-of-pocket expense (Eisenberg et al., 1993). Not all CAM therapies bring about the desired outcomes and may need to be replaced with other options. By identifying patients' CAM practices, health professionals can help patients minimize potential risks by providing the patient teaching and guidance so that both CAM and conventional approaches can be utilized in a way that will most benefit the patient.

PATIENT TEACHING ABOUT COMPLEMENTARY AND ALTERNATIVE MEDICINE

Patient teaching about complementary or alternative methods should focus on safety, informed choice, and shared decision making. Health professionals should not only be solidly grounded in conventional health practices but also possess unbiased knowledge about the value and limitations of complementary or alternative methods.

In initiating the dialogue about patient use of CAM, health professionals should give permission for patients to discuss the topic of complementary or alternative methods by conveying a nonjudgmental, supportive attitude. They should indicate willingness to work with patients, utilizing complementary or alternative methods chosen by the patient in conjunction with conventional therapies when appropriate. Opening discussion of CAM practices might begin with a statement from the health professional such as, "What other things are you doing to stay healthy?" or "Sometimes people have home remedies or other practices they've heard about to treat disease besides those used by their doctor. Have you tried other things to treat your condition?"

Being open and nonjudgmental does not mean that health professionals should condone or refrain from discussion of complementary or alternative methods for which there are safety concerns. Alerting patients to potential hazards, however, should be done in a sensitive manner using sound reasoning and evidence rather than from an emotional basis, which could be construed by the patient as a struggle for authority and control. The goal should be to help patients make an informed choice, not necessarily to have them choose what the health professional thinks is best. As with all instances of patient teaching, informed choice should be based on unbiased, factual information, not coercion. If the health professional disapproves of the patient's choice of a particular type of complementary or alternative method, they should not criticize the patient's use but rather give a rational basis for their concern. The following statement might be used to alert the patient of the health professional's concerns while also informing the patient of safer alternatives: "I have heard of the herbal preparation you are taking, but I have concerns about its safety. You may have read in the paper about of some of the adverse effects several people have experienced. There are some other herbal products, however, that you may consider instead."

In instances where there is no major concern about safety of a method but the health professional feels it is inappropriate, the health professional may explain reasons for objection, without deriding the method or discounting the patient's interest in it. In so doing, the health professional communicates respect for the patient's position while at the same time voicing logical concerns. For example, "Mrs. Clark, although there is no evidence the supplement is harmful, it is very expensive, and I don't think there is clear evidence that its benefits are in keeping with the cost. The final decision, of course, is up to you, but I did want you know my thoughts."

Patients should always be aware that the health professional will continue to care for them despite complementary or alternative use practices. Patients who fear they will be abandoned by the health professional are not as likely to openly share information, which can be important to effective care. By building an open, trusting relationship, the health professional has the continuing opportunity to monitor patient progress.

Helping patients distinguish between legitimate alternative methods and fraud is another important part of patient teaching about complementary or alternative practices. Health professionals should be advocates for patients by helping to diminish the potential that they will be casualties of fraud. When patients are seeking care from an alternative care provider, the health professional can help them determine if the individual has some type of certification or peer oversight, the amount of experience the individual has in working with specific conditions, the cost of each visit or treatment, the length of treatment, and the associated risks and benefits. Health professionals should help patients to be aware of warning signs of inappropriate complementary or alternative products or practices, such as therapies that make claims to exclusivity or products that purport secret formulas or ingredients that cannot be revealed. Products or procedures that claim extravagant effectiveness or only personal testimonials as a way of verification of effectiveness should also be called into question.

If health professionals are unfamiliar with a complementary or alternative method, they should be open about their lack of knowledge. They may say, "I'm unfamiliar with that [method; product]. Could you bring some information in so I can learn more about it, or tell me where information is available?"

TEACHING PATIENTS ABOUT SAFETY ISSUES REGARDING COMPLEMENTARY AND ALTERNATIVE MEDICINE

When patients consider using complementary or alternative methods, they may look to the health professional for guidance in choosing safe and appropriate approaches. By giving patients factual, unbiased information, the health professional can help patients make logical and informed choices for safer use of CAM. Although many complementary or alternative methods can be helpful, in some instances safety concerns may be present. When patients look for information and guidance, there are several issues of which they should be made aware.

Medicinal plants have been used for centuries to treat a variety of conditions and symptoms, often with success. They are the original source of many contemporary synthetic medications, and many offer promise of being a source of new drugs in the future. Although some botanical preparations can help or some may be innocuous, not all methods may be safe and, in fact, can be responsible for adverse health effects (D'Arcy, 1991; Gordon et al., 1996). Some methods may expose patients to potential harm either directly or indirectly. Direct harm, for example, may result from indiscriminate use of herbal medicines. Patients may believe that because many herbal preparations are labeled as "natural" that they are safe. Some herbs have toxic effects and others can interact with other drugs. Herbs or supplements that have a pharmacological effect used in conjunction with conventional medications can either potentiate or negate effects of the prescribed drug or cause adverse drug interactions (Lazar, 1996). Potential adulterants have also been reported in some herbal medications (Slifman et al., 1998). Patients may also be harmed indirectly if use of a complementary or alternative method draws them away from prescribed medical treatment or if they discontinue using prescribed medications without informing the health professional.

Patients should be helped to realize that there may be considerable variation in the same herbs from different manufacturers. Herbal preparations vary greatly in efficacy and results from different manufacturers, even if they are taken in the same dose. Patients may view herbal products as more natural than pharmaceuticals and therefore believe that taking more than the recommended dosage can increase the effects from the preparation with little or no risk. Patients should be encouraged to take the recommended dose of herbal preparations and assisted to understand that results should not be expected as quickly as with prescription drugs. Because patients may associate herbal medications with less potent or less harmful effects, they should be helped to understand that even though medicines are herbal, they should not be taken in larger-than-recommended quantities because of the potential for side effects or interactions with other drugs. Patients should be cautioned to read labels of herbal preparations carefully, paying attention to any warnings.

Herbal preparations should not be taken longer than necessary. Patients should be helped to understand that herbs do not necessarily cure all conditions and that herbal preparations should not be substituted for medications that have been prescribed by their health professional without discussion.

Lack of standardization is also a potential problem related to patient safety in using complementary or alternative methods. For example, herbal products are not closely regulated in the same way pharmaceuticals are. In most instances, they are not required to undergo premarket testing and are not manufactured in standardized fashion, nor does safety or therapeutic effectiveness need to be demonstrated scientifically before outcomes are advertised. Likewise, whereas training standards and credentialing are mandated for practicing health professionals in conventional treatment settings, standards and professional standing of alternative practitioners are not well regulated and competence and training received by CAM practitioners may be inconsistent.

Patients are often bombarded with information about complementary or alternative methods from personal testimony of family or friends, or from advertisements in the media. They may find it difficult to discern scientifically sound data from that which is based on emotion or on fraudulent claims with no empirical evidence. They may be unaware of possible herb–drug or herb–disease interactions or potential harmful effects of some complementary or alternative methods.

Patients should also be helped to understand that what has been reported to be helpful in the case of one patient may not mean that the same alternative method will be safe or helpful to everyone. Patients should be encouraged to consult several reliable sources for information before making the decision to use complementary or alternative methods. Above all, they should be encouraged to talk with their health professional about any complementary or alternative methods they are using and to promptly report any problems or new symptoms they experience after use.

THE HEALTH PROFESSIONAL AND COMPLEMENTARY AND ALTERNATIVE MEDICINE

Health professionals should become familiar with various complementary or alternative methods, especially those that seem to be more prevalent in their particular geographic area. There should be an awareness that patients' use and interest in complementary or alternative methods may change over time. Consequently, checking only once with patients about whether or not complementary or alternative methods are being used may not be enough. Checks for CAM use should be conducted on a regular basis. The following questions can be helpful in determining whether patients use alternative methods:

- "Have you tried anything else to help your symptoms?"
- "What have you tried on your own to treat your condition?"
- "Is there anything else you have tried besides your prescribed medicine?"

When patients ask about or mention use of specific complementary or alternative methods with which health professionals are unfamiliar, lack of knowledge of the product or method should be admitted. Asking patients for additional information or for resources where additional information can be obtained helps patients feel health professionals are interested in learning more and opens up opportunities for more communication. Attempting to gain understanding of patients' rationale for using the alternative therapy also communicates interest and helps build a collaborative relationship.

Patients may use complementary or alternative methods not only for treatment of disease but also for health maintenance. Health professionals can approach the subject with direct statements such as, "Patients use a variety of products and techniques to maintain or improve their general health status. Are you using vitamins, supplements, or techniques such as yoga or meditation to improve your health?"

Health professionals should be aware of patients' unmet expectations for care. Patients' underlying vulnerabilities and past experiences should be considered. Understanding patients' expectations helps health professionals better meet patients' needs by providing information to help them make rational decisions and, when necessary, to enter into negotiation regarding patient choices.

Despite open mindedness and willingness to work with patients' expectations, there may be some instances when patients and health professionals disagree on safety or effectiveness of complementary or alternative treatments. When this situation occurs, decisions should be negotiated. Health professionals should express concern, provide sound rational and evidence, rather than fabrications or coercion, and should not use emotional or psychological force. Patients have the right to make informed choices. Health professionals have the responsibility to provide factual information to assure that choices are informed. Health professionals should recognize and accept patients' desire for empowerment. Patients' choices should be accepted and their need for empowerment acknowledged. Health professionals should communicate their availability to patients should questions or problems arise and emphasize the importance of continuing contact and follow up. Disagreeing without humiliating patients or demonstrating hostility offers further opportunity to explore factors involved in patient choices. Health professionals should avoid deriding the CAM modality chosen by the patient, showing respect for patient choices. Patients should not be threatened or forced to choose between continuing care with the health professional and using CAM.

Whereas health professionals may have some difficulty accepting patient use of questionable CAM methods, they may also find patient use of CAM practitioners or therapies threatening. However, if the CAM practitioner's training and credentials can be verified, they can be a good referral source. Health professionals may find it helpful and informative to meet with CAM practitioners to discuss philosophy, training, experience, and cost, and to ascertain ways in which complementary or alternative care may be integrated into conventional care with individual patients.

INTEGRATIVE APPROACHES TO THE USE OF COMPLEMENTARY AND ALTERNATIVE MEDICINE

Conventional health care has achieved excellence in many realms of preventing, treating, and curing disease. CAM models, however, have also been shown to offer exemplary frameworks for interdisciplinary and holistic health care. Although most health professionals do not want to abandon conventional approaches to health care, complementary or alternative methods can, in many instances, be integrated into conventional health practices, complementing conventional approaches. Complementary or alternative methods used in conjunction with conventional treatments can help patients gain a sense of control over the effects of their condition and maximize the benefit of self-care strategies. When conditions are seen in the context of individual patients and the impact on their lives, complementary or alternative approaches can supplement conventional therapies, helping patients live with their condition.

Regardless of whether health professionals are enthusiastic or critical of complementary or alternative methods, there is a responsibility to be informed of such approaches and to respond to patients' interest. Although teaching patients about complementary or alternative methods requires additional skills and time, exploring patient use of alternative methods provides health professionals with important information that can ultimately increase quality of care. By not approaching the subject with patients, many opportunities for patient teaching are lost. Effective patient teaching about CAM can enrich the relationship between patient and health professional, as well as provide important insights that can help health professionals improve patient care. To effectively teach patients about complementary or alternative methods and to provide guidance that enables patients to make safe decisions about their use, health professionals must also be informed. Utilizing resources for continuing professional development that address different types of complementary or alternative methods and that provide factual information about their use and benefits helps health professionals be better prepared to discuss safety, risks and benefits, and cost-effectiveness of various approaches with patients, as well as to discuss how some complementary or alternative methods may be optimally combined with conventional approaches. A first step, however, may be addressing basic attitudes toward complementary or alternative approaches. By reexamining personal values and theories about health care as well as rethinking how to relate to patients regarding alternative methods, health professionals may find that they are able to more fully adapt to patients' expectations and, consequently, are better able to meet their needs.

REFERENCES

Anderson, W. H., O'Connor, B. B., MacGregor, R. R., & Schwartz, J. S. (1993). Patient use and assessment of conventional and alternative therapies for HIV infection and AIDS. *Acquired Immunodeficiency Syndrome, 7*, 561–565.

Applewhite, S. L. (1995). Curanderismo: Demystifying the health beliefs and practices of elderly Mexican Americans. *Health and Social Work, 20*, 247–253.

Astin, J. A. (1998). Why patients use alternative medicine: Results of a national study. *Journal of the American Medical Association, 279*, 1548–1553.

Berman, B. M., Singh, B. K., Lao, L., Singh, B. B., Ferentz, K. S., & Heartnoll, S. M. (1995). Physicians, attitudes toward complementary or alternative medicine. A regional survey. *Journal of the American Board of Family Practice, 8*, 361–366.

Cassileth, B. R., Lusk, E. J., Strouse, T. B., & Bodenheimer, B. J. (1984). Contemporary unorthodox treatments in cancer medicine: A study of patients, treatments, and practitioners. *Annals of Internal Medicine, 101*, 105–112.

Cohen, S., Tyrrel, D. A. J., & Smith, A. P. (1991). Psychological stress and susceptibility to the common cold. *New England Journal of Medicine, 325*, 606–612.

Crigger, B. J. (2000). Alternative and complementary medicine: What's a doctor to do? *The Hastings Center Report, 30*, 47–48.

D'Arcy, P. F. (1991). Adverse reactions and interactions with herbal medicines. Part I. Adverse reactions. *Adverse Drug Reaction and Toxicology Review, 19*, 189–208.

Dokken, D., & Sydnor-Greenberg, N. (2000). Exploring complementary and alternative medicine in pediatrics: Parents and professionals working together for new understanding. *Pediatric Nursing, 26*, 383–390.

Eisenberg, D. M. (1997). Advising patients who seek alternative medical therapies. *Annals of Internal Medicine, 127,* 61–69.

Eisenberg, D. M. (2005). The Institute of Medicine Report on complementary and alternative medicine in the United States: Personal reflection on its contents and implications. *Alternative Therapy in Health and Medicine, 11,* 14.

Eisenberg, D. M., Davis, R. B., Ettner, S. L., Appel, S., Wilkey, S., & Van Rompay, M. (1998). Trends in alternative medicine use in the United States, 1990–1997. *Journal of the American Medical Association, 28,* 1569–1575.

Eisenberg, D. M., Kessler, R. C., Foster, C., Norlock, F. E., Calkins, D. R., & Delbanco, T. L. (1993). Unconventional medicine in the United States: Prevalence, costs, and patterns of use. *New England Journal of Medicine, 328,* 246–252.

Elder, N. C., Gillcrist, A., & Minz, R. (1997). Use of alternative health care by family practice patients. *Archives of Family Medicine, 6,* 181–184.

Ernst, E., Resch, K. L., & White, A. R. (1995). Complementary medicine: what physicians think of it. A meta-analysis. *Archives of Internal Medicine, 155,* 2405–2408.

Feldman, M. K. (1990). Patients who seek unorthodox medical treatment. *Minnesota Medicine, 73,* 19–25.

Fuller, R. C. (1989). *Alternative medicine and American religious life.* New York: Oxford University Press.

Furnham, A., & Forey, J. (1994). The attitudes, behaviors, and beliefs of patients of conventional vs complementary alternative medicine. *Journal of Clinical Psychiatry, 50,* 458–469.

Gevitz, N. (1988). Three perspectives on unorthodox medicine. In N. Gevitz (Ed.). *Other healers: unorthodox medicine in America* (pp. 1–28). Baltimore: Johns Hopkins University Press.

Goleman, D., & Gurin, J. (1993). *Mind-body medicine: how to use your mind for better health.* Yonkers, NY: Consumer Reports Books.

Gordon, D. W., Rosenthal, G., Hart, J., Sirotan, R., & Baker, A. L. (1996). Chaparral ingestion: The broadening spectrum of liver injury caused by herbal medications. *Journal of the American Medical Association, 273,* 489–490.

Guerrera, M. P. (2007). Complementary and alternative medicine: A new dimension of integrative care. In R. Rakel (Ed). *Textbook of family medicine* (7th ed., pp. 223–242). Philadelphia: Saunders.

Harpham, W. S. (2001). Alternative therapies for curing cancer: What do patients want? What do patients need? *CA - A Cancer Journal for Clinicians, 51,* 131–136.

Horbert, C. P. (1997). Can primary care physicians be a resource to their patients in decisions regarding alternative and complementary therapies for cancer? *Patient Education and Counseling, 3,* 179–180.

Hufford, D. J. (1988). Contemporary folk medicine. In N. Gevitz (Ed.). *Other healers: unorthodox medicine in America* (pp. 228–264). Baltimore: Johns Hopkins University Press.

Hufford, D. J. (1997). Complementary and alternative therapies in primary care: folk medicine and health culture in contemporary society. *Primary Care: Clinics in Office Practice, 24,* 723–741.

Jensen, P. (1990). Alternative therapy for atopic dermatitis and psoriasis: Patient-reported motivation, information source and effect. *Acta Dermato-venereologica, 70,* 425–428.

Josefek, K. J. (2000). Alternative medicine's roadmap to mainstream. *American Journal of Law and Medicine, 26,* 295–310.

Kaptchuk, T. J., & Eisenberg, D. M. (1998). The persuasive appeal of alternative medicine. *Annals of Internal Medicine, 129,* 1061–1065.

Lazar, J. S. (1996). Mind-body medicine in primary care: Implications and applications. *Primary Care, 23,* 169–182.

Lazar, J. S., & O'Connor, B. B. (1997). Talking with patients about their use of alternative therapies. *Complementary and Alternative Therapies in Primary Care, 24,* 699–714.

McGuire, M. B. (1988). *Ritual healing in suburban America.* New Brunswick, NY: Rutgers University Press.

Miller, J. K. (1990). Use of traditional Korean health care by Korean immigrants to the United States. *Sociology and Social Research, 75,* 38–48.

Morgan, D. R., Glanville, H., Mars, S., Very, V., & The British Medical Association. (1998). Education and training in complementary and alternative medicine: A postal survey of UK universities, medical schools and faculties of nurse education. *Complementary and Therapeutic Medicine, 6,* 64–70.

Murray, R. H., & Rubel, A. J. (1992). Physicians and healers: Unwitting partners in health care. *New England Journal of Medicine, 326,* 61–64.

National Center for Complementary and Alternative Medicine (NCCAM). (2000). *Expanding horizons of health care: Five-year strategic plan 2001–2005.* Bethesda, MD: National Institute of Health. Retrieved July 28, 2009, from http://www.nccam.nih.gov/about/plans/2005/.

National Institutes of Health (NIH). (1994). *Alternative medicine: expanding medical horizons.* NIH Report No. 94-06. Chantilly, VA: NIH.

National Library of Medicine. (2005) *Medical subject headings.* Retrieved July 28, 2009, from http://www.nlm.nih.gov/mesh

O'Connor, B. B. (1995). *Healing traditions: alternative medicine and the health professions.* Philadelphia: University of Pennsylvania Press.

Owen, D. K., Lewith, G., Stephens, C. R., & Bryden, H. (2001). Can doctors respond to patients' increasing interest in complementary and alternative medicine? Commentary. *British Medical Journal, 322,* 154–158.

Pachter, L. (1993). Culture and clinical care. *Journal of the American Medical Association, 27,* 127–131.

Panush, R. (2000). *American College of Rheumatology position statement: Complementary and alternative therapies for rheumatic disease.* (Vol. 26, No. 1). New York: Elsevier.

Pelletier, K. R., Astin, J. A., & Haskell, W. L. (1999). Current trends in the integration and reimbursement of complementary and alternative medicine by managed care organizations (MCOs) and insurance providers: 1998 update and cohort analysis. *American Journal of Health Promotion, 14,* 25–33.

Planta, M., Gundersen, B., & Petitt, J. C. (2000). Prevalence of the use of herbal products in a low-income population. *Family Medicine, 32,* 252–257.

Rakel, D. (2007). *Integrative medicine* (2nd ed.). Philadelphia: Saunders.

Rampes, H., Sharples, F., Mai-agh, S., & Fisher, P. (1997). Introducing complementary medicine into the medical curriculum. *Journal of the Royal Society of Medicine, 90,* 19–22.

Richardson, P. H., & Vincent, C. A. (1986). Acupuncture for the treatment of pain: A review of evaluative research. *Pain, 24,* 15–40.

Riesmann, F. (1994). Alternative health movements. *Social Policy,* Spring, 53–57.

Slifman, N. R., Obermeyer, W. R., Aloi, B. K., Mussser, S. A., Correll, W. A., Cichowicz, S. M., Betz, J. M., & Love, L. A. (1998). Brief report: Contamination of botanical dietary supplements by digitalis ianata. *New England Journal of Medicine, 339,* 806–808.

Spigelblatt, L., Laine-Ammara, G., & Pless, I. B. (1994). The use of alternative medicine by children. *Pediatrics, 94,* 811–814.

Thompson, W. G. (1990). Alternatives to medicine. *Canadian Medical Association Journal, 142,* 105–106.

Vincent, C., & Furnham, A. (1996). Why do patients turn to complementary medicine? An empirical study. *British Journal of Clinical Psychology, 35,* 37–48.

Visser, G. J., Peters, L., & Rasker, J. J. (1992). Rheumatologist and their patients who seek alternative care. *British Journal of Rheumatology, 31,* 485–490.

Williams, J. W., Mulrow, C. D., Chiquette, E., Noel, P. K., Aguilar, C., & Cornell, J. (2000). A systematic review of newer pharmacotherapies for depression in adults: evidence report summary. *Annals of Internal Medicine, 132,* 743–756.

Zollman, C., & Vickers, A. (1999). Complementary medicine and the doctor. *British Medical Journal, 319,* 1558–1561.

Zollman, C., & Vickers, A. (2000). *ABC of complementary medicine.* London: BMJ Publishing.

CHAPTER 12

Patient Teaching and Patient Adherence Issues for Older Adults

DEMOGRAPHICS

The number and proportion of older persons living in the United States has increased dramatically during the 20th century. In the early 1900s, people over the age of 65 accounted for 4% of the population. By 2007, this group had grown to 12.6% of the population (US Census Bureau, 2009) with the projection that those 65 and older will reach 17.9% of the total population by 2025 (US Census Bureau, 2008). While much of this growth is a result of the aging baby boom population, the majority can be accounted for by the fact that many other older adults are now living well into their eighth decade and more and more individuals are living to reach 100 years and beyond (National Institute on Aging, 2002). Implications of this growth for healthcare delivery in general and patient teaching in particular are enormous. The increased need for patient teaching both for patients and caregivers is evident, and the need for effective patient teaching is imperative.

Although many principles of patient teaching remain the same for all age groups, there are special needs of older adults that must be addressed. Developing more effective approaches to teaching older adults and their families is an increasing challenge for patient teaching.

UNDERSTANDING AGING

Aging is a complex multidimensional process beginning at conception with continuing changes throughout life. The initial stages of the continuum consist of growth and development, followed in later stages by gradual decline (Schaie & Willis, 2002).

Everyone has their own perception of what constitutes *older age*. Older adults, however, are not a homogeneous group and do not share a distinctive or separate culture. A correlation between chronological and physiological or functional age cannot be assumed. Whereas physiologically, older age has been defined as a time in the postreproductive years when systematic deterioration begins at different rates and degrees of severity (Falvo, 2009), older age can have biological, cultural, social, psychological, political, legal, chronological, and functional connotations. Not all older adults age at the same rate or to the same degree. Wide individual differences exist in individual aging and are determined by physical, psychological, social, and economic factors. Even though much diversity exists among older adults and their experience with later life stages, older individuals are often lumped into one group, a tendency that promotes stereotyping. Attempting to place all individuals above a certain age into one "older age" category is problematic for a number of reasons. In addition to discounting individual differences, such a grouping does not take into account the wide age differences at each end of the spectrum. If an arbitrary age of 60 is established at the lower end of the grouping, a 40-year or more time span could exist between those at the beginning and end of the spectrum. The general profile physically, psychologically, and socially of an individual at the age of 60 is much different from an individual who is 100 years of age.

There is no uniform definition or specification of what constitutes older age. Rather, the definition of older age is often determined by the context in which it is being referenced. For instance, older age may be defined in terms of individual perceptions of what chronological age constitutes older age, with perceptions varying widely. While some individuals may perceive individuals who are 50 years of age as being in the older age group, others may consider the marker for older age to be much later. There are also legal and economic basis for defining older age. Rules regarding the age at which an individual may retire, the age at which more frequent drivers tests are mandated, and eligibility for withdrawing from pension funds are examples. Older age has also been defined legislatively. Legislation such as the Older American's Act and the Social Security Act have yet other specifications as to what constitutes older age (Atchley, 2000). Social groups or organizations can also define old age. The age at which individuals can become a member of the American Association of Retired Persons as well as varying ages at which individuals are eligible for "senior discounts" are examples of other markers of older age.

In addition to defining older age legally, legislatively, or socially, older age can also be defined biologically, based on physical changes. Outward physical changes that are indicative of older age include postural and gait changes, changes in facial features, hair color, or body fat distribution. Less visible internal signs of aging may include changes in stamina, reaction time, alteration of sleep patterns, or increasing susceptibility to pathological changes related to illness. The rate and extent to which these changes occur vary considerably from individual to individual and are determined by a number of factors. Whereas some individuals may show significant signs of outward or internal aging by the time they are 50 years old, others may show only minor aging changes well into their 70s.

Old age may also be defined psychologically. An indication of psychological age is the individual's ability to adapt behaviorally to the demands of the environment. Psychological aging may be related to individuals' expectations for aging and how they compare themselves to most other people their age in terms of appearance, interests, or behaviors. If, for example, an individual feels they look or feel older than those of their peer group, they may label themselves as "old," whereas if they feel more vital and productive than others in their age group, they may denounce the label of "old." For instance, Mrs. Johnson, at age 75, continues to run her own business, enjoys dancing, and remains active in the community. When she was asked to participate at the local Senior Citizen Center she declined, stating that she was not interested in participating because Senior Citizens Centers were for "old people."

Older age can be defined by culture or society in terms of social roles or social expectations for behavior for individuals of a certain age or how they react to life events. For instance, individuals may be expected to dress or act "age appropriately" regardless of their interests, abilities, or energy level. Social pressure based on these standards may compel older adults to "act their age" even though they may be capable of participating in a number of activities they still enjoy, but which are not considered to be age appropriate. Take, for example, Mr. and Mrs. Atkins. They had always been music lovers. They also loved to dance and throughout their lives had frequented clubs and bars that tended to be popular for jazz, reggae, and rock music. As they reached their 60s however, their son was overheard telling his friends, "I wish mom and dad weren't having so much trouble accepting their age. They still try to act as if they're young by going to clubs that are inappropriate for people their age. They should know when it's time to act their age and just stay home." Although attitudes and expectations of what constitutes age-appropriate behavior for older adults are changing, individuals are not immune to social values, customs, and attitudes that formed stereotypes in the past.

TERMINOLOGY OF AGING

Many terms are commonly used to describe individuals who have reached the later stages of life. Terms such as "elderly," "senior citizen," or individuals in their "golden years" are all terms used to describe adults who have reached their later years. Although these terms are a way of identifying an age group, such terms can also create negative images of older adults as individuals who are frail, inactive, or in other ways devalued. Many individuals in later years do not think of themselves as "elderly" or as "senior citizens," and find being lumped into this category offensive. Given the wide range in age that exists in later life stages as well as diversity of the aging experience, terms used to categorize individuals in later stages of life seem outmoded. What term, then, can best be used to communicate that an individual is in the later stage of life? The term that seems least offensive and that has a more positive connotation is the term *older adult*. This term still communicates that someone has reached the later stage in life but does not create stereotypic mental images that many of the other terms engender.

There is no one correct definition of what constitutes an older adult, nor is there a uniform age marker that indicates when older adulthood is reached. Health professionals should not assume that persons after a certain age fit into a stereotypical category; however, to fully assess individual patient teaching needs, health professionals must also be aware of specific factors that can be associated with aging and can influence patient teaching and its effectiveness. Treating persons as individuals and appreciating dimensions that are beyond the physical condition and chronological age are important components in effective patient teaching regardless of the age group. In advancing age, however, social, psychological, and physical domains become more interdependent.

INDIVIDUAL DIFFERENCES IN AGING

Aging is not an illness, but rather a cumulative process resulting from a sum of changes that occur gradually (Christiansen & Grzybowski, 1999). Many changes once associated with normal aging are now known to be pathological conditions rather than part of the normal aging process (Arking, 1998). It is therefore important for health professionals as well as patients to distinguish pathological changes from those changes as a result of normal aging. When pathological changes occur, they become superimposed on changes associated with normal aging. As a result, presentation of many conditions, symptoms experienced, and response to treatment may be different in older adults than in younger adults with the same condition.

All people do not "age" at the same rate. Some people seem physically, mentally, or socially older at 60 years old than others at 80. Aging is an individual process with different types of aging occurring at different rates. How an individual ages depends on a number of individual factors. Psychological and social stress may accelerate deteriorating changes associated with aging. Environmental factors, such as exposure to extreme temperatures, sun, or toxic substances, may also accelerate the aging process.

How individuals age may also be determined by genetic factors. Although how genetics affects aging is not fully known, it may determine individuals' susceptibility to certain illnesses or may influence functioning of various body organs or systems (Timiras, 1997). Socioeconomic status of individuals is also a factor that can contribute to aging because, to a great extent, it determines access to health care, including preventive treatment and treatment of illness, access to adequate nutrition both in terms of quantity and quality, and levels of stress to which individuals are exposed. Social expectations also play a role in the rate of aging. Individuals who have been devalued or coerced into diminishing roles may exhibit observable changes in behavior, feelings, or attitudes related to older age regardless of other parameters of aging.

Although some changes associated with aging are not reversible, others are, or at least can be delayed. Patient teaching directed toward prevention and health promotion (discussed later in this chapter) can diminish changes brought about by the normal aging process. When changes associated with aging do produce permanent functional loss, patient teaching can help alter deterioration and at times ameliorate the problem. For example, individuals who experience hearing loss because of aging may be taught about ways to maximize their hearing capacity and, when appropriate, how to use a hearing aid most effectively. If vision is affected, it may be useful to help patients learn how to maximize their vision and how to minimize accidents because of poor vision.

BARRIERS TO EFFECTIVE PATIENT TEACHING WITH OLDER ADULTS

Attitudes

Attitudes usually consist of beliefs about or labels of people, behavior, or circumstances that determine expectations related to people or events. Attitudes, either positive or negative, are important factors which can shape both the quality and framework of interpersonal interactions, including patient teaching, by affecting communication patterns and responses in both patient and health professional.

Health professionals may have positive or negative attitudes about aging that are based on their experience with older adults or their exposure to attitudes of others about aging. For instance, a health professional whose main experience with older adults has been in a nursing home where most individuals were ill and frail may have a much different perception of older adults than a health professional whose experience consisted of working with active older adults on community projects. Attitudes held by health professionals are transmitted to patients they serve. Older patients' perception of the attitude of the health professional is more of a determinant of help-seeking behavior than awareness of illness or perception of the health professional's competence (Nuttbrock & Kosburg, 1980).

Negative attitudes about aging can hinder the health professional's ability to effectively conduct patient teaching with older adults, and in some instances may contribute to the health professional's avoidance of patient teaching interactions with older patients. Health professionals may have negative prejudgments about older adults, such as beliefs that older adults are incapable of behavior change and that attempts to help them make changes to achieve treatment goals are futile. If the health professional expects that the patient teaching encounter will have limited positive results, then a self-fulfilling prophecy may result. Other examples of how negative attitudes of the health professional can impact patient teaching include the belief that patient teaching with older adults will take too much time and is not cost-effective given the older adult's limited life expectancy. If the older adult experiences chronic illness or has a complex treatment plan, the health professional may feel frustrated because of the complexity of the recommendations, because the condition is incurable, or because problems associated with the patient's ability to follow recommendations seem insurmountable. Health professionals may believe that, because of limited resources, more time and effort should be spent on younger adults who are still in their productive years rather than on individuals in later stages of life. In other instances, health professionals who are uncomfortable with their own aging may limit their interactions with older adults because they view older adults as a reminder of their own mortality, or in some cases, older patients may remind the health professional about conflicts they experienced with their own parents. Negative attitudes, regardless of their origin, can have a negative impact on patient teaching as well as on the degree to which patients follow recommendations.

Positive attitudes about older adults, however, can facilitate effective patient teaching. Viewing older people as individuals with values, beliefs, and preferences and demonstrating respect for them as individuals builds trust and rapport important to the success of patient teaching. Positive attitudes on the part of the heath professional can enhance not only the patient teaching interaction but also the possibility of increased adherence.

Although there has been increased interest in including information about later stages of life in curriculums of health professionals, often information presented focuses on illness processes or on negative aspects of aging, which may result in health professionals developing negative prejudgments about individuals in older age groups.

Although communication skills are important in every patient teaching encounter, even good communication skills cannot camouflage negative attitudes held by the health professional (Engram, 1981). Health professionals must acknowledge and confront negative attitudes before patient teaching can be effective.

Stereotypes

Ageism describes deep and profound bias against older adults that is manifested by feelings of uneasiness, intolerance, anxiety, fear, or revulsion (Butler, 1969). Like racism or sexism, ageism is a prejudice that can result in discrimination or harm to those to which the prejudice is directed (Coe, Morley, & Tumosa, 2006).

Myths and stereotypes about aging are widespread in society despite recent attempts to "normalize" aging. Society emphasizes youth, vitality, and productivity and tends to overestimate the number of older adults who are functionally disabled and unable to live on their own and underestimate the number of individuals who are active and independent. Older adults may be stereotyped as having declining cognitive ability, as having the inability to learn, or as being rigid and incapable of change. Or, they may be stereotyped as having little interest in outside involvement and being content to live passively rather than participating in responsible activities. Common stereotypes related to psychological aging consist of beliefs that older adults are conservative, stuck in their ways, or resistant to change as opposed to a younger psychological state in which there is receptiveness to new ideas or concepts and the ability to be flexible and to adapt. Any of these stereotypes perpetuates prejudice and contributes to failure to view each older adult as an individual with his or her own strengths and limitations.

Myths and stereotypes are perpetuated overtly and covertly through humor, literature, media, and advertisements. Humor often projects negative themes in aging, emphasizing memory loss, aberrant behavior, decline in physical appearance, or sexual dysfunction. Although recently literature as well as films have attempted to portray some older adults as heroes or heroines or as romantic love interests, portrayals of older adults as frail, dependent, disagreeable, and undesirable are far more common. Advertisements directed to older adults also emphasize negative aspects of aging, emphasizing remedies to mask signs of aging through antiwrinkle cream products or products to cover gray hair, while other products are directed toward problems such as incontinence, aches and pains, or constipation. Even birthday cards directed toward older adults often reflect negative stereotypes about aging and consequently reinforce ageist ideas. Sentiments expressed on greeting cards for older adults often refer to declines in physical ability, appearance, or mental abilities, understating positive traits and abilities while fixating on and generalizing negative characteristics.

Stereotypes diminish the value of older adults. Negative views portrayed by mass media and literature influence the views of younger adults and health professionals, as well as of older adults themselves. As a result, older adults may incorporate stereotypes into their own self-image, accepting negative stereotypes of aging as factual. Because they have incorporated negative views of aging into their self-perception, or because they fear ridicule of younger adults, they may participate in perpetuating negative stereotypes through jokes or negative statements about themselves as aging individuals.

Stereotyping results in compartmentalization of people rather than viewing them as individuals. Stereotypes are harmful to all aspects of social interaction, but they are especially harmful when they impede effective patient teaching. Take, for example, Mr. Morris, the patient educator for a local senior health project initiative. He had outlined a number of health promotion and prevention topics to be presented at the Senior Citizen Center. When choosing topics, because of his assumption that older adults did not actively engage in sexual activity or that they would be offended by discussion of sexual topics, he neglected to include information regarding human immunodeficiency virus (HIV)/acquired immunodeficiency syndrome prevention through the use of condoms. He was unaware of the inaccuracy of his assumption about sexual interest and activity of older adults and unaware that several participants at the Senior Citizen Center were living with HIV.

The negative effects of stereotyping on individuals' self-perception also have ramifications for patient teaching. During a routine physical examination, Dr. Jenkins attempted to discuss how to maintain cardiovascular health with Mr. Wylie, an 82-year-old patient. Before Dr. Jenkins could complete the patient teaching, Mr. Wylie interrupted, stating, "Why should I be concerned about this? When you're my age, it's too late anyway." In other instances, patients may be influenced by the negative expectations of others. Dr. Ellington was concerned when evaluating Mrs. Boucher, age 85, at a follow-up visit and found that she had not been following the meal plan for her type II diabetes diet. Mrs. Boucher's daughter, who had accompanied her to the office visit, stated to Dr. Ellington that "You just can't teach an old dog new tricks. Older people are naturally forgetful anyway, so how could you expect her to remember what she should have on her diet." A common misperception and stereotype about aging is that older adults are incapable or less able to learn and remember new material than younger adults. In this case, the stereotype was perpetuated by Mrs. Boucher's daughter, and Mrs. Boucher was living up to her daughter's expectation.

Health professionals should remember that there is wide variation in older adults and should not pigeonhole older adults into one group with shared general characteristics. The impact of stereotyping on patient teaching can be far reaching. Stereotyping can interfere not only with effective patient teaching but also have repercussions on patients' health and well-being as well.

Generational Differences

An outstanding feature of the older population as a group is its continual change in character. The older adult of today has had different experiences than older adults of 50 years ago. These differences create different perspectives on social roles, health, health care, and expectations for aging. Likewise, young adults today will have had different experiences throughout their lifetime, which will in turn affect their attitudes and perspectives when they reach older age.

Each individual has a unique life history, a unique personality, and a unique set of life circumstances, but life experiences are also influenced by the groups within which individuals function as well as by the events and circumstances of the times. Specific historic circumstances help shape individuals' attitudes and perspectives. For example, a person born in 1920 has had different life experiences from someone born in 1945. Events in history, technological advances, and social changes will impact each individual's world view, as well as his or her view regarding health and illness.

Age roles also differ from era to era. Individuals have been socialized regarding appropriate behavior for certain age roles. The expectations the individual born in 1920 has for their role in older age may be much different from the expectations of the individual born in 1945.

Because of the historic period in which people grow up, impressions of aging, as well as impressions of health behavior, may be different in older and younger adults. These factors may distort communication between individuals of different generations. For example, Mr. Byrne grew up during the depression. Because of the influence of the events he experienced during his early years, he believes in self-sufficiency and that he should be able to overcome problems on his own without asking questions or without seeking service of others. Dr. Karnes, a family practice resident working with Mr. Byrne, found it extremely frustrating when she discovered that Mr. Byrne had delayed seeking advice about medical problems he was having on several occasions. Those medical problems, if promptly treated, could have been controlled so that the complications he is currently experiencing could have been avoided. Dr. Karnes neglected to take into consideration that in avoiding medical consultation, Mr. Byrne was not being obstinate but was rather behaving in accordance with the social expectations of his historic past.

In other instances, older individuals may, because of social expectations at the time they were growing up, view the health professional's role as one of authority and paternalism. Consequently, these older adults may have difficulty accepting a more active role in their own health care. In other situations, older adults may be reluctant to talk about emotions, believing that personal and emotional problems are private, not to be shared with those outside the family.

Although generational differences can result in misunderstanding and can interfere with effective communication between patient and health professional, awareness of the possibility of differences can help health professionals adjust their approach to patient teaching, compensating for generational differences to maximize patient teaching effectiveness.

Cultural Differences

Cultural differences and their impact on patient teaching and patient adherence are, of course, important to any age group. Other variables related to culture, which may or may not include ethnicity issues, include social class, nationality, and whether individuals live in a rural or urban environment. Cultural differences can affect patients' views of health and illness, concepts of body function, perceptions of causes of illness, and the use of healthcare services. These differences may be more pronounced in older adults.

How age is defined and how age is marked varies among cultures. Age roles differ from culture to culture. Delineating age groups in different cultures may include not only chronological age but also functions performed by people in different age groups. In some cultures, old age may be defined by altered work responsibilities or retirement. In others, old age may be defined in terms of the status of one's children. For example, in some cultures, becoming a grandparent may be an age marker and bring with it social role expectations for that age.

Older adults, even though they possibly immigrated many years before, may have clung to cultural customs and beliefs, including use of folk remedies for treatment of illness. Older adults may also have clung to their native language, creating potential communication difficulties when interacting with health professionals.

The role of the family in caring for older adults also varies in different cultures. Consequently, how social networks, including family, friends, and neighbors, are used to help older patients mobilize resources and how these are applied to health and health care may be of special significance when working with older adults with culturally diverse backgrounds.

Specific cultural differences related to aging are especially important to effective patient teaching. The chances of developing a chronic illness become greater as individuals become older (Ory & Bond, 1989; Siegler, Bastian, & Bosworth, 2001) regardless of cultural or ethnic background. Cultural or ethnic variations impact on health and well-being in all age groups. Despite mediating factors, such as socioeconomic status, however, some ethnic groups are more prone to development of certain illnesses than others. For example, the rate of diabetes mellitus is higher in Native Americans (Burke et al., 1999), while hypertension and heart disease remains higher in Blacks (Harris et al., 1998). Some differences may be associated with poverty and a history of inadequate health care; however, others are rooted in cultural traditions, such as dietary practices. Consequently, awareness of increased risk for such illnesses requires special consideration for patient teaching to older patients from diverse cultural backgrounds.

Cultural issues should be addressed directly and individual beliefs and values should be respected. Health professionals should be aware that there is significant diversity within cultural groups, with each group containing their own customs and belief systems. These belief systems may extend to how patients view their role in treatment and how they expect to interact with health professionals.

Culture influences the experience of aging, perspectives on health, and relationships. Having an understanding of cultural influences helps health professionals determine potential or actual problems that could interfere with effective patient teaching. Such an understanding also provides a structure through which various solutions to meet these challenges can be devised.

SPECIAL CONSIDERATIONS FOR PATIENT TEACHING WITH OLDER ADULTS

Chronic Illness

Although aging is not synonymous with illness, the incidence of illness and associated disability increases with age (Digiovanna, 2000). With advanced age, several chronic conditions may coexist at one time. Over 80% of all older persons report one or more chronic conditions, such as arthritis, heart disease, hypertension, or diabetes (Ory & Bond, 1989; Stanley, Blair, & Beare, 2005).

As individuals reach later stages of life, chronic and acute illness are superimposed on normal changes of aging, having greater impact on health status, becoming more serious, and resulting in a higher level of functional dependency. The patient's initial condition may lead to a cascading effect of a secondary complication or problem, which then contributes to a yet a third problem. Take, for example, Mrs. Barnes, age 89, who had made a concerted effort to walk and exercise on a regular basis after her myocardial infarction, which had resulted in mild congestive heart failure. Because she also had osteoarthritis of both knees, however, she experienced increasing pain when walking and, as a result, was unable to maintain her exercise program.

Because of her inactivity, she became so constipated and felt so bloated and nauseated, that she no longer consumed adequate amounts of fluid because she felt it increased her bloating. As a result of her decreased fluid intake, in combination with the diuretic she was taking for the mild congestive heart failure, she became dehydrated. Her dehydration resulted in orthostatic hypotension, so that one day when getting up from her afternoon nap, she lost her balance, fell, and broke her hip.

In some instances, one illness may mask or alter the presentation of another. For example, Mr. Roberts, because of his arthritis, was unable to perform major exercise. Because of his decreased level of activity and consequent lack of increased oxygen demand, it was not discovered that he also had angina pectoris until late into the course of the illness. Mild symptoms he had been experiencing because of his coronary artery disease had been attributed to indigestion. He was not aware that his symptoms could be indicators of another illness.

In other instances, one illness may exacerbate the symptoms of the second. Mrs. Little was in the early stages of Alzheimer's disease, although still able to function somewhat independently. Mrs. Little's son, who checked on her daily, mentioned to his neighbor, a nurse, that he was surprised at how quickly his mother's Alzheimer's disease was progressing, stating that one week she was able to function on her own and suddenly she was unable to perform most of the tasks she had still be capable of performing. Mrs. Little's son had not been informed that sudden changes in cognitive function could indicate the presence of another illness. His neighbor encouraged him to consult his physician. When Mrs. Little was evaluated by the physician she was found to have a urinary tract infection that had not been identified, but which was exacerbating her symptoms of confusion.

Standard treatment for illness may also need to be altered because of coexisting conditions. Mr. Simmons underwent coronary bypass surgery. Although part of rehabilitation process would normally include exercise, Mr. Simmons had preexisting osteoarthritis of his left hip and knee, which made walking very difficult. Consequently, patient teaching was directed to helping Mr. Simmons find other ways to increase his exercise tolerance.

Medications

Coexistent chronic illness frequently involves an increased use of medications. In older adults, with increased medication use, patient teaching about medication is especially important. In the United States, it has been estimated that 10% of hospital readmission and 23% of nursing home admissions are related to the patient's inability to take medications correctly (Merkatz & Couig, 1992). Patients may be unaware of the potential for side effects or for drug interactions. They also may be unaware of the potential for inter-actions of their prescription medications with over-the-counter medications. Patient teaching that helps patients identify potential drug interactions as well as alerts them to interactions with other over-the-counter medications can help them avoid adverse effects, complications, and further disability. Older adults, just as younger adults, should be knowledgeable about the medications they take and about the potential side effects. They should be encouraged to check with the appropriate health professional when they have questions or if they experience problems with the medication. Like all patients, older patients should be informed about why they are having the medication prescribed, the anticipated effect of the medication, and possible consequences of taking the medication.

Adherence to recommendations is a major issue for all patients, but espe-cially so with older adults, particularly with regard to medications (Stanley et al., 2005). Conditions such as arthritis, poor eyesight, or memory problems can interfere with older patients' ability to take medications appropriately (Brown, 2007). Patient teaching may need to be directed to devising strate-gies that can make taking medication less difficult. Instructing the patient to ask the pharmacist for medication bottles that are easily opened or to use a magnifying glass for medication identification, or development of charts to assist the patient in keeping track of when to take medications are examples of patient teaching that can maximize the older adult's ability to follow treat-ment recommendations accurately.

Sensory Changes

Sensory changes are well documented in aging (Fozard & Gordon-Salant, 2001). Auditory and/or visual impairments vary in degree in older adults; however, there are declines in both with aging. Hearing loss and loss of visual acuity can interfere with effective patient teaching as well as the patient's ability to follow treatment recommendations, especially if appro-priate assistive devices are not being utilized. Hearing or visual loss may not have been identified or may be denied by the patient. Assessing the presence of these conditions and the degree to which they impact on function as well as on the patient teaching can assist health professionals in altering com-munication approaches as well as guide them in providing patient teaching that helps older patients to maximize function through use of appropriate assistive devices.

Hearing impairment can have significant impact on both patient teaching and adherence at any age, and older adults are no exception. Patients cannot follow recommendations that they are unable to hear. Take, for example, Mr. Jorden. During patient teaching about a test he was to have, the nurse instructed him, "Make sure you take the pill before you come for the test." On the day of the test, Mr. Jorden came to the appointment, but when the technician checked to see if he had taken the preparatory medication as instructed, Mr. Jorden replied, "What medication? The only thing the nurse told me to do before I came was to make sure I paid the bill before the test. I took care of that that very day."

When the patient has a hearing impairment, patient teaching is best conducted in a room free of excessive and background noise. If the patient does not see the health professional enter the room, the patient's attention should be obtained by touch or verbal greeting. Health professionals should talk with the patient in a normal tone of voice, speaking slowly and distinctly. Raising the voice causes distortion, making it more difficult for the patient to hear. Excessive body movements or exaggerated movements should be avoided. Health professionals should face the patient when they speak and look at them directly. Not only is this polite, but it also provides better sound and enables patients to pick up visual cues. Health professionals should also avoid covering their mouth when they speak. Speaking directly into the patient's ear should also be avoided. A comfortable distance should be maintained between the patient and the health professional since being too close can distort sound.

Normal changes in the eyes as a result of aging can affect visual acuity and the perception of color, as well as degree of illumination needed for different tasks (Brown, 2007). Color perceptions may change, making it more difficult for older individuals to distinguish between certain colors. This can affect not only the individual's ability to comfortably read materials with differing color contrasts but can also affect his or her ability to distinguish between medications of different colors.

Patient teaching materials should be evaluated based on their readability, both in terms of color contrasts and size of print. When conducting patient teaching, health professionals should also make sure that sufficient lighting is available, especially if patient teaching involves demonstration of tasks. Lighting that minimizes shadows and reduces glare is optimal. When conducting patient teaching, health professionals should position themselves in light and facing the patient, preferably at eye level.

Cognitive Changes

Although aging per se does not affect intelligence or the ability to learn (Stanley et al., 2005) and not all older adults have severe memory impairment, there are some changes in cognition that have been associated with aging and which could affect patient teaching. Cognitive changes associated with aging include speed with which individuals can process information, and working memory and recall (Park et al., 2002). Older patients may be unable to process complex information as swiftly and efficiently as younger patients and may need more time to conceptualize and organize their thoughts. Health professionals should not interrupt or try to put words into the patient's mouth. More time may be needed to allow patients to process the information appropriately. When conducting teaching with the older adult, the health professional should allow time for the patient to process and understand the information and respond appropriately. While not patronizing the older patient, the health professional should use familiar terms and simple sentence structures as much as possible. Breaking down instructions into sections or small steps may also be useful.

Health professionals should not show annoyance if patients ask questions or ask to have information repeated, but should rather respond to questions appropriately. If patients perceive annoyance on the part of the health professional, they may be more reluctant to ask questions or may pretend to understand even when they do not. Health professionals should look for clues of misunderstanding and restate what they said if needed. If a lot of information is being provided, patients should be given the opportunity to rest, or the patient teaching should be broken up into several sessions.

If memory problems are present, the health professional should assess the degree of memory impairment and tailor patient activities accordingly. If patients become distracted from the topic being discussed, they may need to be gently reminded of the topic at hand before continuing. Repeating and reinforcing information that has been given is important in helping patients absorb patient teaching points. Written materials that the patient can review at home may also be of help. Various prompts may also be used for helping patients remember treatment recommendations.

Involving a Third Party in Patient Teaching

Patient teaching with older adults sometimes necessitates involvement of a family member or caregiver (Brown et al., 1998). Various studies have indicated that between 20% and 57% of older adults are accompanied to healthcare visits by another person (Prohaska & Glasser, 1996). Inclusion of a third person into the medical encounter changes and influences the relationship between patient and health professional and can have both positive and negative effects on outcomes of patient teaching (Brown, 2007; Stewart et al., 2000). The presence of a third party can have a positive effect on the patient teaching interaction if the person helps the older adult understand and remember recommendations. The third party may also serve as an advocate for the older adult, or provide additional information about the patient's symptoms or responsiveness to treatment or potential barriers to following recommendations (Adelman, Greene, & Ory, 2000).

On the other hand, when a third party is involved in the interaction between the patient and health professional, issues of the older adult's autonomy are also present. Discussion may become focused on issues *about* the patient rather than holding discussion *with* the patient. The patient may not be given the opportunity to ask questions or address his or her specific concerns. Likewise, the older adult may become less involved in decision making about his or her own care. Older patients have a right to information about prevention, illness, and treatment and to make decisions about the degree to which recommendations will be followed. This right may be compromised unless the health professional is mindful of the autonomy of the patient. The patient and third party may disagree about the recommendations being made or the extent to which the older patient can carry them out. Family members or caregivers may request to speak with the health professional alone and then attempt to collude with the health professional to withhold concerns or other information from the patient. It can be difficult to respect the concerns of the family member as well as to respect autonomy of the patient; however, older patients should be approached with the same respect and concern that would be given any other patient.

The health professional's primary obligation is to the patient. This means that in some instances, patient teaching may involve helping the family member or caregiver understand the patient's rights to information and to determine treatment. For example, Mr. Jackson, at 82, was shown to have elevated cholesterol. His daughter insisted he follow a strict diet, which he found unpalatable. Ms. Freeburn, the nurse conducting patient teaching, helped Mr. Jackson's daughter see that following the diet in moderation while still allowing Mr. Jackson to have some foods he enjoyed may be more important in helping to lower his cholesterol than strict adherence to the dietary recommendations.

Although it is important to be sensitive to family or caregiver concerns, it is also important to stress patients' rights to be fully informed about their treatment and condition. The Patient Self-Determination Act of 1991 affirmed patients' rights to accept or refuse treatment (Cate & Gill, 1991). Consequently, the older patient's autonomy should be respected as much as is reasonable. Health professionals should address the patient directly, rather than addressing the third party as if the patient were not present. The older patient should be included in discussions about healthcare decisions and allowed to make his or her own decisions as much as possible.

TEACHING OLDER ADULTS ABOUT PREVENTION AND HEALTH PROMOTION

Not all older adults have chronic illness, and older adults who do have chronic illness are often not incapacitated and still believe themselves to be in good health despite their illness (Cockerham, 1997; Meiner & Lueckenotte, 2007). Older adults' assessment of their own health is frequently more related to their ability to maintain activities and independence than to actual diagnosis and treatment of illness. A goal of patient teaching for older adults is to help them maintain or achieve their optimal level of function and quality of life. Therefore, another focus of patient teaching with older adults is preventing development or progression of illness as much as possible, and helping them learn how to avoid acute illness or other events that could result in functional decline or disability.

Negative attitudes about aging and ageism may be a barrier to teaching about health promotion or prevention issues with older adults as a result of the health professional's perceptions about the older adult's future or the value of their future (Kane et al., 2009). Although the incidence of chronic illness increases with age, the focus of patient teaching on chronic illness may overshadow other health promotion and other issues important to older individuals.

A simple example of patient teaching related to prevention may be assessment of the accident potential in the patient's living environment and accompanying instruction to the patient and/or caregivers about how to prevent falls from occurring. Helping patients recognize the potential hazards of throw rugs or cluttered stairs, or encouraging them to use a night light may be simple recommendations that could prevent disastrous consequences.

In some instances, patient teaching might involve helping older adults learn how to avoid overuse of over-the-counter medications by introducing them to alternative techniques for treatment of symptoms other than medication. For example, patients with joint pain may be able to reduce the amount of medication they use if they are instructed about the use of heat and massage as treatment modalities. Or, teaching patients about the importance of fiber, fluids, and exercise to prevent constipation may help them avoid use of laxatives.

A more subtle form of prevention teaching may involve teaching the patient and/or caregiver how to differentiate the normal aging process from treatable illness. Older patients and their families may attribute symptoms they experience to normal aging when symptoms they are experiencing may be associated with illness or medication side effects. Consequently, the older adult may delay seeking medical treatment and as a result develop more serious consequences of illness that might have been contained if treated earlier.

Health promotion is a process of helping people change health practices in order to move to optimal state of health, which can be defined as a balance of physical, emotional, spiritual, and intellectual states of health (Green & Krueter, 1991). Teaching older adults about good health practices can help them to diminish susceptibility to illness, maintain functional ability, and increase overall quality of life.

Sexuality remains an important component of quality of life throughout the lifespan (Morley, 2006); however, issues of sexuality may not be addressed with older adults because of the assumption that older adults no longer engage in or are interested in sexual activity. Sexual activity in older adults can relate to companionship, intimacy, and pleasure and can contribute to self-esteem, a sense of belonging, and overall sense of well-being. Older adults may not bring up sexual issues. Awareness of sexual needs of older adults, whether in illness or in health, helps the health professional to identify teaching needs which may not otherwise be addressed. Health professionals should also not make assumptions about the sexual preferences of older adults and should consider the possibility that the older adult, just as younger adults, may have an alternative lifestyle. Likewise, the health professional should not assume that sexual issues are not of concern if an older adult is single or widowed.

Discussions with older adults about sexuality can include aspects of health promotion as well as prevention. Not only should issues of sexual health be addressed, teaching regarding prevention of sexually transmitted diseases may also be needed. Age is not a barrier for sexually transmitted disease, including HIV (Hess & Ebersole, 2004; Kaiser, 2006).

Physical fitness and exercise are important components of health regardless of age. However, these issues may not be recognized as patient teaching needs for older adults. Not only have studies indicated that changing from a sedentary to a more active lifestyle can decrease mortality in older adults (Singh, 2006), but there is a growing body of evidence that it can also have significant impact on cognitive function (Kramer et al., 2004). In addition, teaching older adults about the importance of exercise as well as appropriate forms of exercise can help them maintain flexibility and stamina, so that normal changes associated with aging, in the absence of pathological conditions, have little impact on functional capacity.

Other issues of prevention include smoking cessation, drinking alcohol in moderation, or safety while driving. Alcohol and drug abuse in older adults is increasing in prevalence (Levkoff et al., 2004). The chances of developing health problems related to drug and alcohol are greater in older adults because of physiological changes that are associated with older age (Naegle, 2008). Consequently, patient teaching regarding alcohol and drug use is an important component of prevention teaching for older adults. Health professionals may be reluctant to approach older adults about these issues because of discomfort regarding how to approach older adults, or because of attitudes of leniency in response to older age (Dufour, 2006).

Other issues that are important to health and well-being, but which may not be routinely addressed with older adults, are oral health and issues of nutrition.

Dental care begins at home, and should be reinforced by the health professional. If reduced dexterity or other problems are noted as interfering with dental hygiene, the health professional has the opportunity to teach patients how to modify usual dental care to accomplish the goals of dental hygiene. If memory is an issue, it may be necessary for the health professional to provide written instruction or reminders that the patient can use to implement their dental care plan. Oral health is important not only to maintain teeth but also to salvage them. Not only can tooth loss have an impact on quality of life (Davis et al., 2000), but it can also contribute to general health, self-image, and social interaction (Griffiths, 2006).

Nutritional issues should also be considered as a potential aspect of patient teaching with older adults. Healthy diet patterns in older adults are related to decreased mortality and illness as well as overall health (Biggs, 2007). The nutritional state of individuals reflects their current and past food practices. Eating habits are developed out of tradition, ethnicity, and religion. Eating habits are also influenced by economic, behavioral, and social issues. It is not enough to merely teach older individuals about good nutritional practices. The health professional must also assess potential barriers that may interfere with the individual's ability to carry out nutritional recommendations.

Attitudes individuals possess regarding life events determine their perceptions of whether those events have a positive or negative influence on their life. Stress may be physical or emotional. Although some events, like illness or death of a loved one are, by their very nature, stressful, the degree of stress experienced by the individual is determined by their individual reaction to it. Ongoing stress can have detrimental effects regardless of age. Older adults may have the decreased capacity to cope with daily challenges, illness, loss, or other life events because of decreased adaptive capacity as a result of cumulative effects of aging (Hess & Ebersole, 2004). Identifying potential sources of stress and individuals' perception of events as well as teaching about stress management techniques are also an important part of patient teaching with older adults in order to help them increase their optimal level of functioning and health.

Other topics important to include in patient teaching of older adults include annual immunizations to prevent occurrence of acute problems such as influenza and pneumonia as well as the importance of routine screening for early identification of diseases, which have been shown to be more prevalent in older adults (Resnick, 2007). As with other recommendations, it is important that the health professional assess the individual's thoughts about participating in screening practices as well as his or her ability to obtain the screening should he or she agree to have them.

BARRIERS TO PATIENT ADHERENCE FOR OLDER ADULTS

Patient teaching recommendations with older adults may range from teaching them about how to prevent illness or complications from occurring to assisting older patients and their families acquire skills in self-management of chronic illness. As with other patients, however, the ultimate measure of effectiveness is the patient's willingness and ability to incorporate the recommendations into their daily life and circumstances. For example, prevention teaching, which may address topics such as fitness, nutrition, stress management, personal healthcare management, or accident prevention, cannot be totally effective unless various other factors are considered. Merely giving older patients information about prevention practices may be insufficient to ensure that the practices can be carried out. Teaching patients about the importance of exercise and encouraging them to obtain exercise by walking may not be adequate without also assessing potential barriers that could preclude patients from following the recommendation. Does the patient have a place in which to walk safely? Do they live in a high-crime area that might place them in jeopardy? Are there sidewalks in their neighborhood, and if so, are they in good repair? If there is a mall nearby in which older adults routinely walk, and does the patient have the means to get there? Does the patient have another condition, such as arthritis or foot problems, that may prevent them from walking as recommended?

Likewise, it does little good to teach older adults how to eat nutritiously without also assessing their ability to afford the foods recommended or their ability to obtain and prepare them. Does a coexisting medical condition makes food preparation difficult? Are assistive devices needed? If the patient lives alone, is eating alone or preparing food for him- or herself an issue? Are there other services in the area, such as transportation services, Meals on Wheels, or communal food programs for older adults that can be used to help patients follow the food recommendations? In addition, if patients are being taught about stress management techniques, it may be insufficient to teach techniques without also evaluating the source of the stress and helping older patients identify ways the source of the stress can be reduced or eliminated.

Health professionals must be aware of social and economic needs of the older adult. Physical handicaps or other factors such as fixed incomes, limited insurance reimbursement, or transportation problems may make it more difficult for patients to follow recommendations given by health professionals. Does the patient have support from family members or friends? Does the patient have transportation to reach healthcare facilities for appointments? Is the older adult able to afford the prescribed medication? Does the patient have physical problems that interfere with following recommendations given in patient teaching? Is there need for modifications to help the older patient compensate for any sensory or physical problems?

To help patients remain at their maximum functional capacity as well as carry out recommendations, patient teaching may be directed toward teaching patients about the availability and use of self-help devices to compensate for physical need. Many simple and inexpensive adaptive devices are available to help promote independence. For example, in the case of arthritis, which can impede manual dexterity, Velcro closures can eliminate the need for buttons or zippers. For kitchens, there are specially designed cooking tools, such as cutting boards with finger guards or sticky materials to hold plates in place. Individuals with visual impairment may find large-print stove dials or magnifying devices useful. All of these devices not only serve as aids to independent living but can also help the older adult follow through with patient teaching recommendations.

Health professionals are not expected to be able to solve all problems related to older patients' ability to follow recommendations, but an understanding of the limitations patients experience and the availability of means to overcome limitations promotes better planning and enhances the opportunity for adherence. Many organizations and devices are available to assist older adults. These services and tools are often the critical factors that enable older patients to maintain maximum independence. Consequently, health professionals' knowledge of the availability of services and devices and ability to pass this information along to patients and their families is an important aspect of providing effective patient teaching to older patients.

MAXIMIZING EFFECTIVE PATIENT TEACHING WITH OLDER ADULTS

The focus of patient teaching is to help individuals function at their optimal level within the confines of illness and/or to maintain good health and independent function in order to live longer and healthier lives (Stanley et al., 2005). When teaching older patients about specific conditions, health professionals should be aware that there are differences in approaches to older adults and younger adults, even though they may have the same diagnosis. The overall health status of every individual, young or old, represents to some degree a synthesis of medical, psychological, and social domains. In older adults, however, these domains become more interdependent. Differences both in physiology in advanced age as well as the patient's life circumstances may not only alter the course of illness but the patient's response to treatment as well.

Older adults, just as all other patients, require patient teaching that considers comprehensive, individually tailored information and takes into account the whole person, including the physical and psychological environment in which they live. Although many older adults remain active and in relative good health, function is compromised to some degree with advanced age or with additive effects of illness. Patient teaching with older adults, then, should be directed not only to prevention or management of any chronic or acute condition they may be experiencing but also toward maximizing functional independence. This means that the approach toward older patients may be more complex. In advanced age, changes that are a result of normal aging, chronic illness, or a combination of both precipitate additional competing risks that raise additional questions of prolongation of life versus quality of life. These factors add to the complexity of patient teaching as well as decision making.

Most older individuals are not institutionalized, and most do remain in their own homes; however, the incidence of chronic disability requiring some type of assisted-living arrangement increases with advanced age. When illness results in functional dependency so that patients are unable to carry out one or more major activity such as eating, hygiene, or dressing, or when safety becomes an issue, alternative living arrangements may be necessary. A realistic assessment of affordability, available support systems, and the patient's physical environment are critical components in determining when a change of living arrangements may be necessary. Although physical and/or cognitive disabilities are not necessarily a normal part of aging, when physical or cognitive limitations make independent living for older adults less feasible, helping patients and families determine when different living arrangements are needed as well as informing them about available housing options are important parts of patient teaching. Choosing a housing option can be confusing and overwhelming for both the patient and his or her family. By helping patients and families identify preferences, recognize the level of need for assistance, and determine resources available, health professionals can assist patients and families choose the living arrangement most appropriate for them.

Maximizing Verbal Communication Effectiveness with Older Adults

Although many principles of patient teaching remain the same regardless of patients' ages, when teaching older adults, a number of factors specific to older age can hinder communication. Attitudes, both on the part of older patients and health professionals, can interfere with effective communication regarding health-related matters. Attitudes of health professionals and the impact on effective patient teaching have previously been discussed. Attitudes of older patients can also play a role. Although older patients should be treated as individuals, rather than as a part of a stereotypical group, there are some commonalities of which health professionals should be aware.

Not all older patients feel "old." Patients may resent being categorized as "old" or having terms such as "senior" applied to them. Consequently, instructions regarding specific safety measures, screening procedures, or other medical interventions that they believe are being directed toward them because they are "older patients" may be rejected.

As discussed previously, generational differences may exist between the patient and health professional, creating differences in beliefs and expectations. The experience of older adults in the context of the social milieu of their younger and middle years may be different from that of a younger or middle-aged adult of today. When the health professional is of a different generation from that of the patient, differences which could affect the teaching interaction must be considered. For instance, the health professional may expect to actively include the patient in determining healthcare decisions, while the older patient may be more reluctant to ask questions or to be active participants in their care, desiring to take a more passive role. Or, they may believe that health professionals should not be bothered with what the patient considers as "trivial concerns" or may refrain from asking questions for fear of offending the health professionals or for fear that their questions will be perceived as a challenge to health professionals' recommendations or judgment. The health professional may expect open and frank discussion of health concerns, while the older patient may be reluctant to share information that they consider to be too private or personal to discuss. This may be especially true of issues such as incontinence, impotence, or other sexual concerns.

Health professionals and older patients may have different perceptions of what constitutes health and illness and may define health differently than health professionals. To older adults, remaining independent and active may be defined as healthy, despite chronic illness and symptoms. They may believe that many of their symptoms are to be expected as a part of aging and may avoid seeking medical attention or following medical advice because they believe symptoms to be a natural consequence of aging. They may fear that by sharing all their symptoms and concerns with health professionals, they will be labeled as hypochondriacs or as complaining old persons. In other instances, they may not mention their symptoms to health professionals because they believe tests or treatment will be too expensive, or that treatment could involve giving up independence and perhaps even being moved from their own home.

Patient teaching information should be provided to patients in a way that they will be able to understand. Health professionals should be alert for clues about the ability of the older adult to comprehend information, whether these clues relate to level of alertness, cognitive ability, or decreased hearing ability or vision.

As much information as possible about the patient should be gathered before the patient teaching intervention. Health professionals should assess patients' general level of alertness. For instance, if patients are sedated, they will be unable to focus attention on the information being presented. Being aware of patients' thought processes can help health professionals assess the detail of information that needs to be given and whether a caregiver should also be present.

Maximizing Effectiveness of Written Materials

Patient education materials that are customized to the unique needs of the individual have been found to be more effective than generic materials that are directed toward patients at large (Kreuter, Wray, & Caburnay, 2007). Although many materials may have not been tested specifically on older adults, attributes that are generally associated with aging, such as changes in vision and cognitive processing, should be considered when choosing materials for use. Materials that have an easy to read typeface, contrasting black and white, and with larger print will be more accessible to older adults than materials with complementary colors and smaller print. Because of older adults' sensitivity to glare, written materials printed on nonglare finishes will also be easier for them to read. Generally, the materials should use short sentences and paragraphs, avoiding jargon.

Web-based tools and their applications offer healthcare professionals a number of options that can be used in patient teaching (Mayer & Villaire, 2007). The Internet is only a useful tool, however, if patients know how to use it. Although in the past older adults were less likely to use the Internet as a source of health information, this is changing rapidly. Stereotypes of older adults' abilities may influence attempts and willingness to inform them about technology and Internet resources (Harwood, 2007). Studies indicate, however, that many older adults are interested in computer use (Hilt & Lipschultz, 2004) and are able to perform competently when provided the appropriate training and motivation (Sterns, 2005). One problem with the Internet as a health information resource is, however, that much of the material generated can lack adequate quality (Wallace et al., 2005). Patients may not have a way to determine the accuracy of information. Helping patients determine valid sources for information on the Internet can be another important point of patient teaching.

Maximizing the Therapeutic Alliance

Because much of the effectiveness of patient teaching is dependent on the therapeutic alliance built between patient and health professional, conveying respect for the patient early on in the intervention is crucial. Health professionals should avoid calling older patients by their first name unless invited to do so. Likewise, terms such as "sweetie" or "honey" should be avoided. Using touch on the hand, arm, or shoulder of the patient can convey reassurance and help put the patient at ease.

Health professionals should be flexible in following the patients' train of thought and pace the patient teaching session. Patients should be given ample opportunity to express concerns, and their most pressing concerns should be addressed even though it may be different from that of the health professional.

Special sensitivities and skills are required for effective patient teaching with older adults. As discussed previously, definition of "older" varies with the individual. Some individuals are relatively healthy and active in their 80s, whereas others have significant functional limitations and consider themselves old in their late 60s. There are no specific rules or definitions of when a person is considered old. The approach to teaching older adults must, therefore, be individualized and based on individual patient needs. Patient teaching should be geared to specific patient circumstances, rather than chronological age.

An evaluation of patient teaching potential should be performed routinely. Patient teaching must be conducted within the context of a multidisciplinary plan that considers additional medical problems, potential side effects of treatment, and special arrangements that may need to be made so the individual has the best opportunity for carrying out the patient teaching plan. As with all patient teaching encounters, the health professional must work to establish a therapeutic alliance with the patient.

Assessing patients' perceptions about their concepts of aging provides health professionals with beginning information that can be helpful in patient teaching. Patients may attribute symptoms to normal aging even though symptoms may be indicative of side effects of treatment or of a specific illness. Likewise, symptoms related to illness may present more subtly in older adults than in younger adults. If symptoms are ignored or unrecognized, a treatable condition may go untreated and complications may result. Older patients may be reluctant to share symptoms because they fear they will be categorized as complaining. Helping patients understand the importance of reporting symptoms and reporting them accurately is an important first step in patient teaching.

Distinguishing acute symptoms from those that are chronic provides important information that can be used as a guideline for patient teaching. For example, if the patient complains of incontinence, patient teaching takes a different approach depending upon whether the problem has existed for years or whether the symptom is new. If incontinence has been ongoing and has been appropriately evaluated, depending on the cause of incontinence, patient teaching may involve teaching patients to use easily removable garments that facilitate toilet use or teaching patients behavior techniques that can help them learn to control their bladder and pelvic muscles. If the condition is new, however, patient teaching may involve teaching patients that incontinence is not a normal part of aging and helping them obtain a referral for evaluation.

Content of patient teaching may be different as well. The need to assess functional status in terms of everyday activity and their ability to carry out recommendations may need to be more detailed in the older adult. For example, teaching younger patients about medications and potential side effects as well as their ability to obtain the medication is important. In older adults, however, depending on circumstances and other illness processes, patient teaching about medication may also include strategies for remembering to take the medication. If visual problems exist, the patient may need to be taught how to distinguish one medication from another, or if physical limitations exist, what devices or solutions may be used to help patients carry out recommendations.

Patient teaching for family members is also important. Although the goal may be to help the patient maintain independence, family members may be overly protective. The health professional may need to help family members accept the patient's feelings and need for maintaining maximum independence while at the same time allaying family members' anxiety by identifying potential services and resources that enhance independence while assuring safety. In other instances, patient teaching interventions for family members may be directed toward helping them reduce their burden of care. Resources regarding respite care or other services can be helpful.

Patient teaching should be structured with problem-focused, well-defined goals. The health professional should emphasize patients' strengths, supporting pre-existing positive coping patterns. Emphasis should be placed on current concerns of the older adult, and practical solutions should be considered. As with all patient teaching encounters, the best predictor of adherence is concordance between the health professional and patient regarding goals. This is especially true when working with older adults because much variability exists in cognitive ability, verbal skills, medical problems, and degrees of social support.

The health professional should be flexible in patient teaching, tailoring teaching to the patient's specific needs and orientation. If the patient's major concern is maintaining independence, this need should be addressed first, even though the health professional may believe another aspect of patient teaching to be more important. Establishing plans for maintaining contact with the health professional through return visits or phone calls for short-term follow-up may be even more important with older patients than with younger patients so problems or concerns can be identified early and appropriately addressed.

Effective patient teaching integrates physical as well as social and psychological aspects of each individual patient in to the teaching interaction. Using an interdisciplinary team approach can increase resources available that support health professionals in working with older patients with a variety of social and interpersonal problems related to their care. The older patient should be an equal member of the team. Continued reevaluation and treatment should be ongoing. Most of all, health professionals should treat older patients as individuals and with respect. The older patient's life as an independent person with unique likes, dislikes, values, and choices should not be discounted.

REFERENCES

Adelman, R., Greene, M., & Ory, M. (2000). Communication between older patients and their physicians. *Clinics in Geriatric Medicine, 16*, 1–36.

Arking, R. (1998). *Biology of aging.* Sunderland, MA: Sinauer Associates.

Atchley, R. C. (2000). *Social forces and aging* (9th ed.). Belmont, CA: Wadsworth.

Biggs, A. J. (2007). Nutritional considerations In A. D. Linton & H. W. Lack. *Matteson & McConnell's gerontological nursing: Concepts and practice* (3rd ed., pp. 169–197). St. Louis: Saunders.

Brown, J. B., Brett, P., Stewart, M., & Marshall, J. M. (1998). Roles and influence of people who accompany patients on visits to the doctor. *Canadian Family Physician, 44*, 1644–1650.

Brown, S. (2007). How older patients learn medical information. In D. C. Park & L. L. Liu (Eds.). *Medical adherence and aging: Social and cognitive perspectives* (pp. 93–121). Washington DC: American Psychological Association.

Burke, J. P., Williams, K., Gaskill, S. P., Hazuda, H. P., Haffner, S. M., & Stern, M. P. (1999). Rapid rise in the incidence of type II diabetes from 1987–1996: Results from the San Antonio Heart Study. *Archives of Internal Medicine, 159*, 1450–1455.

Butler, R. N. (1969). Age-ism: Another form of bigotry. *Gerontologist, 9*, 243.

Cate, F. H., & Gill, B. A. (1991). *The patient self-determination act: Implementation issues and opportunities: A white paper of the Annenberg Washington Program.* Evanston, IL: Northwestern University Press.

Christiansen, J. L., & Grzybowski, J. M. (1999). *Biology of aging: An introduction to the biomedical aspects of aging.* New York: McGraw-Hill.

Cockerham, W. C. (1997). *This aging society* (2nd ed.). Upper Saddle River, NJ: Prentice Hall.

Coe, R. M., Morley, J. E., & Tumosa, N. (2006). Social and community aspects of aging. In M. S. J. Pathy, A. J. Sinclair, & J. E. Morley. *Principles and practice of geriatric medicine Vol 1* (4th ed., pp. 101–114).West Sussex, England: Wiley.

Davis, D. M., Fiske, J., Scott, B., & Radford, D. R. (2000). The emotional effects of tooth loss: A preliminary quantitative study. *British Dental Journal, 188*(9), 503–506.

Digiovanna, A. G. (2000). *Human aging: Biological perspectives.* Boston: McGraw-Hill.

Dufour, M. (2006). Alcohol use and abuse. In M. S. J. Pathy, A. J. Sinclair, & J. E. Morley (Eds.) *Principles and practice of geriatric medicine Vol 1* (4th ed., pp. 157–168). West Sussex, England: Wiley.

Engram, B. E. (1981). Communication skills training for rehabilitation counselors working with older persons. *Journal of Rehabilitation, 47*(4), 51–56.

Falvo, R. (2009). Cell biology and physiology of aging. In C. Arenson, J. Busby-Whitehead, K. Brummel-Smith, J. G. O'Brien, M. Palmer, & W. Reichel (Eds.). *Reichel's care of the elderly* (6th ed., pp. 536–542). Cambridge: Cambridge University Press.

Fozard, J. L., & Gordon-Salant, S. (2001). Changes in vision and hearing with aging. In J. E. Birren (Ed.). *Handbook on the psychology of aging* (pp. 241–266). San Diego, CA: Academic Press.

Green, L., & Kreuter, M. (1991). *Health promotion planning: An educational & environmental approach* (2nd ed.). Mountain View, CA: Mayfield.

Griffiths, J. E. (2006). Oral health. In M. S. J. Pathy, A. J. Sinclair, & J. E. Morley (Eds.) *Principles and Practice of Geriatric Medicine, Vol 1* (4th ed., pp. 279–290). West Sussex, England: Wiley.

Harris, M. E., Flegal, K. M., Cowie, C. C., Eberhardt, M. S., Goldstein, D. E., Little, et al. (1998). Prevalence of diabetes, impaired fasting glucose, and impaired glucose tolerance in U.S. adults: The Third National Health and Nutrition Examination Survey, 1988–1994. *Diabetes Care, 21,* 518–525.

Harwood, J. (2007). *Understanding communication and aging.* Thousand Oaks, CA: Sage.

Hess, P., & Ebersole, P. (2004). Health and wellness. In P. Ebersole, P.Hess, & A. S. Luggen. *Toward health aging: Human needs and nursing response* (pp. 56–78). St. Louis: Mosby.

Hilt, M. L., & Lipschultz, J. H. (2004). Elderly Americans and the internet: E-mail, T.V. news, information, and entertainment web sites. *Educational Gerontology, 30,* 57–72.

Kaiser, F. E. (2006). Sexual function and the older adult. In T. Rosenbal, B. Naughton, & M. Williams. *Office care geriatrics* (pp. 196–206). Philadelphia: Lippincott Williams & Wilkins.

Kane, R. L., Ouslander, J. G., Abrass, I. B., & Resnick, B. (2009). *Essentials of clinical geriatrics* (6th ed). New York: McGraw-Hill.

Kramer, A. F., Bherer, L., Colcombe, S. J., Dong, W., & Greenough, W. T. (2004). Environmental influences on cognitive and brain plasticity during aging. *Journals of Gerontology Series A. Biological Sciences and Medical Sciences, 59A,* 940–957.

Kreuter, M. W., Wray, R., & Caburnay, C. (2007). Customized communication in patient education. In D. C. Park & L. L. Liu. *Medical adherence and aging: Social and cognitive perspectives* (pp. 235–249). Washington, DC: American Psychological Association.

Levkoff, S. E., Chen, H., Coakley, E., Herr, E. C., Oslin, D. W., & Katz, I. (2004). Design and sample characteristics of the PRISM-E multi-site randomized trial to improve behavioral health for the elderly. *Journal of Aging and Health, 16*(1), 3–27.

Mayer, G. G., & Villaire, M. (2007). *Health literacy in primary care: A clinician's guide.* New York: Springer.

Meiner, S. E., & Lueckenotte, A. G. (2007). Overview of gerontologic nursing. In S. E. Meiner & A. G. Lueckenotte. *Gerontologic nursing* (3rd ed., pp. 1–18). St. Louis: Mosby.

Merkatz, R., & Couig, M. (1992). Helping America take its medicine. *American Journal of Medicine, 93*(6), 56–62.

Morley, J. E. (2006). Sexuality and aging. In M. S. J. Pathy, A. J. Sinclair, & J. E. Morley *Principles and practice of geriatric medicine Vol 1* (4th ed., pp. 115–122).West Sussex, England: Wiley.

Naegle, M. (2008). Substance misuse and alcohol disorders. In E. Capezuti, D. A. Zwicker, M. Mezey, & T. Fulmer (Eds.). *Evidence based geriatric nursing: Protocols for best practice* (3rd ed., pp. 649–676). New York: Springer.

National Institute on Aging. (2002). *Aging in the United States: past, present and future. 1960–2020.* Washington, DC: US Department of Commerce.

Nuttbrock, L., & Kosburg, J. I. (1980). Images of the physician and help seeking behavior of the elderly: a multivariate assessment. *Journal of Gerontology, 35*(2), 241–248.

Ory, M. G., & Bond, K. (1989). *Aging and health care.* London: Routledge.

Park, D. C., Lautenschlager, G., Hedden, T., Davidson, N., Smith, A. D., & Smith, P. (2002). Models of visuospatial and verbal memory across the adult life span. *Psychology and Aging, 17,* 299–320.

Prohaska, T. R., & Glasser, M. (1996). Patients: Views of family involvement in medical care decisions and medical encounters. *Research on Aging, 18*, 52–69.

Resnick, B. (2007). Health maintenance, exercise, and nutrition. In R. J. Ham, P. D. Sloane, G. A. Warshaw, M. A. Bernard, & E. Flaherty (Eds.). *Primary care geriatrics: A case based approach* (5th ed., pp. 72–89). Philadelphia: Mosby.

Schaie, K. W., & Willis, S. L. (2002). *Adult development and aging* (5th ed.). Upper Saddle River, NJ: Prentice Hall.

Siegler, I. C., Bastian, L. A. & Bosworth, H. B. (2001). Health, behavior, and aging. In A. Baum, T. A. Revenson, & J. E. Singer (Eds.). *Handbook of health psychology* (pp. 469–476). Mahwwah, NJ: Erlbaum.

Singh, M. A. F. (2006). Physical fitness and exercise. In M. S. J. Pathy, A. J. Sinclair, & J. E. Morley. *Principles and practice of geriatric medicine Vol 1* (4th ed., pp. 123–140). West Sussex, England: Wiley.

Stanley, M., Blair, K. A., & Beare, P. G. (2005). *Gerontological nursing: Promoting successful aging with older adults* (3rd ed.). Philadelphia: F. A. Davis Co.

Sterns, A. A. (2005). Curriculum design and programs to train older adults to use personal digital assistants. *The Gerontologist, 45*, 828–834.

Stewart, M., Meredith, L., Brown, J. B., & Galajda, J. (2000). Communication between older patients and their physician: the influence of older patient physician communication on health and health related outcomes. *Clinics in Geriatric Medicine, 16*(1), 25–36.

Timiras, P. S. (1997). *Physiological basis of aging and geriatrics* (4th ed.). Boca Raton: CRC Press.

US Census Bureau. (2008). 2008 national population projections. Retrieved December 3, 2009, from http://www.census.gov/poplation/www/projections/2008projections.html

US Census Bureau. (2009). Statistical abstract of the United States: 2009 (128th ed). Retrieved July 1, 2009, from http://www.census.gov/statab/www/

Wallace, L. S., Turner, L. W., Ballard, J. E., Keenum, A. J., & Weiss, B. D. (2005). Evaluation of web-based osteoporosis educational materials. *Journal of Women's Health* (Larchmont), *14*(10), 936–945.

CHAPTER 13

Patient Teaching About End-of-Life Issues

IMPORTANCE OF TEACHING ABOUT END-OF-LIFE ISSUES

Patient teaching is usually characterized as a process by which patients are provided with information about causes and treatments of health problems, are counseled about risk factors, or are given information about prevention of disease or complications. The focus on patient teaching is to help patients maintain or improve health by achieving long-range outcomes or lifestyle changes. Another focus of patient teaching is to enhance patients' ability to make informed choices about health and health care.

Patient teaching about end-of-life issues is rarely considered a part of the general concept of patient teaching. However, health professionals have the duty to teach patients and families about end-of-life issues, to encourage discussion of life preferences, and to provide relevant information that would assist patients in making end-of-life decisions (Dahlin & Giansiracusa, 2006; Doran & Geary, 2005). Although less recognized, patient teaching about end-of-life issues is vitally important to assist patients to make informed choices and to enhance quality of life, whether death is imminent or a distant possibility.

As technological advances and treatment interventions that extend the life of those with life-threatening diseases multiply, as the aging population grows, and as awareness of the need for compassionate and respectful care of individuals with terminal conditions increases, the need for effective ways to teach patients and families about end-of-life issues becomes even more important (Friedman, 2007; Schears, 1999).

Discussion of living wills and advance directives is important even when patients are in the best of health because no one can predict when a devastating accident or serious illness may necessitate decisions about approaches to dying and death. Whether preparing for the future in the absence of disease, living with a life-threatening disease, or coping with terminal illness, patients may have distinct preferences about treatment, about procedures they would or would not want to have performed at end of life, and about how, under those circumstances, they would prefer to spend the remaining days of their lives. Information about end-of-life issues can provide patients with a sense of preparedness and control.

Although health professionals have become more aware of the need to employ a holistic, family-centered approach to death and dying, in many instances emphasis still often remains on patients' physical needs. Even when issues of death and dying are addressed from a psychological or social perspective, patient teaching needs of the patient may not be adequately addressed. Addressing patients' medical, psychological, or social needs without also providing them with information and skills needed to make end-of-life decisions or to manage care at end of life thwarts their control and autonomy and inhibits patients' ability to fully participate in their own care and decisions.

Whether engaging patients in proactive planning about end of life before a crisis event or discussing end-of-life issues during terminal stages of disease, health professionals should not make assumptions that their personal beliefs coincide with patients' preferences. It is important for the health professional to understand the patient's core values because these play a large role in the patient's decisions about end-of-life issues (Cacchione, 2007). Given vast differences in individual values related to end of life, the only way to determine patients' preferences is to participate in active discussion with them.

Increasing the patient's state of well-being through provision of complete and honest information underpins all patient teaching. Nowhere is this ideology more important than when discussing issues related to end of life. Quality of life and death can be improved when end-of-life issues are addressed (Black, 2007). In the end stages of life, patients may feel isolated, lonely, and may have misconceptions that cause needless fear and anxiety (Finlay & Dorman, 2006). For instance, patients with cancer may believe that all patients with cancer die in severe pain unless they are helped to understand that not all patients experience severe pain and that if pain does occur, there are many measures that can be instituted to reduce or eliminate pain. In other instances, patients may be informed about services such as palliative care or hospice to assist them at end of life (Hentz & Tabloski, 2006). Patient teaching helps patients gain information that increases their knowledge about and control over the dying process (Moore, 2007). Discussions should be individualized and should be directed toward helping patients gain information that enables them to make informed choices, to maximize quality of life at end of life, and to die with as much comfort, dignity, and freedom from anxiety as possible.

In view of the individual nature of beliefs and feelings about death and dying, health professionals face a special challenge when teaching patients and their families about end-of-life issues. The challenge can be met, however, if there is a basic understanding of pertinent principles and dynamics involved, and if health professionals reflect, understand, and acknowledge their own beliefs and feelings about death and dying.

RELUCTANCE TO TALK ABOUT END-OF-LIFE ISSUES

Discussions with patients about end-of-life issues are not always conducted when opportunities are presented. Health professionals may have feelings of discomfort with the topic or may feel they are inadequately trained to communicate with patients about death and dying (Dahlin & Giansiracusa, 2006; Elder, 1996). Health professionals are often action oriented, having been trained to focus on saving lives, curing patients, preventing disease, and stabilizing conditions. Consequently, accepting and acknowledging the realities and finality of death may be difficult (Dangler et al., 1996). When working with generally healthy patients, health professionals may not view such discussions as being relevant or may not think this type of patient teaching is within the general framework of their role. Consequently, health professionals may neglect to bring up the topic altogether. When confronted with patients with terminal illness, health professionals may also avoid discussion of end-of-life issues because they feel a sense of helplessness or because they believe there is little left that they have to offer professionally.

Death and dying may be perceived as a highly ambiguous issue with no clear reference points. Health professionals who have a low tolerance for uncertainty may experience discomfort in end-of-life circumstances that present complex or contradictory situations (Kvale et al., 1999). In these cases, they may find it difficult to confront their own values, beliefs, and attitudes about death and dying, and neglect to focus on more passive, reflective approaches. When patients have beliefs and values that differ from those of the health professional, the situation may be even more difficult.

Discussing death and dying with patients can be emotionally painful, distressing, and sometimes threatening, especially if the patient's condition is incurable or when death is imminent. Under these circumstances, patient teaching may elicit anxiety in health professionals, hindering their ability to effectively help patients and families cope. High degrees of death anxiety may cause health professionals to distance themselves from discussions of end-of-life issues and to focus on patients' physical needs rather than on the emotional aspects of care (Garfinkle & Block, 1996). In some instances, health professionals may minimize patient contact or avoid interacting with patients with life-threatening or terminal conditions altogether.

Reaching a level of comfort with discussion of end-of-life issues requires health professionals to explore their own feelings and attitudes about death and dying. Just as patients' reactions to death and dying are determined by culture, family attitudes, religion, and past experiences with death, so are reactions of health professionals. Issues of death and dying may engender anxiety in health professionals because these issues arouse thoughts about their own mortality or of the fragility and vulnerability of loved ones who could be lost to death.

Anxiety may be provoked by thoughts of the dying process rather than by death itself. Health professionals may experience feelings of inadequacy or failure when faced with patients with life-threatening or terminal conditions. They may also experience feelings of guilt about whether more could have been done to postpone or reverse the dying process.

Some health professionals may focus on personal experiences with the death of loved ones, projecting feelings and experiences onto patients and their situations. Take, for example, Ms. Lanally, who had provided nursing care for Mrs. George throughout her postoperative course after surgery for colon cancer as well as during chemotherapy. Despite surgery and chemotherapy, metastasis resulted. Mrs. George's physicians informed Mrs. George and her family that her prognosis was grave. They offered her the possibility of additional chemotherapy but also advised her of potential adverse effects she might experience. They informed Mrs. George that despite additional chemotherapy, chances of cure or remission were only slight. After discussion with her family, Mrs. George elected to forgo chemotherapy, choosing to return to her home, enlisting the services of Hospice. Ms. Lanally, although maintaining a professional demeanor with Mrs. George, went to her supervisor and requested a change of assignment because she could not understand Mrs. George's resistance to treatment and did not agree with Mrs. George's "not trying." Although Ms. Lanally was unaware of the underlying cause of her strong feelings at the time, she later realized that she was associating Mrs. George's situation with that of her own mother who had died of colon cancer several years earlier.

Caring for patients with life-threatening or terminal illness can revive memories of unresolved losses health professionals have sustained in their lives. Had Ms. Lanally understood how her own situation impacted on her feelings about Mrs. George's situation, or had she resolved her feelings about her mother's death, she may have been able to use her own experiences to provide information and support to Mrs. George and her family. Resolving prior conflicts can provide health professionals with valuable insights that can be useful and helpful in patient teaching.

In some instances, reluctance to discuss end-of-life issues with patients may be a result of fear of the inability to maintain emotional composure or fear of losing control in front of the patient. Although maintaining a professional demeanor with patients is important, displaying a cold, unfeeling exterior in the face of news that is devastating to the patient can do more harm than good. Patients are often touched and feel solace when health professionals demonstrate sincere emotion and concern when discussing serious issues with patients and their families (Buckman, Byrock, & Fry, 2000).

Health professionals may also fear that discussion of end-of-life issues will be upsetting to patients and their families and consequently avoid such discussions altogether. Avoiding discussions, especially in the case of life-threatening or terminal conditions, can cause even more anxiety in patients who may not know what to expect or feel they have lost control of their own destiny. Frank and compassionate discussions with patients during this time can be a source of empowerment and help patients to more fully participate in their own care and decisions.

For health professionals to reach a comfort level that would enable them to initiate and conduct effective dialogue with patients about end-of-life issues, feelings and attitudes about death and dying must first be explored. Examining these feelings and attitudes assists health professionals to recognize their limitations as well as areas of strength in conducting patient teaching about end-of-life issues. Through awareness of their own feelings related to death and dying, health professionals will be better able to approach patients' feelings and preferences about care at the end of life with sensitivity and compassion.

Awareness of personal beliefs, feelings, and attitudes about death and dying is an important first step to effectively conducting patient teaching about end-of-life issues. Despite self-exploration and awareness, however, resolution of all personal issues may not be reached. Not everyone can work adequately with all types of patients with life-threatening conditions. Ms. Janis a fourth year medical student, lost her own child to leukemia before entering medical school. The event was devastating for Ms. Janis, who went into medicine with the hope that she could help others who had been touched by life-threatening conditions. When choosing the medical field in which she wanted to specialize, she determined that pediatrics would not be a good choice for her. Despite her desire to help others, she was aware of potential difficulties her own experiences might cause if she were providing care for children with life-threatening conditions. She realized, however, that by choosing a specialty such as internal medicine, she could use her own experiences and insights to offer support and understanding to adult patients should they be confronted with a situation similar to what she had experienced in the past. Ms. Janis was able to recognize not only her limitations but her strengths in dealing with end-of-life issues and was able to use this knowledge productively.

When health professionals feel unable to provide appropriate information or support to patients regarding end-of-life issues, referrals should be made.

Health professionals can still convey concern to patients without compromising their own feelings and without causing patients to feel abandoned. Statements such as the following can help patients feel that the health professional is still providing the support they need but not deserting them when making a referral: "In this situation, I want to make sure that you have the very best support possible. Although I will continue to be a resource for you, I would like to refer you to Mr. Walker, a social worker, who has special training in helping with these issues and, consequently, may be better able to meet your specific needs right now."

CULTURAL VARIATIONS IN DEATH AND DYING

Culture is more than race or ethnicity. It can be broadly defined as a common social experience containing a shared belief system, shared expectations, and shared behaviors and rituals (Hallenbeck, 2001). Cultural differences have an impact on all aspects of health care. Because culture permeates life, all aspects of end-of-life issues have a cultural component. Cultural beliefs, rituals, and attitudes impact on concepts and reactions to death, and on end-of-life care and decision making regarding preferences to care. Whereas Eastern philosophies tend to accept death as part of the natural rhythm of life, Western cultures tend to view death as an event to be postponed as long as possible (Klessig, 1998). Concepts of death in our society often focus on Euro-American and Judeo-Christian values rather than incorporating beliefs of other ethnic and religious groups. Some cultures encourage truth telling, whereas other cultures expect the truth to be hidden from the patient. Some cultures value individual autonomy in decision making, whereas other cultures traditionally view families as the decision makers.

Racial, religious, and cultural differences influence views of end of life held by health professionals, as well as those held by patients and their families (Vincent, 2001). Therefore, basic understanding of cultural issues involved in death and dying and sensitivity to interpersonal relations in the context of culture are key to effective patient teaching about end-of-life issues.

When the patient's skin color, mode of dress, facial features, or language are different from those of the health professional, the possibility of cultural differences is easy to recognize. Cultural differences may be discounted, however, when patients share many of the same cultural attributes with health professionals even though their cultures may still differ in significant ways. Not only are there variations within the same culture, but every individual within the culture is unique (Safonte-Strumolo & Dunn, 2000; Stanley, Blair, & Beare, 2005). Sensitivity to individual differences related to culture, even in situations where culture differences are not immediately recognized, helps health professionals avoid misunderstandings and cultural conflicts and facilitates communication about end-of-life issues.

Before initiating patient teaching about end-of-life issues with the patient from a different culture, health professionals may find it useful to inquire about concepts and practices about death and dying within the patient's culture. Some cultures have taboos against direct, verbal communication about death related to a specific individual. There may be fear that discussion of death and dying increases the chance of death for the patient or that talking about death will have unfortunate consequences for family members (Hallenbeck, 2001). If this is the case, patient teaching interventions that include end-of-life discussions may be resisted by patients. Health professionals can still introduce the discussion while respecting patients' beliefs with a phrase such as, "I am unfamiliar with your culture, but would like to learn more. Talking in general terms, what is your culture's belief or practice surrounding end of life?"

Such an inquiry helps health professionals approach the subject and learn more about cultural beliefs of the patient while avoiding direct discussion of death related to a specific patient.

If patient teaching involves a situation in which death is imminent, but discussion of death and dying remains a sensitive issue, health professionals may ask the patient or family members if there are specific concerns about activities or procedures health professionals may carry out at this time that could violate cultural taboos. By asking for specific ways in which the patient's cultural integrity can be maintained, health professionals communicate concern and respect for the patient and family's cultural priorities.

Cultural differences about the role of family in end-of-life decision making varies greatly. Some cultures focus mainly on the family, protecting it from outsiders (Vincent, 2001). In these instances, participation by health professionals in end-of-life discussion or decision making may be viewed as an intrusion or violation of family privacy. Family members may be reluctant to discuss end-of-life issues for fear of appearing to be disloyal to the family unit. Approaching the family in a nonjudgmental and nondefensive way builds trust and shows regard for the patient's cultural concerns.

Some cultures value individual participation and involvement in end-of-life issues, whereas other cultures prescribe that close relatives, rather than patients themselves, are involved in decision making and given details about the patient's condition. When health professionals are from a culture that values patient autonomy as an important part of medical care, withholding information from the patient may seem like a violation of patient rights. Under these circumstances, health professionals may approach the family request for withholding information by clarifying reasons for the request with statements such as, "I know different people have different beliefs about how situations such as this should be approached. In my country, we generally believe that it is the patient's right to know about their condition and to participate in decision making about their care. Could you tell me more about your culture's beliefs?"

If family members confirm that it is appropriate in their culture to allow family members to be given medical information about the patient and to make decisions without patient input, health professionals need to confirm this belief with the patient. The patient may be approached with a statement such as, "I've been trying to understand more about your culture so I can provide care that does not violate your beliefs or values. I understand that in your culture details about a patient's medical condition as well as decisions about how care should be managed is discussed with the family and that the family, rather than the patient, and usually makes decisions. Is this the way you would like for me to handle this in your case?"

If the patient agrees, his or her wishes should be respected. If the patient confirms that this is the practice in the culture, but also acknowledges that he or she would prefer to understand his or her own condition and be involved in making his or her own decisions, the health professional should honor the patient's wishes. In this instance, further discussion with the patient about how he or she would like this situation to be approached with the family, as well as further discussion with the family, should be undertaken.

Patients can be from a different culture but still share a common language with health professionals. In instances where there are language differences, however, a significant barrier to communication exists. Unless information can be translated competently and completely, patient teaching interventions will be ineffective. If possible, services of a professional medical translator should be requested. Health professionals should be aware that translations can be skewed, misinterpreted, or filtered when family members or others who only have a working knowledge of the language are utilized as translators.

Cultural history can also influence patient teaching about end-of-life issues, especially where there has been a history of inequities and conflict between cultural groups or where mistrust, prejudice, and discrimination have existed. For example, in discussions about advanced care planning and end-of-life decision making, patients in some cultures may be more likely to desire full and prolonged life support for fear of premature termination of life based on prejudice, whereas individuals in other cultures who have not experienced the same degree of prejudice or discrimination may prefer limited intervention or withholding treatment when death is imminent.

Health professionals must always be aware of cultural influences and how these have shaped their lives and practices. They should also be aware of possible differences between their own beliefs and those of patients from cultures different from their own. In addition to awareness of cultural differences, health professionals should be aware of intergenerational differences in beliefs, reactions, and adherence to traditions about end-of-life issues, even within the same culture. Culture is not stagnant but rather is continually evolving. Consequently, health professionals should not assume that values, beliefs, and traditions that a culture held relevant many years ago are necessarily still prevalent today. Patient teaching about end-of-life issues with individuals from different cultures should focus on respect for individual differences, promoting mutual understanding.

Even when individuals from other cultures have become acculturated into a new society, it is important to note that in death, people often revert to their own cultural roots. Health professionals should not assume that individuals who have apparently incorporated beliefs and values of a new culture into their own life have necessarily abandoned their own cultural beliefs, especially in discussions of death and dying. Clarification of values without making assumptions helps health professionals avoid misunderstanding in these instances.

Although maintaining cultural sensitivity is important, individual variations exist within each culture. Factors such as educational and socioeconomic status as well as other individual factors can impact a patient's cultural beliefs and values. The same approach may not be appropriate to all patients, even when they are from the same culture. Consequently, approaches to patient teaching about end-of-life issues should be adapted to fit the patient's cultural norms and individual needs.

UNDERSTANDING END-OF-LIFE ISSUES IN THE CONTEXT OF THE PATIENT

Health professionals' awareness of their own personal feelings about death and dying is an important component of effective patient teaching about end-of-life issues; however, another important consideration is health professionals' understanding the meaning death and dying has to individual patients (Bone, 1997). Not everyone shares the same concept of the meaning of death. Likewise, not everyone's outward report of their concept coincides with their unconscious or internal beliefs.

There is no standard meaning of death. Each patient brings a unique perspective to death and dying. This individual perspective is dependent on culture, religion, past experiences, and general philosophy of life. When conducting patient teaching about end-of-life issues, health professionals must be ever mindful of individual differences, considering the patient's perspective. To be maximally effective, patient teaching information about end-of-life issues should be presented within that context.

Reactions to Bad News

Receiving news of a life-threatening or terminal condition is an individual experience. However, it has multiple dimensions that also involves the patient's family and friends, as well as health professionals. Not all patients react to the diagnosis of life-threatening or terminal illness in the same way, nor do they progress in their reactions to the diagnosis in predictable stages (Peteet et al., 1991). Although the way patients react to bad news is individual, most patients experience cognitive, emotional, behavioral, and physical reactions to the information. Health professionals should remember, however, that "bad news" is contextual—it is not interpreted in the same way by everyone. How news is interpreted may depend on the nature of the news and the meaning the individual attaches to the news. Take the following case as an example.

Ms. Bridger had been having vague symptoms for the past 8 months. Sometimes she felt dizzy; sometimes she felt weak and tired; other times she experienced loss of appetite. She made an appointment with her physician, but there were no physical findings that accounted for her symptoms. Her symptoms would subside for a while but then reappear. She sought opinions from a number of physicians, all of whom could find no reason for her symptoms. One physician suggested that her symptoms were results of work-related stress, although she insisted she loved her job as a teacher. Her family also began to doubt the physical nature of her symptoms, suggesting that it appeared her symptoms seemed to flare up only when there was something she didn't want to do. Ms. Bridger became very discouraged and withdrawn. Finally, she decided to attempt one more time to solve the mystery of her symptoms, seeking an opinion from yet another physician. After listening to her symptoms and history, conducting an examination, and ordering a series of diagnostic tests, the physician finally discovered that Ms. Bridger had non-Hodgkin's lymphoma. In preparing to tell Ms. Bridger of the diagnosis, the doctor told a colleague, "I really dread giving this type of diagnosis. I never like giving bad news." The physician was surprised, however, when Ms. Bridger responded to the news with relief. "I am so relieved that there is a physical cause for what I've been experiencing. Not knowing why I felt like I did, and having everyone think I was crazy or that I was making the symptoms up was really getting to me. Now I know the cause, even though it is a serious condition, I can at least plan accordingly."

Ms. Bridger's condition was a serious one, and the news still implied potential loss. Despite the potentially life-threatening nature of her condition and losses she could be expected to experience, she felt relief now that she knew the diagnosis and could plan accordingly. Although different reactions and issues may be associated with a diagnosis of a life-threatening or terminal condition, patients may react in a way similar to Ms Bridger, putting energy into planning for the future.

Fear

A natural first reaction to a diagnosis that threatens one's existence is fear. Patients may fear death, but also, more than death itself, they may fear the process of dying. Fear may lie in the uncertainty of what the process of dying holds. Many patients fear the potential pain and discomfort associated with dying. Assuring patients that all measures will be taken to keep them as comfortable as possible and providing them with practical information about how symptoms they may be experiencing can be controlled can help decrease fear.

Patients may also fear being deserted by family, friends, or perhaps even by health professionals. Although there is no way of predicting reactions of family and friends, promoting active inclusion and participation of those individuals to whom the patient feels close helps strengthen relationships and bonding between individuals. Active collaboration and building a partnership between patient and health professional also helps to decrease fears and reassures the patient that help will be provided when they need it most.

Fears of loss of dignity and/or loss of control can be lessened by encouraging and respecting patient autonomy and authority in their own care and by exploring and maintaining as many areas of control for the patient as possible. If the patient had previously addressed end-of-life issues through a living will or advance directives, reassuring patients that their wishes will be adhered to can also reduce fear.

Patients may fear that medical costs could jeopardize continued medical care or treatment, or could cause significant financial burden to family. Referrals to appropriate personnel and social agencies can help patients sort out their concerns and help them determine how financial concerns can be addressed.

Denial

Some patients react to the life-threatening or terminal nature of a condition through denial of implications of the diagnosis. Denial, especially in the initial stages, can be one of the most pervasive and persistent responses to dying. Denial, however, expresses itself in different ways. Individuals may totally avoid admitting anything is wrong, or they may acknowledge the seriousness of their diagnosis but deny the terminal nature of the condition. This reaction is not uncommon, especially initially. Patients may be unable to accept or assimilate the seriousness of their condition, such as was the case of Mr. Kottke. After undergoing a liver biopsy, Mr. Kottke was found to have end-stage nonalcoholic fatty liver disease. Liver transplantation was recommended. He declined the procedure, stating, "Oh, I'm sure that can't be a correct diagnosis; I just had a physical exam last year and everything was fine."

Patients may also react by distorting the facts and placing a more favorable prognosis on the diagnosis than is warranted. Mrs. Jameson's physician informed her that she had an inoperable malignant tumor of the brain. When she told family and friends about her diagnosis, however, she was heard to say, "The doctor said I have a tumor on the brain, but luckily didn't say I had cancer, so although it's serious, I think I'll be alright."

Denial can be a protective mechanism when the diagnosis causes more stress than the patient can cope with at the time. Unfortunately, denial can also result in avoidance of medical care and treatment that could prolong life or make life more comfortable for a longer period of time. In some instances, although the seriousness of the condition is not denied, the terminal nature of the condition may be, causing patients to frantically seek other medical or nonmedical options, which can be costly and at times harmful, causing additional suffering or even earlier death.

Patients who deny the terminal nature of their condition may be unable to cope with the pain and anxiety associated with the reality that accompanies the threat of loss of self. Acceptance of patients' feelings builds trust and provides time for patients to begin to assimilate the diagnosis and work toward acceptance. Forcing patients to face the reality of the diagnosis before they are able to accept it only increases anxiety, causes alienation, fractures trust, and potentially delays the possibility of helping patients accept their diagnosis. By expressing care and concern as well as offering patient support, health professionals provide patients the opportunity to gradually accept the threat of the diagnosis so they may adjust to the terminal nature of their illness.

Anxiety

Anxiety is a universal reaction to threat and is a common reaction to a diagnosis that implies potential or imminent threat to life. One source of anxiety is related to loss. Health professionals can help patients deal with their sense of loss by being available to them and understanding what loss means to them and how it affects them.

No one knows exactly what it is like to die. Death is an unknowable and irreversible experience. A major source of anxiety about death in some patients may stem from loss of the unknown. Questions of what lies ahead, the thought of nothingness, or the concept of ceasing to exist can all be sources of anxiety for the patient. Health professionals can reduce patient anxiety by demonstrating willingness to listen to patients' fears and concerns. Approaching patient concerns in a nonjudgmental manner creates an atmosphere of trust and confidence, thereby decreasing anxiety.

In other instances, patients' anxiety may be related to fear of separation from loved ones or loss of the comfort and self-esteem such relationships provide. Exploring the significance of patients' relationships and acknowledging their importance helps establish a sense of continuity and meaning. Fostering interactions between patients and those they hold dear, as well as encouraging involvement in life and with other people, can be a source of strength for all concerned. If conflicts between the patients and family members exist, helping patients identify resources that enable them to explore opportunities for resolution can also allay anxiety.

Patients' anxiety, in some instances, may not be caused by their realization that they will lose contact with loved ones, but rather because of fear about the consequences their death will have on those they care about. Patients may perceive their death as loss of ability to provide assistance or support to family members. Take, for example, Mr. Pearson. At the age of 90, he stated he felt he had lived a successful, productive life, and did not fear his own death per se. He did, however, relate that he felt considerable anxiety because after his own death he feared what would happen to his wife who had dementia.

Another example is that of Mr. Appleton. Mr. Appleton's wife and three children appeared to have accepted the terminal nature of his condition and offered him support and consolation. Despite his close-knit family, Mr. Appleton continued to experience anxiety. He stated that he worried constantly about the impact his death would have on his family's financial stability. In the case of both Mr. Pearson and Mr. Appleton, identifying and acknowledging their fears and then assisting them to identify resources that could be used to help them plan for the future could provide a mechanism through which potential solutions can be reached, thus decreasing anxiety levels.

Other patients experience anxiety when confronted with end-of-life issues because of fear of loss of dignity and integrity. They may fear loss of control of their life, of their self, of their body, or of the ability to master their own fate. Patients can be helped to explore remaining areas in which they do have control or in which they can take more control. Providing patients with information about how to control symptoms, as well as collaborating with patients in the management of their care, can help them gain a sense of control and consequently reduce anxiety. By respecting and encouraging patient autonomy and authority in those matters in which they can make choices, a sense of control and freedom can be fostered.

If patients have not planned advance directives, helping them outline specific wishes and assuring them of cooperation and support of health professionals in carrying out their wishes can also be a means of reducing anxiety. If the patient has already prepared advance directives, reviewing the directives with the patient and providing reassurance can also bring a measure of peace.

Grief

Grief is a normal reaction to loss. It is to be expected that patients who experience a life-threatening or terminal illness will also experience grief to some degree. Grief can be manifested in a number of ways, from physical symptoms to psychological symptoms including depression. Health professionals can help patients through the grieving process by acknowledging grief and exploring ways to deal with it. A first step is to listen and acknowledge patients' expressions of feelings. Teaching patients that grief is an expected reaction to loss helps them to recognize symptoms that may be related to grief as well as helps them normalize reactions they may be experiencing. The following types of statements may be helpful: "Grief is a natural and normal reaction to loss. We've just talked about some of the losses you feel you will be experiencing because of your diagnosis. Grief is a reaction to those experiences and feelings that you have in response to the losses. As painful as grief is, however, it can be used to learn new approaches to living and to relating. There is no one right way to grieve and there is no timetable associated with it. It is an individual process that each person experiences differently."

Health professionals can help patients identify sources of support, such as family, friends, church, or other social groups. Patient support groups can also help patients be in touch with others with similar experiences. Sharing feelings in an atmosphere of understanding can help patients work through their grief and reach acceptance.

Helping patients review and identify their strengths and abilities can also promote confidence in their ability to cope. Other interventions that can help patients cope are providing written information, acknowledging reactions and feelings, and providing opportunities for patients to express feelings. Some patients may find it helpful to record their thoughts and experiences in a journal. Writing out thoughts can help patients express feelings as well as clarify issues that they may otherwise find difficult to bring into focus or to express verbally.

Anger

When threatened with the potential or imminent loss of life, patients may react with anger. Angry outbursts may be directed toward those individuals closest to the patient or toward health professionals most involved in an attempt to help.

Take, for example, the case of Mr. Lovelace. Mr. Lovelace was unaware he was living with human immunodeficiency virus (HIV), although he had had significant weight loss and had begun to experience other symptoms that he couldn't explain. When he was admitted to the hospital for elective surgery, results of routine preoperative surgical lab tests showed him to be HIV positive.

In conducting the preoperative interview, it was noted that he had begun to experience symptoms consistent with the diagnosis of acquired immunodeficiency syndrome (AIDS). When the physician discussed the diagnosis with him, Mr. Lovelace became extremely angry. His anger was directed not only toward his physician but also toward the nurses responsible for his care. He insinuated that they were incompetent and threatened to sue the physician for defamation of character.

Mr. Lovelace's expressions of anger, although directed at health professionals, were actually a reflection of anxiety related to his diagnosis. Although his physician and nurses were not responsible, nor could they cure his condition, Mr. Lovelace's anxiety about the condition caused him to lash out at those most readily available to help.

Reactions of hostility, anger, or defensiveness may be difficult for health professionals to accept. Hostility or anger, however, should be viewed as a symptom with meaning that should be explored, not ignored or avoided. Communicating understanding of the distress brought about by the situation helps patients gradually come to grips with their anger and reach acceptance of the situation at hand. Although communicating understanding may not help patients immediately resolve their anger, it affords patients the opportunity to work through their anger in a supportive atmosphere, increasing the likelihood that a helping relationship can be established.

Retreat

Patients may also react to bad news through retreat. Ms. Castilano, who had surgery for breast cancer, underwent radiation and chemotherapy after surgery. After treatment, she was relieved to hear that the physician was 95% sure that all cancer cells had been eradicated. When Ms. Castilano began experiencing symptoms several years later, she was again evaluated by her physician. The cancer was found to have metastasized to the extent that only palliative treatment could be of benefit. Ms. Castilano accepted the diagnosis calmly and returned to her apartment where she stayed for weeks, refusing to go out, refusing to answer the phone, and refusing to answer the door.

Reflection

Other patients may use the diagnosis of life-threatening or terminal conditions to reexamine goals and values, altering both to reach a higher level of growth. Such individuals may become more acutely aware of their environment and those in it. They may become more compassionate and caring, directing their life toward the needs of others.

For example, Mr. Fang experienced severe heart disease. He received a heart transplant but was told that in all likelihood the transplant would help him survive no longer than 5 years. "I feel like I have a new lease on life," he told friends. "All the things I once thought were important, such as my social status and advancing in my profession, no longer seem so important. I may have limited time, but I'm going to make the best of it. I want to spend more time with my children. I want to volunteer at the Senior Citizen Center, helping others; things I never took time to do before."

Humor

Individuals who have used humor as a coping mechanism in their healthier life or who see humor as a way of maintaining a sense of self may react with humor in face of adversity, a reaction some health professionals may interpret as inappropriate. Patients using humor in this way should not have their efforts thwarted but rather should be encouraged to continue to use humor as a coping mechanism, if it is appropriate for them. As an example, Mr. Andreasi, upon learning from his physician, Dr. Lawrence, that he had amyotrophic lateral sclerosis responded by saying, "That sure won't do much for my golf game." Dr. Lawrence was shocked by the response and later said to the nurse, "Mr. Andreasi obviously is denying the seriousness of his condition," when in fact, Mr. Andreasi was well aware of the seriousness and implications of his condition and was merely using humor as a way to cope with news, which he found devastating.

Humor should not, of course, be imposed on the individual by health professionals. Health professionals should be sensitive to the patient's needs, taking cues from the patient and participating in humor to the extent the patient continues to do so. Health professionals should be cautious, however, that patients are not made to feel they have to continue to approach their condition in a humorous way to keep up appearances or for the sake of others. Being available, open, and sensitive to patients communicates willingness of health professionals to accept them as they are, whether or not humor is used.

UNDERSTANDING END-OF-LIFE ISSUES IN THE CONTEXT OF THE FAMILY

In an attempt to approach patient teaching about end-of-life issues from a holistic point of view, health professionals may tend to think of families as a single entity, as if all members of the family share the same views and values. Health professionals should be continually mindful, however, of individual differences regarding adaptation and coping with crisis in general and in issues related to death and dying in particular. Consequently, assumptions about shared values within a family should not be made. It may not be possible to approach all family members in the same way. By considering individual differences, health professionals can better help family members understand and appreciate each other's perspectives as well as the perspective of the patient. Sensitive intervention can increase family members' tolerance for variation of perspectives among family members.

Each family member is involved, to some degree, in the overall functioning of the family, whether financially, emotionally, or by merely being a physical presence. The roles and contributions each family member makes to the overall functioning of the family is determined to a large part by the age of the individual as well as other factors. When a family member becomes ill, and especially if illness is life-threatening or terminal, family roles are disrupted. The family member who has the life-threatening or terminal condition may have decreased ability to contribute to the family emotionally and may be unable to participate in daily tasks once associated with their role. They may also be unable to contribute financially to the family. Consequently, other family members may need to assume additional responsibilities, thus potentially increasing stress on individuals within the family unit.

Not only does the patient's illness affect the family, but how the family responds also affects the patient (Davies, 2006). Families may react to a diagnosis of life-threatening or terminal illness in a myriad of ways. Some reactions are determined by personality or temperament of individual family members. Reactions may also be determined by the role the patient played within the family unit. For example, if the patient was the authority figure and decision maker of the family, family members may experience insecurity and instability if the patient is no longer able to function in the leadership role.

Intergenerational differences, integrated with gender and cultural factors, can also alter views of end-of-life issues. It is important for health professionals to affirm values of protection, respect, and loyalty, and identify with the family to enhance the ability of the family to accept and understand individual differences, thus facilitating positive communication about issues of death and dying.

How family members react to the diagnosis can impact on their response to the patient and, in turn, to the patient's response to their diagnosis. While some families may be supportive and open in communication with the patient by helping them process and accept the information, other families may attempt to shield patients from what they consider trauma of the news. They may play down the serious nature of the condition or attempt to withhold additional information from the patient. In some instances, families become angry, blaming the patient for the diagnosis. At times, because of their own fear and anxiety, family members may withdraw from the patient completely. In other instances, withdrawal is a result of family members' perceived inadequacy of no longer knowing what to do or what to say.

Health professionals, sensitive to family members' needs, can help families cope by providing information related to reactions to life-threatening and terminal conditions, by helping them learn how to assist in the care of the patient, and by increasing their awareness that it is often not what they say or do but merely their very presence that is the most important to the patient.

Although the presence of family members can offer solace to patients, health professionals should not make the assumption that family members are a source of strength and support for the patient. At times, depending on the relationship and the patient's and family members' reactions to the diagnosis, family members can cause the patient additional stress. Relationships that were strained before the illness can become more strained because of the diagnosis of a life-threatening or terminal condition. Family members with strong, opposite preferences can cause increased conflict. Patient preferences regarding involvement of family members should be assessed and their wishes should be respected.

Just as patients have rights and responsibilities that should be respected, so do family members. Health professionals can help family members recognize that they have the right not to be blamed for the patient's diagnosis and that they have a right to maintain as normal a family life as possible. By helping family members gain information about illness and treatment, as well as helping them understand what might be expected, health professionals enable them to cope with the situation at hand. Health professionals should remain nonjudgmental when working with family members of patients with a life-threatening or terminal condition. The goal should be not only to help family members accept the patient and his or her diagnosis but also to help the family members accept the patient's rights to his or her own preferences and decision making, especially should those preferences and decisions differ from those of the family.

COMMUNICATION SKILLS IN TEACHING ABOUT END-OF-LIFE ISSUES

Good communication skills are essential to forming an open and trusting relationship with the patient. Also important is demonstrating sensitivity to individual patient needs. These skills are the foundation of all effective patient teaching. Never are these skills more critical, however, than when discussing end-of-life issues with patients and their families (Soriano, 2007). Patients who feel accepted as individuals are more likely to divulge feelings and thoughts about issues and preferences surrounding death and dying. They will also be more receptive to information they are given (Detmar et al., 2001).

When teaching about end-of-life issues, it is important to use responses that communicate that the health professional both hears and understands what the patient is saying and experiencing. Patients should not be interrupted when they are attempting to express feelings or explain their views; however, health professionals should convey a sincere desire to grasp what patients are saying. This can be accomplished by clarifying the meaning of what the patient is expressing. For example, if the patient makes a statement such as, "I'm just not sure I can tell my mother about the serious nature of my diagnosis," the health professional may respond with a statement such as, "Do you mean you're afraid of how you might respond when telling her, or that you are afraid of how she will react?" By making such a response, the health professional communicates the desire to understand the patient's concerns by asking for additional clarification. If, however, in the same scenario, the health professional knows from previous interactions that the patient's main concern is the emotional fragility of the mother, the health professional may respond with a statement such as, "You're really concerned that this may be very hard for your mother." This statement conveys not only the health professional's desire to understand but that he or she actually does understand the meaning of what the patient said.

Responses that restate and reflect feelings the patient has expressed communicate both understanding and caring. For example, if a patient were to make a statement such as, "I feel so self-centered because it seems all I do is think about my future right now," an appropriate response may be, "It sounds like you're feeling selfish, when in fact it is perfectly natural to have feelings of concern. That's really important for you to do right now." Such a response communicates acceptance, gives reassurance, and encourages the patient to further discuss feelings and concerns. Health professionals who actively listen to patients, observing both verbal and nonverbal cues, increase effectiveness of patient teaching about end-of-life issues.

TEACHING ABOUT ADVANCED PLANNING

Patient teaching about advanced planning regarding end of life is a collaborative effort between the patient, his or her family, and the health professional. The purpose of advanced planning is to help the patient clarify goals, values, and preferences for future medical treatment (Tulsky, 2005). Included in advanced planning are advance directives and living wills.

An advance directive is a legal document in which patients exert their right to accept or refuse medical care even if they should be incapacitated and unable to make their own decisions (Levenson & Feinsod, 1998). The document came out of a Supreme Court ruling, which was followed by the Patient Self-Determination Act. Under the Patient Self-Determination Act, healthcare facilities are obligated, among other things, to educate patients about advance directives and about their right to accept or refuse treatment (Lynn, Miles, & Olick, 1998).

There are several types of advance directives, but the most common are the living will and durable power of attorney for health care (Emanuel et al., 2000; Parkman & Calfee, 1997). Living wills enable patients to describe the type of health care they would or would not wish to receive in certain medical situations. Durable power of attorney for health care enables patients to specify what type of care they would or would not want to receive in certain medical situations, as well as to appoint an individual or proxy to make decisions for them if they are unable to do so.

The ultimate goal of advance directives is to provide patients with autonomy to make their own decisions about end-of-life care and to communicate these choices clearly to family, friends, and healthcare providers (Arenson et al., 1996). Having advance directives can help to ward off potential disagreements between family members who may have different perceptions about what they think the patient wants. Advance directives can also ease the burden of decision making for the family.

Patients may not be aware of the importance of engaging in end-of-life discussions, especially if they are not currently faced with a life-threatening or terminal condition. They may be unaware that they have the right to be involved in end-of-life decision making. Patients may also be reluctant to initiate discussion of end-of-life issues because they believe health professionals do not have the time or are unreceptive to taking time for this type of discussion. Raising patients' awareness of their right to be active participants in end-of-life decisions, and creating an atmosphere that conveys receptivity on the part of health professionals to this type of discussion, can be done easily. Information about advance directives can be obtained from local, state, and national organizations. Flyers, brochures, or posters that encourage patients to ask their healthcare provider about advance directives or other end-of-life issues can be displayed in waiting rooms of physician offices, health clinics, or hospitals. Information can also be disseminated when patients are discharged from the hospital, at health clinic checkouts, or with regular mailings patients receive. Actively attempting to provide patients with information conveys the importance of this type of planning and communicates openness and willingness on the part of the health professional to engage in discussion about end-of-life issues.

Ideally, patients initiate end-of-life discussions on their own from interest in and willingness to attend to practical issues in the event they are faced with a life-threatening or terminal situation. In many instances, despite efforts to communicate with patients about end-of-life issues, patients may be unaware of the importance of advance planning. In these cases, the health professional may choose to instigate the discussion. Health professionals can take the initiative and approach the subject with the patient with a statement such as, "We all have the right to participate in making decisions about medical care and treatment at end of life. The best time to make those decisions is before the situation occurs, when we can discuss possibilities rationally. Even though you aren't currently faced with a life-threatening situation, none of us know when we could be faced with a disease or an accident in which end-of-life decisions need to be made. If that situation would occur, have you thought of how you might like things handled, or what you would or would not want to have done medically?"

Discussion about advance directives can be directive or nondirective. Directive approaches to discussions focus on problem solving, helping patients identify or clarify specific problems and issues, and on identifying how those problems and issues might be resolved. Nondirective approaches facilitate communication with the patient. Patients should be encouraged to express concerns and questions freely so that a clear understanding of what advance directives mean can be reached.

Patients may not have given thought to their values, beliefs, and priorities should they be faced with a life-threatening situation. In these instances, it may be useful to help patients explore their attitudes about life and death, identifying what is important to them. Although patients can be helped to clarify their values through discussion, several "values history forms" are also available to help patients clarify values (Doukas & McCullough, 1991). Values history forms contain a list of values from which patients can identify the ones that are most consistent with their own definition of quality of life. Whether engaging in discussion with patients about their values or using a values history form, in all instances patients should be allowed to set the pace and agenda.

The focus of communication about end-of-life issues should be on developing a mutual understanding between the patient and health professional so that patients' preferences about end-of-life care are identified and correctly interpreted (Kassirer, 1994). Reaching this type of understanding helps to prevent potential conflict between patients, family, and health professionals when a life-threatening or terminal condition does occur. Patients should be encouraged to discuss their values and preferences with their family. If there is a religious affiliation, patients may also want to discuss end-of-life issues with members of their religious community.

At times, advance directives can be so general that their content is open to wide interpretation (Siegler & Levin, 2000). For instance, an advance directive that states that "no extraordinary means should be taken" can be interpreted in a number of ways, depending on individual perceptions of the meaning of "extraordinary." To be useful, advance directives should address patient preferences specifically, in language that is clear, concise, and free of multiple interpretations. Patients should be taught about life-sustaining measures such as cardiopulmonary resuscitation, artificial ventilation, hydration, and nutrition. They should be helped to understand that they have the right to refuse all of the treatment or only some of it.

Health professionals should ensure that patients have a clear understanding of the meaning of what the advance directive means. The health professional should also make sure that he or she understands exactly what the patient means when the patient states his or her wishes. For example, Dr. Adams had engaged in a long discussion with Mr. Hadley about advance directives. Mr. Hadley was adamant about wanting everything done for him during end-of-life care. Dr. Adams interpreted this to mean that Mr. Hadley wanted life-support measures instituted. At a later visit, the nurse discovered, in reviewing the advance directives with Mr. Hadley, that by "everything," Mr. Hadley meant he wanted to be kept as comfortable and pain free as possible, not to be kept alive by artificial means. In another instance, Mrs. Coleman told Ms. Donnley, the nurse, that she wanted no artificial life support. As Ms. Donnley further questioned Mrs. Coleman, however, it became evident that Mrs. Coleman only meant mechanical ventilation when referring to life support, not nutrition and hydration.

Teaching patients about end-of-life issues may take place over several visits. When patients are unfamiliar with advance directives or living wills, they may be sent home with sample copies as well as with information explaining advance directives, living wills, and their purpose. Patients may need time to reflect on preferences for end-of-life care, on who they would name as a durable power of attorney, and whether different disease scenarios may warrant different procedures. More detailed discussion can then take place during subsequent teaching sessions after patients have had the opportunity to read the material, think about their values, and clarify their preferences for end-of-life care.

Patients' treatment preferences and priorities regarding end-of-life issues may change over time. Periodic review of advance directives, preferences and priorities, and specifications for durable power of attorney for health care helps assure that the type of care the patient has specified is current with their current wishes.

Teaching patients about advance directives and helping them clarify their values so they can make decisions about life-sustaining treatments before a crisis is an essential skill for health professionals. Health professionals should have an understanding of legal and ethical issues as well as practical issues involved in individual situations. They should also be aware of specific laws in their state regarding withholding or withdrawing life-sustaining treatments.

In all instances, plans should be customized to the patients' individual needs and desires.

DELIVERING BAD NEWS

Giving patients bad news is a difficult task for most health professionals. From patients' perspectives, receiving news about progression of a chronic condition, a diagnosis of a life-threatening condition, or news that they have a terminal condition is a traumatic event. The extent of the negative impact of bad news is often related not to the information itself but to how the information is delivered. How the news is presented can impact the way patients respond to recommendations for future care and treatment and can set the tone for how the entire illness experience is handled by patients and their families (Ptacek & Eberhardt, 1996).

What constitutes bad news is subjective (Ambuel & Mazzone, 2001). Bad news can be defined as news the patient does not want to hear. Patients and health professionals may have differing views as to the meaning of the news. News considered as benign by health professionals may be considered catastrophic by the patient and visa versa. Take, for example, Mrs. Lopez, who had come to the health clinic for a pregnancy test. The nurse, assuming that a positive test would be joyous news for Mrs. Lopez excitedly announced to her that the test was positive and indeed she was pregnant. Mrs. Lopez burst into tears, obviously upset with confirmation of the diagnosis. Because of different meanings news may have for patients and health professionals, health professionals need to be sensitive to patients' perspectives and reactions before making assumptions about the impact. Health professionals should be ready and available to tend to patients' emotional needs and reactions, no matter what they are.

The amount of information patients want about their condition, especially if the diagnosis is unfavorable, is frequently underestimated by health professionals (Covinsky et al., 2000). Most patients want to be given information about their condition even if the news is bad (Peteet et al., 1991). Evidence suggests that although patients may initially experience a negative emotional impact from bad news, they generally adjust well in the long term.

Because breaking bad news can be a difficult task, providing patients with bad news may be delayed, or the responsibility for giving bad news may be passed from health professional to health professional. As a result, patients receive scattered, and at times inconsistent, information. Generally, the health professional who delivers the bad news should be an individual who has had or who will continue to care for the patient. In some instances, more than one health professional may participate in relaying the information, especially if there have been several health professionals closely involved with the patient. Information should be presented in a manner appropriate to the individual patient and should be presented in a compassionate, direct manner.

In most instances, patients should be given the news directly and in person. In most cases, giving patients or family members bad news over the phone should be avoided. There may be circumstances, however, in which giving bad news over the phone is the only option. Under these circumstances, information should be provided in the same sensitive way as if it were being given to the patient or family member face-to-face. It is especially important under these circumstances to determine that patients have access to support in their location. Take the example of Mrs. Saunders and her daughter, Ms. Flint. Mrs. Saunders, an 85-year-old woman living in her own home, fell, breaking her left hip. Ms. Flint, who lived several states away, immediately came to be with her mother during surgery and the postoperative period. Mrs. Saunders appeared to be progressing well and was transferred to an extended care facility for recovery and rehabilitation. Her daughter returned home, planning to return periodically to monitor her mother's progress. Shortly after Ms. Flint returned home, Mrs. Saunders unexpectedly experienced a pulmonary embolus and died. The nurse had no choice but to relay the news of Mrs. Saunders death to her daughter over the phone.

Before beginning discussion with patients, health professionals should be sure they have all the information needed, including potential resources that patients may find useful. When giving bad news, timing should be considered. The time chosen for delivering the news should be convenient for the patient and when they are relatively comfortable. Sufficient time should be allowed so that information is not presented in a rushed manner and so that there is time for patients to vent feelings and to ask questions. Patients should be given the option of having a family member or a friend present; however, if patients prefer no one else to be present, their wishes should be respected. If the patient chooses to have a friend or family member present who is unfamiliar to the health professional, the health professional should introduce him- or herself before beginning the discussion.

News should be delivered in a comfortable, relatively quiet location where there are no interruptions, and in which the patient has privacy. Presenting information to the patient in a hallway, waiting room, or the patient's hospital room where another patient is present should be avoided. If news is being given to the patient in an examining room, they should be allowed to dress before the discussion begins.

In most instances, health professionals should sit close to the patient and make sure no physical barriers, such as a desk, are separating them. This enhances health professionals' ability to monitor patient reactions and to use touch, when appropriate, for reassurance or comfort. Health professionals should be aware of their own body language while delivering the information, attempting to look as at ease as possible. Nonverbal cues should be used to convey warmth, sympathy, encouragement, or reassurance. Cues such as eye contact, rather than looking at the floor or out the window, and giving the patient full attention are crucial. Flipping through the chart or other materials, writing notes, or checking the clock should be avoided during the discussion.

Rather than giving the news immediately at the beginning of the session, it is usually helpful to begin with a statement that gives patients warning so that there is some preparation for bad news. Compare the differences in impact on Mr. Mason a patient returning to a clinic after being tested for HIV infection.

> *Scenario I*: The health professional walks into the room, sits down, looks at Mr. Mason, and says, "Your test show that you are HIV positive."
> *Scenario II*: The health professional walks into the room, greets Mr. Mason, sits down, then looks at Joseph and says, "We are here today to discuss the results of your lab tests. I'm afraid they didn't turn out as well as we had hoped. . . ."

In the first scenario, Mr. Mason has no time to prepare emotionally for the news he is about to receive, potentially causing him to be overwhelmed. The second scenario allows Mr. Mason time to ease into the notion that bad news is about to be given and to mobilize coping mechanisms that will make him better able to withstand the shock.

News should be delivered in a direct, nontechnical way. Although information should be honest and direct, it should also be presented in a hopeful way. Rather than saying, "You have a terminal condition and nothing can be done," a more appropriate statement may be, "Although currently there is no cure for your condition, there is much that can be done to help assure that you continue to be as comfortable as possible."

After patients have received bad news, health professionals should remain silent, allowing patients to absorb the news they have received, to ask questions, or to react. Time should be provided for exploration, expression of concerns, and review of the circumstances. Patients and their families should be allowed to express emotions freely. Reactions may consist of crying, silence, or anger. Regardless of feelings expressed, health professionals should convey a presence and acceptance of patients' feelings. By observing patients' reactions, health professionals will be better able to know how they can best lend support.

By listening to patients, health professionals can also determine how they are interpreting the news given. Patients' most immediate concerns can then be assessed and health professionals can then tailor their response to match patients' reactions. In Scenario II above, after hearing that he was HIV positive, Mr. Mason's first statement was, "You mean I'll be dead soon?" The health professional was able to explain to Mr. Mason that there are now a number of medications available that can help people who are HIV positive from developing symptoms of AIDS, thereby enabling them to continue to live productive lives with their diagnosis. The information given by the health professional did not provide false hope, but helped to correct misinterpretation of the information given, addressing Mr. Mason's most immediate concern.

After receiving bad news, ample time should be provided for patients to talk and to ask questions. After responding to patients' immediate concerns after receiving bad news, health professionals should assess the extent to which patients understand the information presented and their knowledge and understanding about the condition. In this way, patient teaching needs are identified and any misinformation present may be corrected. Before providing additional information, health professionals should assess patients' ability to absorb information. If the patient seems overwhelmed, additional information is better given at a later time. Patients are often in a state of shock after first hearing bad news and may not be able to immediately process additional information (Eden et al., 1994). In most instances, providing patients with additional, detailed information is better done at a later date when patients are more likely to hear and comprehend the information presented.

After being given bad news, patients may be emotionally devastated and consequently unable to carry out regular tasks safely. For example, if the patient has received bad news while at an outpatient facility, is unaccompanied, and is driving him- or herself home, the patient should be asked if there is someone who could be called to drive him or her home or if alternative means of transportation could be arranged. Other supports and resources available to the patient should also be assessed.

At subsequent patient teaching sessions, health professionals should be open to expression of emotional experiences and help patients and families gain a sense of personal control by encouraging them to be actively involved in treatment decisions. Pacing information and presenting it gradually over several patient teaching sessions in clear, understandable terms helps patients adapt and to incorporate information. Health professionals should be prepared to offer resources as needed such as support groups or other resources such as clergy or social service.

Arrangements for follow-up should be made. Additional questions may arise as patients have time to come to full realization of their diagnosis and its implications. Need and desire for additional information may also change. As patients adjust to the news, facts may need to be repeated or revised. Follow-up visits also enable health professionals to monitor patients' adjustment and provide additional assistance as the need arises.

TEACHING PATIENTS LIVING WITH
LIFE-THREATENING ILLNESS

End-of-life discussions may be precipitated when patients are living with a life-threatening condition (Cherny, Coyle, & Foley, 1996). Although patients may not be in the terminal stages of disease, the nature of the condition or its expected progression may necessitate discussion about the potential for death.

The prospect of dying raises many practical issues, and patients may look to health professionals to provide information that helps them address these issues. Resolving practical matters can help patients focus on issues of living with a life-threatening condition, thus enabling them to enhance their overall quality of life.

The nature and focus of patient teaching in end-of-life discussions with patients with life-threatening conditions should be based on patients' individual needs and priorities. Many of the same principles used in teaching patients with other conditions also apply to teaching patients with life-threatening illness. Timing of patient teaching, assessing specific learning needs, evaluating supports and barriers, appraising patients' social situation and life circumstances, and considering patients' abilities and willingness to follow recommendations are all crucial regardless of the patient's condition. The difference in patient teaching results from the emotionally charged potential of loss of life.

Under these circumstances, patients and their families need honest, realistic, and accurate information about the condition and general status of the patient, options for treatment, and prognosis (Shields, 1998). Only with clear, concise information can patients make informed choices about treatment and care. Having straightforward information about the condition and its prognosis also enables patients to establish priorities regarding personal or relationship issues or regarding business concerns they need to put in order.

Part of establishing patient priorities is to determine patient goals, which also help determine specific treatment preferences. Some patients may have a major goal of maximizing quantity of life, while others focus on quality. In either instance, patients' definition of terms should be clarified because concepts of quality and quantity of life can be broadly and individually defined. Although it is difficult to predict patients' reactions to life-threatening illness, open discussions help alleviate fears and build a sense of collaboration and support.

After diagnosis, patients may initially have extreme concern for the well-being and future of their family. They may have concern about abandonment and isolation. Financial issues in the face of increasing medical bills or potential loss of income if they are no longer able to work may be a major concern. There may be concern for the completion of various work-related projects. In other instances, patients may have major concerns about pain, discomfort, or loss of function as their condition progresses.

Patient teaching with patients with life-threatening conditions extends beyond teaching about their condition and treatment (Laury, 1987). In these circumstances, patient teaching should also be directed toward helping patients increase awareness and acceptance of their condition, and helping them frame their condition as a positive, life-promoting event. The manner in which patients are given information about a life-threatening illness is crucial so that a facilitative relationship can be established with the health professional.

In addition to providing patients with factual information about their condition and treatment, discussion may also include explorations of patients' underlying values, which can help them when faced with decisions to choose or decline various treatment options. In some instances, patients may choose end-of-life options because they fear the cost of ongoing medical care or that family members will view them as a burden. Although these reasons may be valid to the patient, the health professional can encourage the patient to further discuss his or her feelings and options, ascertaining that the patient has not been pressured to make decisions that are not within his or her value framework.

Information about treatment options should be provided in small pieces, with frequent pauses to assess patients' understanding of the information and the context in which specific treatment decisions might apply. Patients should be helped to determine how treatment options relate to their general goals or values. Although the amount of information patients want may vary, information provided should address potential consequences and implications for selecting as well as not selecting treatment options.

PATIENT TEACHING IN TERMINAL STAGES OF DISEASE

Personal care for patients in terminal stages of disease is an appropriate and expected part of the health professional's role (Engle, 1998). Even though treatment and cure may no longer be possible, active care of patients who are terminally ill is important. Effective patient teaching with individuals with terminal conditions needs a broader perspective than other patient teaching interactions. Although helping patients manage pain and increase physical comfort are essential tasks, helping them achieve emotional comfort is equally important (Perron & Schonwetter, 2001). Helping patients and families acknowledge the prospect of death gives patients the opportunity to focus attention on living the remainder of their life to the fullest extent possible. The last stages of life offer patients the opportunity to clarify priorities and values and to seek a stance most consistent with their own sense of self. Facilitation of this type of self-exploration as well as identifying practical considerations and patient priorities can help patients make informed choices, stay in control of their life as long as possible, and view death as an opportunity for growth.

Effective patient teaching in all situations depends on appropriate assessment of patient and family characteristics and needs and tailoring information to the individual. The same is true for patients with terminal illness. Assessment information provides a framework on which to base patient teaching activities and establish priorities for patient teaching. Helping patients learn to make adjustments in the last stage of life should be based on identifying patients' needs and priorities rather than those perceived by health professionals.

Health professionals should assess the patients' family system, identifying family members and specific roles they play within the family unit. Both formal and informal support networks should be identified. Information regarding previous family crises or losses and methods family members used to cope provides information that can be used to help patients and their family cope with the current situation. Identifying experiences patients and families have had with the healthcare system in the past can also help health professionals determine attitudes that can help or hinder care in the future. Take, for example, the case of Mr. Schmidt, who had been hospitalized in the final stages of AIDS. Mr. Schmidt's older brother had died of AIDS several years earlier. Mr. Schmidt's mother became very demanding of the nurses, berating them for not answering his light promptly enough or not adequately straightening his bed, and finding fault no matter how much they tried. Mrs. Dewitt, the nurse, approached Mr. Schmidt's mother one evening and said, "This situation must be very difficult for you, especially since you have already lost one son. How has that experience impacted how you deal with your son's current illness?" Mr. Schmidt's mother broke into tears. "When my first son was dying, everyone just ceased to care. No one checked on him. No one provided adequate care for him. He deserved more. I wasn't there to advocate for him. I won't let the same thing happen to my son now. Although we can't prevent him from dying, we can see to it that he has an appropriate death in which he is comfortable and at least treated with respect and concern."

For many people, dying an "appropriate" death means dying in a way consistent with their concept of self, maintaining values and ideals that guided them through life. Receiving a diagnosis of terminal illness places thoughts of death and dying at the forefront. Issues and concerns the patient and his or her family have about the patient's illness, and about death and dying, must be addressed. Patients may place priority on continuity of relationships with significant others. They may place priority on maintaining dignity and control. Many patients place priority on a death that is peaceful, relatively free of pain, and free of conflict.

When patients are terminally ill, concerns take on different meaning because dying, in this instance, is imminent and real. Although patients with conditions that are not terminal may still face alterations in perceptions of self and identity, patients with terminal illness face loss of self in addition to other things they hold dear such as family, job, or experiences they will not have in the future. Issues that health professionals may consider mundane may be of utmost importance to patients and may need to be addressed before patients are able to actively participate in other patient teaching activities.

Spiritual components of health and illness are imbedded in all aspects of health care (Anandarajah & Hight, 2001). Although spirituality may be part of an individual's religion, religion and spirituality are not synonymous. The health professional should not assume that a patient's spiritual needs or concerns are necessarily related to a religious affiliation. There are many dimensions of spirituality (Taylor, 2006). Regardless of religious affiliation, terminal illness, especially, adds a spiritual dimension that must be addressed and should not be underestimated or ignored. Although spiritual dimensions of experience should not be imposed on individuals, health professionals should be open to allowing patients to express their needs. If health professionals are uncomfortable discussing spiritual topics with patients, they should at least ask if the patient would like to speak with a clergy or other professional about these issues. Whether the referral takes place, and to whom the patient is referred, should, of course, be the patient's choice. When patients express spiritual needs, it is often a comfort for them to know that their needs were acknowledged and that the health professional took steps to help them meet those needs, even if it was in the form of a referral.

Patient teaching with patients with terminal illness can help individuals learn to live with a terminal illness. The focus of patient teaching under these circumstances should be on issues the patient deems important. A crucial part of patient teaching in terminal illness is identifying and confronting concerns, developing interventions to deal with those concerns, and helping patients and families learn how to cope with the diagnosis (Reichel, 1999). Information needed will vary with individual patients. Some patients may need information that will help them make appropriate financial arrangements. Others may need information about burial or cremation, bequest of body or specified organs, or distribution of personal items. Patients may need information about hospice or about other services they can utilize at home. In some instances, they may need information about hospital care. In each of these instances, patient teaching information can be provided to the patient in the form of written material, or they may be given information about appropriate resources that can provide information they are requesting.

Patients' terminal conditions may take away their ability to control their environment as well as their ability to function effectively within it. This inability, in turn, can affect self-concept. Many of the values attached to self-concept are specific to the stage of development of the patient. Consequently the individual's stage of development and its impact on their perceptions and acceptance of their experience with death and dying must be considered. Patients should be helped to gain as much control as possible. Although the diagnosis or outcome cannot be changed, providing opportunities to explore their experience and options through patient teaching can help patients with terminal illness recognize that they still have choices and that they can control how they live in the terminal stages of their illness (Caloras et al., 2000).

Symptoms experienced by patients with terminal illness cause physical problems that require patient teaching to help patients achieve maximum relief from symptoms (Bruera & Byock, 2000; Frederich, 2001). Again, however, when teaching patients about control of symptoms, health professionals should clarify patients' values and preferences. For example, does quality of life during the terminal stages of illness mean being pain-free even though level of consciousness is affected as the result? Does quality of life mean staying alert and aware despite pain that may be experienced? Does the patient measure quality of life by functional capacity and independence, or is merely sanctity of life of the utmost importance?

Helping patients gain emotional comfort can also be addressed in patient teaching. One aspect of loss experienced by patients with terminal illness is the sense of self. By helping patients review their past, there may be a consolidation of sense of self and a validation of their sense of being. Patients can be encouraged to write journals outlining important events, reaffirming what they have been, or to jot down current thoughts and feelings. Journal writing can provide patients with a sense of completion. It should be noted that, although this activity may be helpful for some, it may not be appropriate for all patients with terminal illness. Health professionals still must remain sensitive to the needs and priorities of the individual.

When, in the terminal stages of illness, the patient is unable to speak for him- or herself, the person designated by the patient to make medical decisions should be asked about the patient's values and goals for care at end of life. Take, for example, Mrs. Carter, whose husband was in the terminal stages of cancer and in a coma. Dr. Jones approached Mrs. Carter with the following statement: "Your husband is dying. He is now unconscious so he can no longer make decisions for himself. We can insert a feeding tube into his stomach, which will keep him alive longer; however, it is uncertain at this point whether it will increase his quality of life. In fact, the tube may cause additional discomfort. What do you think he would want to do?"

Family members may not fully understand, or be ready to accept, the terminal nature of the patient's condition. In some instances, family members may understand the terminal nature of the condition but not the impact or implications of maintaining or continuing treatment. There are also situations in which disagreements about end-of-life decisions arise among family members. In each of these instances, health professionals should approach the family in a nonjudgmental way and should facilitate further exploration and explanation. Take, for example, the case of Mr. Bower.

Mr. Bower, an 84-year-old widower, experienced a massive stroke and was placed on a ventilator. Dr. James called the family together to discuss the gravity of Mr. Bower's condition and the limited chance of recovery. His three children had been emotionally close to Mr. Bower, although only his eldest son lived close by and saw him frequently. Because of geographic distance, Mr. Bower's other son and daughter visited him only once a year. When discussing the situation with the family, given the status of Mr. Bower's condition, Dr. James discussed the option of removing life support. Mr. Bower's eldest son, who saw his father more frequently and was more aware of his father's daily circumstances as well as his wishes and desires, was in favor of this option, but his other children, who saw their father infrequently and had no indepth understanding of his wishes were vehemently opposed. Dr. James said, "This type of decision is a very difficult one, I know. I wonder if we could explore each of your views a bit more and see if we can identify your expectations of the consequences and implications of taking your father off life support or leaving the life support in place." By encouraging family dialogue and exploration of feelings and beliefs about consequences of their decision, Dr. James enabled family members to voice their concerns and clarify their own realities regarding the decision. By further exploring the family's beliefs, Dr. James was also able to identify misinformation or unrealistic expectations family members may have and consequently address these issues. Such was the case of Mrs. Nance.

Mrs. Nance was in the terminal stages of pancreatic cancer. Although she was unresponsive, her children insisted that they wanted the doctor to "do everything." In this situation, it might be appropriate for the physician to make a statement such as, "Your mother is dying. There is no treatment we can provide that will prevent her death. We can, however, do much for your mother by keeping her as comfortable as possible." This statement helps clarify the situation for the family, while at the same time providing comfort in the knowledge that although there are not treatment options for cure or reversal of the condition, "something" can be done.

Some family members may find it helpful to be given general guidelines for caregiving. Teaching family members specific techniques for meeting patients' personal needs such as mouth care, skin care, nutrition, and elimination provides family members with a sense of confidence in providing care for their loved one. Helping family members learn how they can help patients with other specific needs such as pain management, control of nausea and vomiting, or breathing difficulties can help reduce anxiety and frustration when symptoms occur. Of course, not all family members are able to accept responsibility for this type of personal care, and if this is the case, patient teaching about personal care should be limited to their wishes and capabilities.

Effective patient teaching with families of patients with terminal illness depends to a great extent on their response to the diagnosis itself. Family members' responses throughout the dying process are determined by a number of factors, including the emotional make up of the family, the degree of family cohesion, and the role of the patient within the family structure. There may be unfinished emotional business with the patient that can alter family members' reactions to the diagnosis as well as to the patient.

Part of patient teaching should involve helping family members understand that as the patient's illness progresses, both physical and emotional needs will change. A major focus of patient teaching should include helping family members learn how they can be of help to the patient without taking away the patient's sense of independence and control. Providing families with information about resources and services available in the community can also help them feel a sense of control by helping them learn ways specific needs can be met.

Teaching family members specific things they can do to help patients manage their condition and how to maintain a relatively low-stress environment can also be helpful. Patients and family members should be encouraged to communicate so that family unity and mutual support is facilitated. Family members and the patients can be encouraged to talk openly about the diagnosis and to discuss experiences they are having. They can also be taught how to provide feedback to individuals within the family unit about specific behaviors and their impact.

Family members may begin the grief process while the patient is still alive. This type of grieving may be confusing for both the family and the patient. While family members are attending to the patient, they may also be beginning to anticipate their life without them. In some instances, family members may begin to divest emotional energy from the patient, investing it instead in preparation for life after the patient dies. Some divestment may be healthy and necessary for continued function. In instances where family members reach a state of emotional depletion, they may naturally begin to withdraw. Helping both the patient and family members understand this reaction helps to avoid misunderstanding and to facilitate future communication and understanding.

Family members should be helped to understand that they too have physical, emotional, and spiritual needs and that building time for self-care is crucial. Helping families balance attending to their own needs while still offering care and support to the patient are important aspects of patient teaching with patients who have terminal conditions.

CONDUCTING A FAMILY CONFERENCE

When advance directives are not available and the patient's condition has progressed so that decisions about withholding or withdrawing medical treatment must be addressed, detailed and complex dialogue with family members is appropriate. Such discussions are usually held in the context of the family conference. Although most states have a hierarchy regarding decision making and the legal next-of-kin retains responsibility for decisions, the ultimate goal in talking with family about these decisions is to gain consensus, if possible, among family members (Curtis et al., 2001).

The family conference should be approached with the same care and planning as other patient teaching activities. The conference should occur in a private room that provides little likelihood of interruption. Who will be present at the family conference should be decided in advance. Family members attending the family conference should be prepared for what to expect during the conference. They should be instructed that the purpose of the conference is to review the patient's status and to make decisions regarding the extent to which medical interventions should continue.

At the beginning of the family conference, the health professional should review the family's understanding of the patient's current situation. The patient's illness and treatment should be reviewed in terms the family can understand, avoiding medical jargon. Family members should be allowed to maintain hope even in a poor prognosis. This does not mean providing unrealistic or false information. Rather it means that the health professional helps the family to redirect their hope from cure to hope for maintaining as much comfort and dignity for the patient as possible. Discussion of the patient's values and goals should be encouraged by asking the family to speculate what the patient may want if they were able to participate in the decision-making process. Spending time reminiscing about the patient with the family can also put the family at ease and bring them comfort in the decision-making process.

During the family conference, family members should be given the opportunity to discuss their own feelings as well as spiritual, religious, or cultural needs. Feelings of the family should be acknowledged and action should be taken to address any unmet needs that have been expressed (Clary et al., 2000).

The family should be assured that even if treatment is withheld or withdrawn that the patient will not be abandoned and that he or she will continue to be cared for (Ackermann, 2000). After the patient's current medical situation and treatment options have been discussed, information should be reinforced by putting information and decisions into perspective. Questions family members raise should be addressed and family reactions to information discussed should be explored. If family members express strong emotions, these emotions should be acknowledged and explored. At times, family members may find expression of emotion difficult. In this case, health professionals should be respectful of the difficulty the family member is experiencing. Periods of silence should be tolerated while family members struggle to express feelings and emotions.

Before completion of the family conference, information discussed should be briefly summarized. Family members should then be offered a private place where they can engage in discussion among themselves and take time to agree on a decision if a decision has not yet been reached. After family members have had sufficient time to discuss the situation, the health professional should again convene the family and explore their feelings. Any disagreements that exist between family members regarding how to proceed should be identified. Decisions made by the family should be supported by the health professional. After making a decision, family members should be encouraged to visit, touch, and talk with the patient. Most importantly, if the decision to withhold or withdraw treatment has been made, the health professional should make a point of being available and checking on the patient and family frequently.

IMPACT OF END-OF-LIFE TEACHING

Patient teaching about end-of-life issues involves more than giving information. When talking with the patient about issues surrounding death and dying, the emotional bond between the health professional and patient and their family transcends information exchange. Patient teaching about end-of-life issues can be a meaningful and significant experience, bringing both the health professional and the patient to a deeper understanding of their own values and crucial life decisions.

REFERENCES

Ackermann, R. J. (2000). Withholding and withdrawing life-sustaining treatment. *American Family Physician, 62*(7), 1555–1560.

Ambuel, B., & Mazzone, M. F. (2001). Breaking bad news and discussing death. *Primary Care: Clinics in Office Practice, 28*(2), 249–267.

Anandarajah, G., & Hight, E. (2001). Spirituality and medical practice: Using the HOPE questions as a practical tool for spiritual assessment. *American Family Physician, 63*(1), 81–89.

Arenson, C. A., Novielli, K. D., Chambers, C. V., & Perkel, R. L. (1996). Models of ambulatory care: The importance of advance directives in primary care. *Primary Care: Clinics in Office Practice, 23*(1), 67–82.

Black, P. (2007). End-of-life care. In B. White & D. Truax. *The nurse practitioner in long-term care: Guidelines for clinical practice* (pp. 533–549). Sudbury, MA: Jones and Bartlett.

Bone, R. C. (1997). End-of-life issues: The physician's role. *Critical Care Medicine, 25*(6), 1083–1084.

Bruera, E., & Byock, I. (2000). Management of pain and other discomfort. *Patient Care, 34*(21), 38–45, 49–50, 52, 55–56, 59–62, 65, 69–71.

Buckman, R., Byrock, I., & Fry, V. L. (2000). Talking with patients and families. *Patient Care, 34*(21), 16–18, 20, 29, 33–36.

Cacchione, P. J. (2007). End-of-life care of the older adult. In: A. D. Linton & H. W. Zach. *Matteson & McConnell's gerontological nursing: Concepts and practice* (3rd ed., pp. 712–735). St. Louis: Saunders.

Caloras, D., Coloney, M. J., Kangas, C. A., & Wegryn, R. L. (2000). The virtues of hospice. *Patient Care, 34*(21), 72–74, 76–78, 80–81, 85–88, 91.

Cherny, N. I., Coyle, N., & Foley, K. M. (1996). Pain and palliative care: Guidelines in the care of the dying cancer patient. *Hematology/Oncology Clinics of North America, 10*(1), 261–286.

Clary, P. L., Ogle, K. S., Plumb, J. D., & Prendergast, T. J. (2000). The role of life prolonging technology. *Patient Care, 34*(21), 113–116, 119–126, 129.

Covinsky, K. E., Fuller, J. D., Yaffe, K., Johnston, C. B., Hamel, M. B., Lynn, J., et al. (2000). Communication and decision-making in seriously ill patients: Findings of the SUPPORT project. *Journal of the American Geriatrics Society, 48*, S187–S193.

Curtis, J. R., Patrick, D. L., Shannon, S. E., Treece, P. D., Engelberg, R. A., & Rubenfeld, G. D. (2001). The family conference as a focus to improve communication about end-of-life care in the intensive care unit: Opportunities for improvement. *Critical Care Medicine, 29*(Suppl 2), N26–N33.

Dahlin, C. M., & Giansiracusa, D. E. (2006). Communication in palliative care. In B. R. Ferrell & N. Coyle (Eds.). *Textbook of palliative nursing* (2nd ed., pp. 67–93). New York: Oxford University Press.

Dangler, L. A., O'Donnell, J., Gingrich, C., & Bope, E. T. (1996). What do family members expect from the family physician of a deceased loved one? *Family Medicine, 28*(10), 694–696.

Davies, B. (2006). Spiritual assessment. In B. R. Ferrell & N. Coyle (Eds.). *Textbook of palliative nursing* (2nd ed., pp. 545–560). New York: Oxford University Press.

Detmar, S. B., Muller, M. J., Wever, L. D. V., Schornagel, J. H., & Aaronson, N. K. (2001). Patient–physician communication during outpatient palliative treatment visits: An observational study. *Journal of the American Medical Association, 285*(10), 1351–1357.

Doran, M., & Geary, K. (2005). End of life. In K. D. Melillo, & S. C. Houde (Eds.). *Geropsychiatric and mental health nursing* (pp. 347–362). Sudbury, MA: Jones and Bartlett.

Doukas, D. J., & McCullough, L. B. (1991). The values history: The evaluation of the patient's values and advance directive. *Journal of Family Practice, 32*, 145–153.

Eden, O. B., Black, I., MacKinlay, G. A., & Emery, A. E. (1994). Communication with parents of children with cancer. *Palliative Medicine, 8*, 105–114.

Elder, N. C. (1996). Dealing with death in patients and families. *Family Medicine, 28*(10), 692–693.

Emanuel, E., Goold, S. D., Hammes, B. J., Lynn, J., & Tonelli, M. (2000). A detailed examination of advance directives. *Patient Care, 34*(21), 92–94, 97–98, 101–102, 105–108.

Engle, V. F. (1998). Care of the living, care of the dying: Reconceptualizing nursing home care. *Journal of the American Geriatrics Society, 46*(9), 1172–1174.

Finlay, I. G., & Dorman, S. (2006). Management of the dying patient. In M. S. J. Pathy, A. J. Sinclair, & J. E. Morley. *Principles and practice of geriatric medicine. Vol 2* (4th ed., pp. 2001–2016). West Sussex, England: Wiley.

Frederich, M. E. (2001). Non-pain symptom management. *Primary Care: Clinics in Office Practice, 28*(2), 299–316.

Friedman, S. (2007). Loss and end-of-life issues. In S. E. Meiner & A. G. Lueckenotte. *Gerontological nursing* (3rd ed., pp. 411–426). St. Louis: Mosby.

Garfinkle, C. L., & Block, P. (1996). Physicians' interactions with families of terminally ill patients. *Family Medicine, 28*(10), 702–707.

Hallenbeck, J. L. (2001). Intercultural differences and communication at the end of life. *Primary Care: Clinics in Office Practice, 28*(2), 401–413.

Hentz, R., & Tabloski, P (2006). Care of the dying. In P. A. Tabloski (Ed.). *Gerontological nursing* (pp. 294–325). Upper Saddle River, NJ: Pearson/Prentice Hall.

Kassirer, J. P. (1994). Incorporating patients' preferences into medical decisions. *New England Journal of Medicine, 330*(26), 1895–1896.

Klessig, J. (1998). Death and culture: the multicultural challenge. *Annals of Long-Term Care, 6*(9), 285–290.

Kvale, J., Berg, L., Groff, J. Y., & Lange, G. (1999). Factors associated with residents' attitudes toward dying patients. *Family Medicine, 31*(10), 691–696.

Laury, G. V. (1987). Sexuality of the dying patient. *Medical Aspects of Human Sexuality, 21*(6), 102–105, 109.

Levenson, S. A., & Feinsod, F. M. (1998). Obtaining instructions for care. *Annals of Long-Term Care, 6*(9), 295–300.

Lynn, J., Miles, S. H., & Olick, R. (1998). Making living wills and health care proxies more useful. *Patient Care, 32*(9), 181–182, 185–186, 189–192.

Moore, C. D. (2007). Advance care planning and end of life decision making. In K. K. Kuebler, E. Heidrich, & P. Esper (Eds.). *Palliative and end of life care: Clinical practice guidelines* (2nd ed., pp. 49–62). St. Louis: Saunders.

Parkman, C. A., & Calfee, B. E. (1997). Advance directives: Honoring your patient's end-of-life wishes. *Nursing, 27,* 48–53.

Perron, V., & Schonwetter, R. (2001). Hospice and palliative care programs. *Primary Care: Clinics in Office Practice, 28*(2), 427–440.

Peteet, J. R., Abrams, H. E., Ross, D. M., & Stearns, N. M. (1991). Presenting a diagnosis of cancer: patients' views. *Journal of Family Practice, 32*(6), 577–581.

Ptacek, J. T., & Eberhardt, T. L. (1996). Breaking bad news: A review of the literature. *Journal of the American Medical Association, 276*(6), 496–502.

Reichel, W. (1999). End-of-life care and family practice. *American Family Physician, 59*(6), 1388, 1395–1396.

Safonte-Strumolo, N., & Dunn, A. B. (2000). Consideration of cultural and relational issues in bereavement: the case of an Italian American family. *The Family Journal: Counseling and Therapy for Couples and Families, 8*(4), 334–340.

Schears, R. M. (1999). Ethical issues in emergency medicine: Emergency physicians' role in end-of-life care. *Emergency Medicine Clinics of North America, 17*(2), 539–559.

Shields, C. E. (1998). Oncology: Giving patients bad news. *Primary Care: Clinics in Office Practice, 25*(2), 381–390.

Siegler, E. L., & Levin, B. W. (2000). Communication between older patients and their physicians: physician–older patient communication at the end of life. *Clinics in Geriatric Medicine, 16*(1), 175–204.

Soriano, R. (2007). Overview of palliative care and non-pain symptom management. In R. Soriano (Ed.). *Fundamentals of geriatric medicine: A case based approach* (pp. 547–572). New York: Springer.

Stanley, M., Blair, K. A., & Beare, P. G. (2005). *Gerontological nursing: Promoting successful aging with older adults.* Philadelphia: F. A. Davis.

Taylor, E. J. (2006). Spiritual assessment. In B. R. Ferrell & N. Coyle (Eds.). *Textbook of palliative nursing* (2nd ed., pp. 581–594). New York: Oxford University Press.

Tulsky, J. A. (2005). Beyond advance directives: Importance of communication skills at the end of life. *Journal of the American Medical Association, 294*(3), 359–365.

Vincent, J. L. (2001). Cultural differences in end-of-life care. *Critical Care Medicine, 29*(2 Suppl), N52–N56.

CHAPTER 14

Ethical Issues in Patient Teaching and Patient Adherence

All health professionals have a code of ethics by which they are to abide. Ethics is a system of values that guides health professionals in their behavior toward patients in a variety of situations. Although each profession's code of ethics provides a statement of responsibilities for members of that profession, the code alone is not adequate for every decision and action with which health professionals may be confronted (Cottone & Tarvydas, 2007). Some situations confronting health professionals in the healthcare setting are straightforward; however, other situations raise ethical issues that involve questions not so easily resolved.

Health professionals sometimes perceive ethical decisions made in one situation as applicable to all similar situations. However, a more appropriate description of ethical decision making is determining what is better or best in a particular situation under the given circumstances. Ethical principles do not determine absolute, eternal law. What is considered ethical in one situation may not necessarily be considered ethical in a similar situation that is under different circumstances. Ethical principles provide guidelines by which health professionals can reach decisions about what should be done in a particular situation after considering all relevant factors.

ETHICAL THEORIES

Ethical theories provide a broad framework of rules and principles that serve as a foundation for judgments or courses of action. There are two major types of ethical theory: (1) teleologic and (2) deontologic.

Teleologic theory, sometimes called utilitarian theory, pertains mainly to consequences or results of action. Using this theory as a basis for ethical problem solving would mean that health professionals would consider the consequences of performing or not performing an act and base their decision on which course of action would bring the greatest good to the greatest number of people.

Consider the following example of applying teleologic theory to patient teaching. A health professional developed new patient teaching materials that he was interested in marketing to a publisher of patient teaching materials. Before approaching the publisher, however, the health professional was interested in testing the effectiveness of the materials with regard to enhancing patient adherence, to have a means of comparison. In so doing, the health professional decided to give one group of patients, the patient teaching materials that were of lesser quality and that did not contain all the relevant information about their condition and the potential side effects of treatment. In determining whether this practice was ethical or not, the health professional reasoned that the action was justified because a greater number of people would benefit in the long run by knowing which material would produce the greatest results.

A problem with this approach, of course, is that it is often difficult to measure or to reach general agreement on what is the "greatest good." "Good" may be based on an individual's values, which may differ significantly from the values or perception of good held by others.

The other major type of ethical theory, deontologic, sometimes called formalist theory, pertains to duty or obligation. In this case, health professionals would consider their own motivation when justifying an action rather than considering the consequences of the action itself.

For instance, consider the same preceding example, but with deontologic theory applied instead. In this case, the health professional would consider his motivation for giving the patients the patient teaching materials that had incomplete information. If, in self-evaluation, the health professional believed that the real reason he was giving the patients the inferior materials was not to form a valid comparison, but rather to be assured that his materials would look better (making it more likely that the publisher would accept the brochure, thus resulting in financial profit for him), he may determine that the action is unethical.

ETHICAL PRINCIPLES

Autonomy

Autonomy is the degree to which individuals are allowed to make their own choices and choose their own destiny. To be autonomous, people must be self-governing, having the ability to exercise control over their own actions and circumstances. This means that to be autonomous in decision making, individuals must make decisions voluntarily without coercion and without undue influence. Autonomy is, however, based on a presumption of the individual's competence to understand information needed to help him or her make decisions and on his or her ability to understand fully the consequences of the decisions.

In patient teaching and patient adherence, the principle of autonomy is used when health professionals allow patients to make their own choices about which instructions they will follow and the extent to which they will follow them. Health professionals are, at times, reluctant to afford patients autonomy, believing that patients do not have the full range of knowledge that would allow them to make reasonable decisions. In other instances, health professionals allow their own values to affect those of patients in deciding what is best. There are limitations to autonomy. No principle is absolute. When allowing patient autonomy would threaten the autonomy or well-being of others, patient autonomy does not take precedence. Take, for example, an individual who has been diagnosed with active tuberculosis but refuses to take the medication needed to treat the disease. To allow the patient complete autonomy in this decision and not attempt to influence him or her to take the medication would not be responsible on the part of the health professional, since actions of not following the treatment protocol could impinge on the health or well-being of others.

Beneficence

Most health professionals hope to do what is ultimately best for the patient to further enhance the patient's welfare or well-being. In holding this view, the health professional is guided in promoting the patient's best interest by preventing harm.

Beneficence is in conflict with autonomy, and like autonomy, it is not absolute. Beneficence is ethically applied if, in so doing, the individual generally believes that what is done will cause more benefit than harm. It is not justified, however, if the individual applying the principle of beneficence has an ulterior motive, such as his or her own gain, or if the benefit would not be experienced by the patient but by others. Although beneficence, when applied appropriately, can be noble, it must be applied with caution so as not to infringe on the patient's rights.

Nonmaleficence

Nonmaleficence can be defined simply as "do no harm." Although it may be difficult to see how providing patient teaching information could ostensibly harm an individual, the information could cause harm if it encouraged the patient to engage in behavior that was ultimately harmful, or if information was withheld from a patient, harm could be caused because he or she was denied information that could have prevented harm.

Health professionals would not, of course, deliberately give patients information or withhold information knowingly that would cause patients harm. However, when determining if or to what extent health professionals should attempt to coerce patients to follow treatment recommendations, or to what extent information should be withheld or emphasized for this purpose, awareness of this principle is important.

Take the case of Mrs. Raines, admitted to the hospital because of chest pain. Mrs. Raines underwent a series of tests indicating no permanent myocardial damage, but tests did demonstrate compromise of oxygen to her heart upon exercise. Believing that a more thorough evaluation of her coronary arteries and cardiac function should be obtained, the physician recommended that she undergo cardiac catheterization. The nurse spent considerable time explaining the procedure to Mrs. Raines, including risks and benefits. Mrs. Raines became quite frightened at the information and declined to have the procedure done. The physician and nurse continued to talk with her, insisting there was nothing to fear from the procedure, but also alluding to a scenario that unless she had her condition evaluated so she could be properly treated, she could put herself at considerable risk of sudden death. The doctor also talked with Mrs. Raines' family members, encouraging them to influence her to have the procedure done, emphasizing that not doing so could have grave consequences. Finally, Mrs. Raines consented to the procedure, only to suffer a cardiac arrest from which she could not be resuscitated during the procedure.

When encouraging patients to follow recommendations, health professionals must keep in mind that they have no way of knowing all the potential risks of treatment or whether side effects or risks will occur if the recommendations are followed. Therefore, providing factual, truthful information that enables patients to be aware of all potential risks, and consequently to weigh risks and benefits based on their own values, helps to ensure that the principle of nonmaleficence is not violated.

Although the basic assumption of nonmaleficence underlies all patient teaching activities, it is not often made explicit. Giving information is at times taken for granted as an innocuous activity that has the potential for influencing behavior and enhancing well-being but has little potential for causing harm. As illustrated in the case above, patient teaching has the potential to do both.

Justice

Justice is a principle that implies fairness and consistency. In other words, justice implies equality in all cases. More broadly, justice may be viewed in terms of how decisions should be made when the interest of one person or group competes with the interest of another person or group. Whatever decision is made, the principle mandates that individuals should be treated impartially and not in a capricious manner. An example of application of this principle to patient teaching may be found in a situation in which there are limited resources, so patient teaching is not available for all patients. In this situation, of course, a decision about which patients will receive patient teaching would need to be made. If, in making the decision, the health professional based his or her reasoning on patients' ethnic or religious background alone, the principle of justice would be violated, and the process used by the health professional to make the decision would be considered unethical. If, however, the health professional made the decision based on a process in which there were equal criteria applied to determine distribution of patient teaching, the principle of justice would be appropriately applied.

CONFIDENTIALITY AND PRIVACY

Confidentiality relates to the concept of privacy. Privacy is a broader concept that relates to the right to be free from interference from others (Grace, 2004) and to decide what information will or will not be shared with others. Confidentiality refers to protection of individual information and specifically of healthcare information (Grace, 2009). Most health professionals understand that information gained from the patient is to be considered confidential and not to be shared with others without the patient's expressed consent. The Health Insurance Portability and Accounting Act took effect in 2003 and protects patients' health information in practice as well as research (Olsen, 2003). In practice, this means that patients' health information, such as information about their mental or physical health, any care they have been provided, or any other related health information that identifies them may not be disclosed without their written consent. As applied to research, this means that attaining information from patients' record, or sharing information for research purposes without their expressed written consent is forbidden. Even with the patient's consent, patient information must not be readily identifiable.

In the case of patient teaching, however, this principle may at times be overlooked. Take, for example, the case of Mrs. Wells, who had recently referred her husband for Alzheimer's disease screening at a local medical facility. As part of the screening protocol, patients and families were asked to participate in a patient teaching program in which they learned about Alzheimer's disease. A few weeks after they had participated in the patient teaching session, Mr. and Mrs. Wells returned to the medical facility to receive results of the screening that Mr. Wells had undergone. The nurse, Ms. Lee, who had conducted the patient teaching session, saw Mr. and Mrs. Wells in the waiting room and approached them, asking for feedback regarding the patient teaching program on Alzheimer's disease they had attended. Mrs. Wells became visibly upset and later complained to Ms. Lee's supervisor for what she considered to be a breech of patient confidentiality. Mrs. Wells had felt very ill at ease taking her husband for Alzheimer's screening, fearing that the possibility of such a diagnosis may have some social stigma for them in their community. One of Mrs. Wells' neighbors had been in the waiting room. Overhearing Ms. Lee's comment, the neighbor later began questioning Mrs. Wells about why she had attended the patient teaching session about Alzheimer's disease. What Ms. Lee had considered a harmless comment, Mrs. Wells considered a breech of confidentiality, which caused her considerable discomfort.

VALUES

Health professionals' assumptions about the nature of patient teaching are based to a great extent on their own values. These values in turn have a direct impact on how they conduct patient teaching. This includes goals considered to be important, techniques and methods used, and the degree of responsibility shared by both health professional and patient. It is important to distinguish fact from value (Rich & Butts, 2005).

The question of values permeates patient teaching. Health professionals' values inevitably affect patient teaching. Health professionals should be clear about their own values and understand how their values influence patient teaching. Being aware of his or her own values does not, however, mean that the health professional should attempt to persuade a patient with different values to accept the values purported by the health professional.

Not all health professionals involved in patient teaching would accept this view. Some health professionals believe that their role in patient teaching is to exert influence on patients to adopt health professionals' values. These health professionals use patient teaching to direct patients toward attitudes and behaviors that health professionals judge to be best. There is a delicate balance between providing information that, in the judgment of the health professional, is considered best and being so concerned about protecting patient autonomy that the health professional is lax in presenting information.

Patient teaching is not a form of indoctrination or a method to make patients conform to what the health professional believes to be an acceptable form of behavior. No health professional has absolute wisdom regarding what is best for the patients he or she serves. Health professionals have no way of knowing how adhering to all the recommendations provided will affect the patient's life or the extent to which adherence to recommendations may be helpful or harmful.

However, patients do learn in both direct and indirect ways. If health professionals remain open to patients' values that may be different from their own, presenting objective information that has basis in fact, an atmosphere of respect and trust is created. In so doing, health professionals not only demonstrate respect for patients' autonomy while also practicing beneficence, but also increase the possibility that patients will, through informed choice, choose the behavior that is in their own best interest.

Health professionals who, on the other hand, attempt to be purely objective without introducing their own personality may appear to be mechanical and routine in their approach to patient teaching, which can diminish patients' sense that the health professional has interest in them as individuals and their particular needs and circumstances, thus making patient teaching less effective. Patients generally expect more involvement from their health professional than merely providing rote information. They want to know that the health professional is concerned for them as individuals and often want to know the health professional's opinion in order to test their own thinking. Since trust is an important factor in patient teaching, it is important that health professionals be honest but tactful about their own values when they are relevant to questions that arise. If health professionals do relate their values to the patient, they should always make it clear they are presenting their personal opinion, based on their own values and circumstances that may be totally different from those of the patient and that may have entirely different consequences.

Health professionals convey values to patients in a number of ways other than verbally. In patient teaching, whether intended or not, health professionals give patients positive and negative reinforcement with behavior as well as words. A frown, a grimace, or a look of approval in response to a patient's statement or behavior all communicate something about the health professional's values. Consequently, health professionals should be aware of their own values and how those are demonstrated to patients both covertly and overtly.

It must be remembered that values are often culturally inherited and determined. This may include religious beliefs and values imbedded within the cultural milieu. Therefore, what one individual considers ethically correct based on his or her own standards or values may not apply universally to all other individuals. Likewise, overreliance on cultural and/or religious principles alone to determine an ethical course of action is not always sufficient to reach an ethical decision acceptable or applicable to all individuals. The same cultural traditions or religious beliefs may not be held by all parties. Consequently, using commonly shared principles rather than personal, cultural, or religious values alone is a more reasonable approach to ethical decision making in situations when a common view is not shared by all.

Religious beliefs and practices affect many dimensions of personal life as well as health and health care. Differences in religious values, in particular, between patient and health professional can be a barrier to effective patient teaching. Health professionals should examine their own religious values and be sensitive to how they influence the way they teach patients. If health professionals have no religious affiliation or are hostile to organized religion, they should be aware of how their own views may affect patient teaching of patients who hold strong commitments to the beliefs of certain religions. It is important that health professionals maintain awareness of the extent to which they understand their patients' religious beliefs and their meanings, and if different from their own, how this affects their relationships with patients during patient teaching.

Take, for example, Mrs. Brown, a migrant worker who came for an individual prenatal teaching session with the nurse, Mr. York. Mrs. Brown was expecting her ninth child. Both Mr. and Mrs. Brown were obviously excited about the pregnancy in anticipation that the baby may be a boy, given that six of their eight children were girls. Mr. York knew that the financial situation of the family was poor, although the children appeared well nourished and well cared for. During the teaching session, Mr. York brought up the issue of birth control and the possibility of sterilization after the birth of the baby. When Mrs. Brown seemed reluctant to accept the idea, Mr. York became more coercive in his presentation, implying that under the circumstances, to have more children would be irresponsible. Mrs. Brown looked shocked and attempted to explain that she and her husband believed strongly that God would provide for any children that would be born. She said they believed that to do anything to prevent pregnancy would be interfering with nature and a demonstration of lack of trust in God.

Mr. York shook his head in despair and said coldly, "I see." He put away the teaching material and said to Mrs. Brown, "Then I guess that will be all. You obviously are not prepared to listen to reason. I need to devote my time to patients I can help." Mrs. Brown, although not saying anything, left with sadness, reluctant to bring up other issues with Mr. York in the future.

Mr. York had, essentially, influenced Mrs. Brown's behavior, but not necessarily in a positive way. Health professionals must determine the extent to which they can remain true to themselves and at the same time allow patients freedom to select their own course of action, even if it differs sharply from the action the health professionals would choose. Health professionals should conduct patient teaching and present information in such a way that patients are enabled to make an informed choice in accordance with their values. Referral to another health professional should be made in situations where the health professional's values are in conflict with those of the patient to such a degree that the health professional believes his or her own ethical principles would be compromised. Under these circumstances, referral should be approached with the patient in a respectful manner.

Health professionals who have liberal values may find themselves working with patients who have more traditional values or vice versa. By questioning these values or imposing their own, health professionals do not show respect for patients' beliefs and consequently lose credibility. In some instances, health professionals may have a strong commitment to values they do not even question, promoting their views at the expense of providing unbiased information that would help patients to reach their own informed choices. Health professionals should be clear about their own values and how these affect patient teaching.

Values may also be related to personal characteristics of individuals. Health professionals should be aware of their own biases and prejudices. For instance, the health professional may have a bias about individuals who are elderly, who are from different racial or ethnic groups, who are physically disabled, who have a criminal record, who abuse substances, or who are obese. Any of these biases, whether positive or negative, can affect the content of or manner in which patient teaching is conducted. Take, for example, the situation described below.

Mr. Slavinsky was a 72-year-old man scheduled for an appointment for a consultation with Dr. Penn. When calling for the appointment, Mr. Slavinsky had been reluctant to tell the appointment clerk the purpose of the visit, saying only that it was "a personal matter." At the office visit, Mr. Slavinsky began by saying that he had not felt well lately and that he had been tired with a slight cough. Dr. Penn examined Mr. Slavinsky briefly and concluded that she could find nothing wrong. Mr. Slavinsky said shyly, "I've been hearing a lot about AIDS lately and I just thought I should get checked out. I don't know very much about it." Dr. Penn smiled and said, "Oh, I don't think you have to worry about that at your age. You haven't had any blood transfusions, so it's unlikely that you would even have been exposed to the virus that causes AIDS."

When Mr. Slavinsky became more insistent about receiving information, Dr. Penn said gently, "Mr. Slavinsky, we have a very busy practice here. Although I would like to have the time to talk with patients about all kinds of things, I have to limit my time to giving them information that is most relevant for them realistically. At your age, you should be more concerned about keeping your blood pressure under control."

Dr. Penn not only made some assumptions about Mr. Slavinsky that she did not attempt to explore for their validity, she also imposed her own values on Mr. Slavinsky based on her bias regarding age and not on Mr. Slavinsky as an individual.

There are many value-laden patient teaching situations. In all instances, it is important that health professionals be clear about their own values and how they influence patient teaching. Values can affect not only the way health professionals conduct patient teaching, but also in the end, how effective patient teaching interactions will be.

IDENTIFYING ETHICAL ISSUES IN PATIENT TEACHING AND PATIENT ADHERENCE

Not every patient teaching situation has ethical ramifications; however, it is important that health professionals be aware of potential ethical problems related to both patient teaching and patient adherence. As health care becomes more complex, so do ethical issues related to patient teaching and patient adherence. Advances in technology in medical care as well as economic issues have brought about significant changes in the healthcare delivery system and subsequently in the amount of responsibility patients are expected to assume for their own health and health care. Patients are often discharged from the hospital earlier and expected to manage more complicated treatment regimens at home. Likewise, as more is learned about the role of lifestyle in the development of chronic disease, issues of prevention have become more prevalent. Ethical issues related to lifestyle and prevention occur in situations in which health professionals and patients have conflicting views about the consequences of lifestyle decisions.

Theoretically, the purpose of patient teaching is to enable patients to make choices that will maintain or improve their health status. Often, this may involve behavior change. Behavior change may involve living a healthier lifestyle to prevent disease or complications from occurring, or it may involve managing a disease or condition by following specific treatment recommendations.

The underlying assumption of patient teaching is that the goal of both the health professional and patient is to help the patient to attain his or her optimal degree of health. The patient and health professional may have differing views, however, about what constitutes optimal health and what methods are best used to achieve it. Take the example of Mr. Lopez.

Mr. Lopez was a serious jogger, running several miles every day. In addition to jogging for health reasons, jogging also constituted a major portion of his social life, since he jogged with friends every morning and was involved with a jogging club, which met for jogging followed by brunch every Sunday morning. During an examination, Dr. Diego instructed Mr. Lopez that he must relinquish jogging because continuing it would only further injure his knee, which had been previously injured. Mr. Lopez, however, continued to jog, a choice made based on his own priority, believing that the other physical and psychological benefits he received from jogging made the risk of continuing to jog worth the benefit, despite Dr. Diego's instructions. Dr. Diego's view was, of course, much different, believing that the increasing damage from jogging would be a future impingement on Mr. Lopez's well-being, having the potential to cause disability and potentially more aggressive treatment.

Looking at the situation described above from a patient adherence perspective, it would appear that the patient teaching was ineffective, given that Mr. Lopez did not change behavior and therefore might be labeled as non-adherent. Although this situation does not present an ethical dilemma per se, it might have if, for instance, Dr. Diego had exaggerated his description about the degree of risk involved if Mr. Lopez continued to jog, or if Dr. Diego had taken other steps to coerce Mr. Lopez into changing his behavior to coincide with his point of view.

The degree to which the health professional interjects his or her own personal bias into patient teaching has ethical implications. Bias of the health professional may be reflected by the type of information provided, what information is stressed, and what, if any, alternatives are discussed. In this situation, after learning Mr. Lopez's values and, consequently, that he would continue to jog despite recommendations to the contrary, Dr. Diego may have provided Mr. Lopez with information relating to how he could minimize the chance of further injury.

The degree to which the health professional uses specific techniques in patient teaching with the specific goal of increasing patient adherence also has ethical implications. Adherence does not always ensure the patient's well-being. Not only is the health professional's ability to predict outcomes not exact, nor is any treatment always 100% effective, but also the patient's sense of well-being itself is often subjective. Even though the health professional may perceive the patient's well-being as being improved because of treatment, the patient may not share this view. Health professionals who impose their values on patients with little respect or attention to the patient's own subjective preference, may, although increasing adherence, actually decrease the patient's quality of life rather than improving it. Such was the case of Mr. Ford.

Mr. Ford was an 84-year-old patient who was very active. He had undergone exploratory surgery because of abdominal pain. The surgery revealed a malignancy, which was removed. There was little evidence of metastasis, but chemotherapy was strongly recommended. Dr. Arnold, Mr. Ford's physician, recommended that he undergo chemotherapy. Mr. Ford seemed resistant to undergoing treatment, stating that he had concerns that the medicine used in the treatment might make him worse. Both Dr. Arnold, and the nurse, Ms. Larkin, spent considerable time and effort providing detailed information about chemotherapy, including the possibility of side effects. However, they minimized the likelihood of occurrence of side effects and the discomfort that might result if they were to occur. Both Dr. Arnold and Ms. Larkin held firm beliefs that chemotherapy could extend Mr. Ford's life and that any side effects and subsequent discomfort he may experience would be well worth it. When Mr. Ford continued to be reluctant to have chemotherapy, Dr. Arnold stated that he would then be forced to withdraw from the case, because if Mr. Ford would not cooperate with his recommendations, then he could be of no further help. Feeling frightened of losing a physician he had grown to know and trust, Mr. Ford agreed to the treatment.

Unfortunately, with the first treatment, Mr. Ford experienced more serious side effects than Dr. Arnold or Ms. Larkin had anticipated. Mr. Ford had severe nausea, hair loss, and general malaise. When Dr. Arnold and Ms. Larkin talked with him later about scheduling the second series of chemotherapy, they were surprised to hear him state with conviction that he refused to undergo any more treatments. Ms. Larkin and Dr. Arnold examined ways in which they could convince Mr. Ford of the necessity of continuing chemotherapy, emphasizing how important the treatment was to his well-being and longevity. They assured him that the discomfort would subside after treatment was completed.

Continual attempts to get Mr. Ford to change his mind were unsuccessful. Mr. Ford finally said, "You don't understand that when you reach my age, every day becomes very precious. I've wasted some of my precious days being sick from the treatments. I want to live out the rest of my days in as much peace as possible. I want to enjoy my grandchildren. I don't want them to remember me like this. Besides, how can you be sure that the treatment will extend my life? Even if it does, at my age, I could just as easily die tomorrow of something else. Then my last days would have been wasted. Not everyone may place the same value on long life as you do."

Dr. Arnold and Ms. Larkin had assumed, mistakenly, that Mr. Ford had the same values and priorities they held. Their perception of what constituted well-being and health was not shared by Mr. Ford. Because Mr. Ford was not given complete information about the potential side effects of chemotherapy, which he could have used in making his decision, his autonomy was thwarted. Dr. Arnold applied coercion when he threatened to withdraw from the case, which in turn influenced Mr. Ford's decision. Dr. Arnold and Ms. Larkin both imposed their own values about extension of life on Mr. Ford. Even though they were both acting out of beneficence, believing that having chemotherapy was ultimately in Mr. Ford's best interest, Mr. Ford's perceptions differed.

Although health professionals may have difficulty understanding patients' views, ultimately, each patient has the right to make his or her own decisions. It is frequently difficult for health professionals dedicated to the idea of effective patient teaching to accept patients' basic rights and responsibilities for determining their own course of action related to the extent to which they will or will not follow recommendations. The zealous health professional may believe that he or she knows what is best for the patient and therefore have the responsibility to influence the patient into following that course of action. This view contains several assumptions. First, it assumes that the diagnosis is correct and that the treatment prescribed is appropriate. Although this may be true for the majority of patients, there have been instances in which patients were misdiagnosed and/or received the wrong treatment. If, during patient teaching, steps are taken to pressure the patient into following the recommendations, but the diagnosis and/or treatment is inaccurate, the results could be harmful if not disastrous. Such is the case of Mrs. Jackson, described below.

Mrs. Jackson received prescription for medication to treat her heart condition. She had the prescription filled at her local pharmacy, but at follow-up with Dr. Peters, her physician, she admitted that she had not taken the medication as directed. Mrs. Jackson complained that the medication made her "feel strange." Rather than questioning Mrs. Jackson more closely about her symptoms, both Dr. Peters, and the nurse, Mr. Parker, began assessing ways they could motivate Mrs. Jackson to follow her medication regimen more closely. Mr. Parker conducted additional patient teaching, stressing the importance of taking the medication as prescribed and emphasizing possible consequences of not taking the medication as directed. During the teaching session, Mr. Parker became quite forceful in his attempt to convince Mrs. Jackson to adhere to recommendations. Unfortunately, neither Dr. Peters nor Mr. Parker had listened closely when Mrs. Jackson had tried to explain why she was not taking the medication as directed. Neither Dr. Peters nor Mr. Parker had explored her reported symptoms of "feeling strange" after taking the medication, nor had either of them actually examined the medication that Mrs. Jackson was taking. Had they done so, they would have noted that Mrs. Jackson had actually been given the wrong medication at the pharmacy. Instead of the prescribed medication, she had actually received an oral antihyperglycemic agent. The mistake was finally discovered when Mrs. Jackson was taken to the emergency room with hypoglycemia.

This case illustrates not only the importance of not coercing patients into following instructions, but also the importance of taking time to interact and listen to what the patient says. Although patients may not always be able to explain feelings or symptoms in sophisticated terms, they do have valuable information to give if the health professional takes the time to listen.

Underlying the assumption that health professionals have the responsibility to coerce patients into following recommendations is the belief that it is the health professional who is the expert in the situation. This assumption does not acknowledge, of course, that patients have expertise regarding their own bodies and can make a valuable contribution to the interaction which could, in fact, help make outcomes of patient teaching more effective. Although the health professional may be an expert in medical or health-related matters, the patient is the expert in his or her own feelings, symptoms, values, and circumstances.

The same recommendations may not be appropriate or in the best interest of all patients even when they have the same condition. Providing standardized information and recommendations without considering the patient as an individual makes patient teaching a rigid, technical exercise rather than a process in which patients are helped to internalize recommendations and apply them to their own circumstances.

The two examples of Mr. Ford and Mrs. Jackson may seem extreme; however, similar principles apply no matter what type of recommendations and information are provided. Effective patient teaching is not so much a matter of persuading patients to do what the health professional wants, but rather a process in which possible courses of action and consequences of each course of action are communicated to the patient. Patient teaching thus becomes a matter of outlining facts so that patients and health professionals can work together to devise a plan that will be most beneficial to patients. Although some patients may be reluctant to accept this type of responsibility in decision making, the health professional has the responsibility to leave the option open and to consider patients' individual needs when providing information and recommendations.

Rather than having the responsibility to promote patient adherence through patient teaching, health professionals have the responsibility to communicate effectively with patients, making sure that the advice and recommendations patients receive are based on fact rather than prejudice. Too often when patients fail to adhere to recommendations, they are viewed as uncooperative, difficult, or as not fully understanding of the consequences of their actions. Health professionals have the responsibility to present the full range of information and options, and for ensuring that patients have the opportunity for self-determination in matters related to their own health and health care. Given this approach, health professionals then have the duty to assist patients to carry out mutually determined recommendations.

The mutual participation approach to patient teaching assumes that effective outcomes are the shared responsibility of patients and health professionals. In many patient teaching situations, patients are vulnerable and distressed by their illnesses, symptoms, or the impact the conditions have on their lives. Health professionals are in a position to help patients deal with these issues and to attain maximum benefit from recommendations provided. This is accomplished by offering not only accurate information but also support and guidance based on the individual patient's needs.

A truly ethical approach to patient teaching, then, demands mutual participation by both patient and health professional to attain the most beneficial outcomes. To do so, however, health professionals should have an understanding of ethical principles that are used as a basis for ethical decision making. Problems may relate to how much or what type of information patients should be given or to what extent strategies should be implemented to increase patient adherence.

A number of specific problems and questions can arise. The first relates to the amount of information the patient should receive. Does the patient have the right to complete information, or are there instances when the health professional has the right to determine how much and what type of information the patient should be given? For example, if the health professional believed that giving the patient complete information about remote side effects or risks of a certain treatment would cause the patient to not follow recommendations, and thus, not receive the potential therapeutic benefits, is the health professional justified in withholding that information from the patient in his or her own best interest? Take the example of Ms. Queen.

Ms. Queen had made an appointment with Dr. Abernathy for healthcare advice regarding an overseas trip she was to take. The area she was to visit had a high prevalence of malaria. Dr. Abernathy had cared for a number of patients with malaria and concluded that taking medication prophylactically is crucial. Although the medication he chose to prescribe for preventing malaria had some potentially serious side effects, Dr. Abernathy concluded that having malaria would be a greater risk than the side effects, which may or may not occur. Consequently, he advised Ms. Queen to take the medication but did not share with her the serious nature of potential side effects. Dr. Abernathy's assumption was, of course, that knowledge of potential side effects may influence Ms. Queen's decision of whether or not to take the medication, so he made the decision to withhold information. Was Dr. Abernathy justified in withholding information from Ms. Queen, or, in so doing, did he violate her right to self-determination? Under what circumstances would withholding information be justified?

Another issue relates to situations where information contains half-truths or untruths judged by the health professional to be in the patient's best interest. Is telling a "therapeutic lie" ever justified, whether that involves withholding the truth, giving an incomplete truth, or outright lying? Take, for example, the case of Mr. Dubois, who had insulin-dependent diabetes. Dr. Little had spent considerable time giving Mr. Dubois information about his condition and treatment, and was pleased at the extent to which Mr. Dubois's blood sugar seemed to be under control. One day at an office visit, Mr. Dubois said the following, "Although I don't find following the diet and insulin protocol easy, I'll continue it as long as I know it makes a difference. I know the complications of diabetes can be serious, and I'd do anything to prevent them. But if I thought that

I might develop complications anyway, I sure would have to think twice about how carefully I would continue to follow the protocol. Will good adherence ensure that I won't develop complications?"

Although Dr. Little recognized that there were no guarantees that complications would not develop despite good adherence and blood sugar control, he was also aware of the risks of not maintaining good control. Based on this judgment, he turned to Mr. Dubois and said, "You just keep doing as well as you are, and you'll do fine." Dr. Little decided if Mr. Dubois knew about the potential of complications despite good adherence, he may fail to follow the diet and insulin protocol as carefully and thereby jeopardize his well-being. Consequently, Dr. Little elected to withhold information from Mr. Dubois. In so doing, was Dr. Little infringing on Mr. Dubois's right to know, or was his action justified to preserve Mr. Dubois's well-being?

On the other hand, does the patient have the right not to know? Should patients be coerced into hearing information they do not want to hear? There are instances in which patients may not want information about their condition or treatment. In these instances, do health professionals have the duty to give the patient information anyway, or should they respect the patient's right to refuse information? Take the example of Mrs. Bowland, who had been diagnosed with pancreatic cancer. Although Mrs. Bowland was given full information about her condition, possible palliative treatments, and the gravity of her prognosis, and appeared to understand the seriousness of her condition, she continued to remain hopeful that she would "beat the odds" and continued to make plans for the future. In this situation, when there appeared to be little indication that the condition could be treated or that life could be extended, to what extent should the health professional be "insistent" that the patient recognize the implications of her condition for the future? When a situation presents in which the patient must be given information he or she does not want to hear, the health professional should refrain from tactless truth, but rather provide the information with gentleness and sensitivity. Projected outcomes should only be given as they can be predicted accurately.

Another issue involves the extent to which the health professional is obligated to share all treatment alternatives with the patient. Does the health professional have the duty and responsibility to provide the patient with information about alternative forms of treatment, even though the health professional might not favor them? Is there more than one course of action or treatment that may be recommended? Can the health professional be absolutely sure that the course of treatment he or she prefers over the one the patient prefers is actually in the patient's best interest? Obviously, when considering treatment alternatives, the health professional has the responsibility to endorse only those treatments that are medically sound. For example, a patient with rheumatoid arthritis who proposes being treated with injections of snake venom rather than the nonsteroidal anti-inflammatory drugs the health professional had recommended may need additional counseling regarding treatment choice. In some instances, there are alternative choices of treatment that may be reasonable and that may be more palatable to the patient than those the health professional has recommended. In these instances, the health professional should keep an open mind and at least consider that there are other treatment alternatives.

The final issue of concern involves the degree to which health professionals implement strategies to increase patient adherence. Is the role of patient teaching to convince patients to acquiesce to health professionals' beliefs about the best course of action, or is it to enable patients to make their own informed decisions based on factual information and their own values and priorities? Although health professionals have the responsibility to offer information, reinforcement, and strategies that can assist patients in following treatment directives, when these approaches become coercive with the expressed purpose of coercion, the ethical justification of such actions is questionable.

Additional ethical questions arise around the issue of who should be involved in decisions regarding what and how much information patients should be given. Are there instances when individuals close to the patient, who fear that information may cause the patient undue anxiety or have other deleterious effects, have the right to request that information be withheld? How do patient factors such as severe pain, limited intellectual capacity, or emotional strain affect the amount or type of information given or strategies used to affect patient adherence with treatment recommendations?

There are no absolute answers for any of these questions. Health professionals must judge each situation individually, considering the specific circumstances in that particular situation. Although some may argue that this means that health professionals could use any rationale to justify any action, for the most part, individuals should be guided by a set of principles on which to base moral judgments. In so doing, however, health professionals must also be honest about their own motives and basis for their decisions, realizing that no one is infallible, nor any decision always right in all circumstances.

In addition, patient teaching generally takes place in some type of institution, whether inpatient or outpatient. Each of these settings also has constraints or regulations that may influence the type of decisions and how certain decisions are made. Institutional constraints may be beyond the control of the health professional who is conducting patient teaching. The goal of ethical decision making for health professionals in these settings is to remain true to their personal ethical standards and values while working within the limits of the institution, while at the same time maintaining some degree of freedom within those limits both for themselves and for the patients they teach.

ETHICAL ISSUES IN THE HEALTH PROFESSIONAL–PATIENT RELATIONSHIP

Effective patient teaching is built on a partnership between patient and health professional. Although a partnership implies equality, the relationship between patient and health professional is, by its very nature, not equal. Patients enter the relationship with greater vulnerability. Health professionals must remain mindful that in the context of the professional relationship, not only is there the potential to do good but also the potential to do harm, even if unintentional. Demonstrating empathy, compassion, and respect for the patient should remain within the professional relationship so that the health professional, while being an advocate for the patient, also maintains appropriate boundaries and does not become overly involved. Health professionals have a legal and ethical responsibility to provide information and base decisions on patients' interests and needs, not on their own. This means that health professionals have a duty to approach patients in an unbiased, fair, and honest manner. Examples of ethical breaches of the professional relationship would include actions such as cultivating patient dependency, treating patients in a paternalistic way, providing patients with limited information that promotes the health professional's views, or terminating services if the patient fails to comply with recommendations.

Take, for example, the case of Mr. Norton who had been Dr. Nash's patient for 20 years. When Mr. Norton was being seen for his annual physical exam, Dr. Nash noted that Mr. Norton, who had just turned 50, had never had screening for colorectal cancer. Dr. Nash believed strongly in prevention and believed flexible sigmoidoscopy to be the most effective type of screening for colorectal cancer. He began to talk with Mr. Norton about the importance of the screening exam.

Dr. Nash: "Now that you've had your 50th birthday you'll need to be screened for colorectal cancer. I know you have no family history of colorectal cancer, but it's good for everyone over 50 to be screened. I would like to schedule you for a flexible sigmoidoscopy."

Mr. Norton: "Well, I'm not too worried about colon cancer. I've never had any problems and I'm not at high risk. I think I would like to wait for a while."

Dr. Nash: "Do you know that colorectal cancer has one of the highest incidence rates of all cancers, with well over 100,000 people being newly diagnosed each year? Last year, almost 60,000 people died of colorectal cancer. The sad thing is that if it's found early it is highly curable. I really believe you need to be screened."

Mr. Norton: "That sounds like a lot of people. I'm still not sure at this point that I want to go through a screening though. I've heard that sigmoidoscopy can be really uncomfortable. If you insist that I be screened maybe I could have one of those fecal occult blood tests instead."

Dr. Nash: "The occult screening isn't nearly as effective, and there is a lot of preparation involved. With flexible sigmoidoscopy, we can actually visualize the intestine and see small growths that may be precancerous and wouldn't even been found on an occult blood test. The flexible sigmoidoscopy only has to be done every few years or so, only takes about 20 minutes, and is safe. You should only have minimal discomfort. Isn't that worth it when you consider it could save your life? I've known you for a long time. I would hate to see you develop a disease that could have been so easily prevented."

After more discussion, Dr. Nash finally convinced Mr. Norton to have the test. Unfortunately, Mr. Norton experienced intestinal perforation during the test and developed peritonitis. Dr. Nash, although well intentioned, used his power in the relationship to pressure Mr. Nash into having a procedure that he was reluctant to have performed and one that ended with unforeseen harmful consequences. In the case of Dr. Nash and Mr. Norton, there was conflict over the definition of the problem, the goals, and the priorities in treatment. Had Dr. Nash worked within the framework of partnership in the relationship and not exerted the power of his position, the two might have come to some agreement or compromise that would have proven to be satisfactory to both and would have prevented what became a disastrous end.

ETHICAL ISSUES IN RESEARCH AND EVALUATION IN PATIENT TEACHING, PATIENT EDUCATION, AND PATIENT ADHERENCE

Although research and evaluation in patient education and patient adherence is important, the health professional conducting it has the obligation to protect the rights and dignity of patients participating. Health professionals should not assume that the research they are conducting is so innocuous that it could cause no potential harm, nor should they attempt to coerce patients into participation. Likewise, health professionals should not assume that the importance of the research they are conducting justifies violating the rights of patients. In terms of evaluation, whether it is evaluation of an intervention or of a program, evaluation must be grounded in facts. Evaluation implies application of values which define the perspective from which the evaluation is made and interpretation of results is reached. Health professionals conducting evaluation should be clear about what values are being incorporated into the process. Information obtained from evaluation may be used as a basis of appraisal and planning for the future; consequently, results from evaluation must be objective. When conducting evaluation, the health professional should consider why the evaluation is being conducted and what decisions may result.

Most institutional settings have a human subjects research review board, which consists of people whose responsibility it is to review research projects involving human subjects before they are conducted in order to ensure that the research protocol does not violate patient rights or present a hazard or danger to patient well-being. When conducting research, the health professional is responsible for ensuring that the research is conducted ethically. One of the first responsibilities is to make sure that patients are fully informed of all features of the research that might influence their willingness to participate. This means that, except under very special circumstances, information regarding features of the study cannot be withheld. Patients should be given complete information so that they can make a free choice about whether or not they want to participate. Patients should not be included in a study without their knowledge, and they must have complete information about the study. For example, a health professional who is interested in monitoring the effect patient teaching about epilepsy has on patients' adherence rates of taking antiepileptic medication cannot have the patient return for weekly blood levels at the patient's expense if the blood work is only for research purposes, if the patient has not been informed, and has not agreed to pay for the lab work.

Patients participating in any research project must also be ensured the freedom to discontinue their participation at any time. It is particularly important to be sensitive to this issue since patients may feel that if they decline to participate or discontinue their participation, their future health care would in some way be threatened. Patients must understand that failure to participate or withdrawal from the study in which they are participating will not influence the quality or quantity of health care they receive at the facility in the future.

Complete disclosure can be a problem when conducting patient adherence research. Informing patients of the complete research protocol may affect the results of the study so that conclusions drawn cannot be considered valid. If, for example, patients know that the degree to which they follow recommendations is being studied, any behavior change observed may actually be a function of the patients being monitored, rather than a function of the strategy designed to improve patient adherence. To draw a conclusion that the intervention itself changed adherence would, under these circumstances, be inaccurate, unless the intervention to increase adherence was merely telling patients that their adherence behavior would be monitored.

In situations where fully informing the patient might influence results, alternatives should be considered. If deception or incomplete information about the nature of the study is used, health professionals have the responsibility to inform patients at the completion of the study and to reveal the conditions and the true intent of the study, so that any misconceptions are dispelled. It is important for health professionals to conduct this debriefing in a sensitive manner, since in some instances, patients may feel that their trust has been violated or may become angry or embarrassed when they find they were deceived. Before deception or incomplete information about the study is considered, health professionals should carefully consider and weigh the possibility of harm or risk to patients and the justification of the research protocol under those circumstances.

In all instances, patient confidentiality should be maintained. Steps should be taken to protect patient identity and to maintain patient anonymity. This includes review of patient records. If, as part of data gathering, information from patients' records prior to or after the intervention is necessary, patients should be made aware of this fact and should be told who will have access to the chart and any other subsequent information.

ETHICAL PATIENT TEACHING PRACTICES

Patient teaching and especially patient adherence can be value-laden concepts. Patient teaching, depending on the content of information provided and the manner in which it is presented, can interject bias of the health professional, which may infringe on patients' ability to make their own free choices about the degree to which they will follow recommendations. Implicit in patient teaching is the assumption that information health professionals give to patients is what the patients need to know for their own benefit. Health professionals must be mindful, however, of patients' rights to determine what constitutes benefit for them. The term adherence itself implies a certain degree of authority on the part of the health professional and cooperation on the part of the patient. The health professional must keep in mind that if adherence is to be an outcome measure of effective patient teaching, the most successful outcome will be based on patient participation in decision making and collaboration between patient and health professional in making those decisions. Likewise, although research is important to both patient teaching and patient adherence, health professionals must be ever mindful that patients' rights must be protected. Whether conducting patient teaching, or conducting research about it, the following concepts should be kept in mind.

1. Information provided should be accurate, should reflect the most current theory or view, and should be evidence based as much as possible.
2. Adherence to recommendations should cause the patient more good than harm.

3. Information should be presented in a factual way, without distortion or exaggeration of facts and without falsification.
4. The health professional should avoid inadvertently introducing bias.
5. Patients' values, beliefs, resources, and barriers regarding following recommendations should be identified and addressed.
6. Any intervention designed to assist patients to follow recommendations should not be coercive.
7. Any research conducted with patients should protect patients' right of freedom to choose to participate and should be based on informed choice.
8. Patient confidentiality should be protected.

REFERENCES

Cottone, R. R., & Tarvydas, V. (2007). *Counseling and ethical decision making* (3rd ed.). Upper Saddle River, NJ: Pearson/Merrill Prentice Hall.

Grace, P. J. (2004). Ethical issues. Patient safety and the limits of confidentiality. *American Journal of Nursing, 104*(11), 33–37.

Grace, P. J. (2009). *Nursing ethics and professional responsibility in advanced practice.* Sudbury, MA: Jones and Bartlett.

Olsen, D. P. (2003). HIPAA privacy regulations and nursing research. *Nursing Research, 52*(5), 344-348.

Rich, K. L., & Butts, J. B. (2005). Values, relationships, virtues. In J. B. Butts & K. L. Rich. *Nursing ethics across the curriculum into practice* (pp. 29–52). Sudbury, MA: Jones and Bartlett.

CHAPTER 15

Informed Consent

Previous chapters have emphasized the need for a relationship between the patient and health professional in which there is a genuine effort by the health professional to provide information that is relevant to the patient to clarify uncertainties, to identify problems, and to work together to arrive at a mutually satisfactory course of action based on the information at hand.

This type of shared decision making is ideal for effective patient teaching and upholds the ethical principles of autonomy and beneficence discussed in the previous chapter. Although informing the patient about care and treatment is ethically desirable, it is also legally incumbent on the health professional in the form of informed consent (Miola, 2009; Pera, 2005).

Beginning in the early 1900s, the courts asserted that, based on the principle of self-determination, patients have the legal right to make decisions regarding their medical care. Historically, informed consent has been the major responsibility of the physician, the law having been developed in the context of claims against physicians who neglected to adequately inform their patients before initiating treatment. However, as other health professionals have assumed increasing responsibility as independent providers of care, the legal requirements of informed consent apply to them as well. The legal doctrine of informed consent requires the health professional not only to obtain consent from patients before treatment is initiated but also to engage in a meaningful exchange of information and discussion with patients so that their consent is actually "informed."

THE MEANING OF INFORMED CONSENT

Informed consent, although a legal doctrine, involves fundamental values. Informed consent is based on respect for individuals and their rights and abilities to determine their own goals based on their own values and to decide how they will achieve the goals they have established (Dickey, 2006).

The concept of informed consent is viewed in the context of the relationship between patient and health professional in which the health professional provides patients with sufficient information so that they are able to make to make informed judgments and decisions. In addition to being based on patients' rights of self-determination as specified in the Patient Self-Determination Act of 1991 (Koch, 1992), informed consent is strongly rooted in the value that patients should be active participants in their own health care.

The legal aspects of informed consent are related to the concept of battery, which consists of physical contact for which one has not given consent. In other words, theoretically, before patients submit to a treatment, procedure, or examination, they must give their consent or authorization for the action in question to be performed. Unfortunately, in the past, this type of consent was often based more on patients' trust and faith in the health professional than on the quality of information they had been given.

During the past years, there has been increasing interest not only in obtaining patient authorization before performing various procedures but also in the quality of the information provided by the health professional, which underlies the patient's informed consent. There is general consensus that informed consent is a process involving more than merely obtaining the patient's signature on an informed consent form. The patient's signature only serves as an indication that this process has taken place. It cannot be equated with the process. For the process to be valid, information provided to the patient must be adequate, the patient must understand the information, and the decision to agree to the treatment or intervention must be voluntary. Health professionals are, therefore, held responsible not only for what they do to the patient but also for what they say to the patient. Information provided to patients by health professionals must be clear, accurate, and in terms the patient can understand. This responsibility can be extended to information given to the patient by the health professional in the form of written patient teaching materials as well. If information contained in written materials is inaccurate or insufficient, and as a result of receiving the material and following the advice provided in it the patient suffers harm, the health professional could be held responsible. As an example, consider the case of Mr. Samuel.

Mr. Samuel was a 64-year-old patient who had been admitted to the hospital because of circulatory problems in his lower extremities as a result of arteriosclerosis. He was well educated and widely read. His physician, Dr. Clark, felt that an arteriogram of the lower extremities was indicated in order to explore the extent of the circulatory problem. The procedure was discussed with Mr. Samuel, and the nurse, Ms. Terrance, was asked to give

Mr. Samuel the patient education booklet on arteriograms, which had been prepared by the hospital patient education staff.

Ms. Terrance gave Mr. Samuel the booklet, leaving him alone for some time while he read over the information it contained. The booklet specifically outlined the nature of the arteriogram, what the procedure consists of, and what it can show. Upon returning, Ms. Terrance asked Mr. Samuel if he had any questions and highlighted certain information contained in the book. Mr. Samuel subsequently signed the consent form to have the procedure performed. Unfortunately, information contained in the booklet neglected to address possible risks associated with the procedure, and, in fact, stated that the procedure was a safe and efficient way of gaining the type of information needed to help physicians in further diagnosis and treatment. Neither Dr. Clark nor Ms. Terrance mentioned the possible risks of the procedure to Mr. Samuel.

During the procedure, Mr. Samuel experienced a complication in which there was occlusion of the vessels to his lower extremities. Although blood flow was partially restored, Mr. Samuel experienced irreparable damage to his left leg, necessitating a below-the-knee amputation. It is quite likely that he, as well as the courts, could question the extent to which his consent to the procedure was actually "informed," since he had not been told about the potential risks involved. Neither Dr. Clark nor Ms. Terrance could assume that Mr. Samuel was already knowledgeable about arteriograms and the possibility of risk simply because of his apparent sophistication and educational level. Likewise, Dr. Clark could not assume that Ms. Terrance would discuss possible risks of the procedure with Mr. Samuel. In addition, Dr. Clark had not reviewed the educational material given to Mr. Samuel, and consequently was unaware of its failure to include potential risks of the procedure.

Before patients can make reasonable informed consent, they must understand not only the procedure to which they are consenting but also any risks involved, as well as alternatives to the procedure that might be available. Informed consent, then, hinges not only on the accuracy and clarity of the information given to patients but also on patients having sufficient information on which to base a truly informed decision.

MISPERCEPTIONS ABOUT INFORMED CONSENT

Although the issue of informed consent has received increased attention and support, many health professionals, as well as patients, continue to have misperceptions as to what informed consent actually is. In a classic study conducted by the President's Commission for the Study of Ethical Problems in Medicine and Biomedical and Behavioral Research, a group of patients and physicians were asked what the term informed consent meant to them (President's Commission for the Study of Ethical Problems in Medicine and Biomedical and Behavioral Research, 1982). Twenty-one percent of the public said they did not know the meaning of the term informed consent. The majority of the rest of the public samples defined informed consent in terms of being informed or agreeing to treatment, but usually agreement to treatment was put in the context of whatever the health professional, in this case the physician, thought best. Only 11% of the public recognized that informed consent included information about risk or alternatives.

In the physician group, most stated that informed consent consisted of generally informing patients about their condition and treatment. Only 34% of physician respondents recognized that informed consent included patient understanding of the information provided, and even fewer mentioned patient understanding of risks as part of the concept. Few physicians mentioned treatment alternatives or that informed consent involved patient choice or preference about treatment.

VALIDITY OF INFORMED CONSENT

Initially, a valid informed consent was taken to mean that the patient had given written authorization to have a procedure performed. The validity of informed consent has been expanded over the years through legal precedent because of individual cases brought before the courts. Consequently, the term is much more broadly defined now than initially, when it was concerned mainly with a patient's authorization to have a procedure performed. To be valid, patients' consent must be informed. In general, information required to make a consent informed currently consists of:

- The diagnosis
- Explanation of the proposed treatment and its purpose
- Risks or consequences of the proposed treatment
- Probability that the proposed treatment will be successful
- Treatment alternatives available
- Consequences of not receiving the proposed treatment

All information must also be provided to patients in terms they can understand. An awareness of the meaning of informed consent is extremely important for all health professionals, especially for those involved in patient teaching. Through their own awareness of its meaning, health professionals may also serve as patient advocates in educating them about the type and extent of information that informed consent requires. Without a clear understanding of what informed consent involves, neither patients nor health professionals can use it to its optimal intent.

THE FUNCTION OF INFORMED CONSENT

The primary purpose of informed consent is the protection of individual autonomy. Autonomy is a form of personal freedom of action in which patients determine their own course of action according to a plan they have chosen. No matter what the health professional thinks may be best for the patient, informed consent puts patients in a position that promotes and protects their right to make decisions concerning their own welfare. Informed consent protects patients from being placed in a position where decisions are based on values and views of the health professional rather than their own. Through informed consent, patients are given information about the procedure itself, as well as the risks and consequences of having or not having the procedure performed. If patients have obtained all the information they feel necessary to make a decision, then they are theoretically protected from submitting to procedures that, according to their own value structure, they may not feel are in their best interests.

Although the function of informed consent seems fairly straightforward, there has been significant confusion about the nature and scope of information that is required to be disclosed and discussed. Some argue that providing patients with too much information and detail can be overwhelming and actually limit the patient's ability to make an informed choice about whether or not he or she will give consent to have the procedure performed. Consider, for example, Dr. Yang, who was conducting preoperative teaching with a patient, Mr. Hall, prior to asking him to sign the informed consent form.

Dr. Yang: "Mr. Hall, tomorrow morning before surgery you will first receive an injection of Demerol, which is a narcotic that will help you to relax and decrease your anxiety level. The Demerol will be mixed with another drug called atropine, which will dry up the secretions of your mucous membrane. This is important because when you go into surgery, we will insert a tube down your throat called an airway that will keep your air passages open and that will allow us to give you the anesthetic. If your mouth is full of saliva, then you could choke when we put the tube in. The tube will be attached to a respirator, which will help you breathe. This is important because we will also inject you with a drug that is actually a poison called curare, which will completely paralyze all your muscles from head to toe. This obviously includes your chest muscles. Since you won't be able to breathe on your own as a result and there must be air exchange in order to keep you alive, the respirator will breathe for you. In the unlikely event that there is a power shortage during surgery, which would cause the respirator to fail, the hospital has an emergency generator that will be used to maintain the respirator's function. Also rarely, but on occasion, people for some reason react to the anesthetic and their hearts stop. The surgery team is ready for such emergencies and, in the rare event that this happens, would be ready to resuscitate immediately, meaning that they would attempt to restore your heart to begin beating again on its own."

Obviously, if Dr. Yang went into this much detail, in all likelihood, the patient may well decide to leave the hospital. Although perhaps an extreme example, this explanation or others that include excessive detail may be considered "information dumping" rather than giving patients information which would help them make an informed decision about whether or not to authorize the procedure, and whether or not they feel the procedure would be in their best interests. Although reason and judgment prevail, there are still circumstances in which it may be unclear how much information is sufficient and when the amount of information is insufficient to enable the patient to make an informed choice.

STANDARDS FOR INFORMED CONSENT

The first requirement of informed consent is that the information given must be adequate so the patient has sufficient information on which to base consent. The standards for what constitutes informed consent are based on the *professional community standard* and the *reasonable person standard.*

The professional community standard is based on what would be considered as customary information that most professionals in that professional community would provide. This standard can apply to local, regional, or national levels, depending on the circumstances. For example, it would be expected that most health professionals would disclose the potential risks of an experimental drug for the treatment of human immunodeficiency virus before prescribing it and that health professionals' failure to do so may be considered negligence.

The professional community standard was determined legally in the case of *Natanson v. Kline* (1960). The case involved a patient, Ms. Natanson, who had undergone a radical mastectomy for breast cancer. After surgery, her physician referred her to Dr. Kline for cobalt radiation therapy. As a result of the radiation therapy, Ms. Natanson experienced sloughing and necrosis of tissues at the site of treatment and subsequently sued Dr. Kline for malpractice and failure to disclose risks of the procedure prior to instigating treatment. The court determination of outcome of the case was the basis of Professional Standard of Disclosure, which states that the amount of information disclosed should be based on what a reasonable medical professional would provide the patient, taking into account the physician's judgment of what is in the patient's best interest.

Opponents of the court's decision argued against the Professional Standard of Disclosure on the grounds that it usurped the patient's right to self-determination. Opponents claimed that the standard should be based on information that any reasonable person would need in order to make an informed decision about whether or not to have a procedure performed.

The second standard, *the reasonable person standard*, is more patient centered than the professional community standard. It is based on the premise that sufficient information should be provided and given in such a way that a reasonable person (defined as one who is competent and capable of systematic reasoning in reaching decisions about his or her treatment), could make an informed choice. The reasonable person standard was determined by the 1972 case of *Canterbury v. Spence.*

In the case, Mr. Canterbury, at 19 years of age, experienced severe pain between his shoulder blades. Despite numerous medical consultations and treatments, he received no relief. Consequently, his physician referred him to Dr. Spence, a neurosurgeon. Dr. Spence obtained a myelogram, which showed a defect in Mr. Canterbury's vertebrae, and a laminectomy was recommended. When discussing the procedure with Mr. Canterbury's mother over the phone, she asked whether the surgery was serious, to which Dr. Spence replied that it was no more serious than any other surgery. In surgery, Dr. Spence found more serious abnormalities in Mr. Canterbury's spine than he had anticipated. The day after surgery, Mr. Canterbury was left unattended as he went to the bathroom. He fell and became paralyzed from the waist down. Mr. Canterbury and his family sued the hospital for failure to provide assistance, and failed Dr. Spence on the grounds that Mr. Canterbury and his family had not been adequately informed about the potential risk of surgery. The court determined that there is a duty to disclose risks based on the right of each individual to determine what is done to his body.

A third standard that was an outcome of the *Canterbury v. Spence* (1972) case is the *subjective standard*, which takes into account the personal needs and values of the patient. This is so that the amount of information and the time it is disclosed are based on the patient's personal circumstances and need to know. This standard implies that appropriate diagnosis, treatment, and informed consent cannot be obtained without the health professional's knowledge of the patient, their circumstances, values, and preferences, and that this knowledge cannot be obtained without adequate open discussion with the patient about their personal views.

The question, however, may still remain: "How much and what type of information should a 'reasonable' patient be given?" In making this determination, it is important to remember the function of informed consent. The health professional should discuss facts and uncertainties with patients that would help them gain a working understanding of their condition, treatment, alternatives, and possible consequences of agreeing or not agreeing to treatment, so that they can make a decision that best suits their own needs and values. The amount, type, and way patients are provided information should be based on health professionals' knowledge of the patient as an individual, along with his or her personal circumstances.

This would imply, then, that in determining what type and how much information to give the patient, the health professional must be able to assess the individual and tailor the presentation of information to the individual according to his or her particular needs. This means that the health professional must gear provision of information to a tactful discussion of facts, remaining sensitive to the individual's needs, intellectual capability, and emotional state at the time, and that the information must be presented in terms that the patient can understand. Although the patient's questions and concerns about the proposed treatment or procedure must be addressed, the health professional cannot depend on the patient's questions to indicate how much he or she wants to know. The patient may not know what to ask or may be too intimidated to ask questions or state concerns. The stress of the condition or illness itself may preclude the patient's thinking of questions that may otherwise seem obvious.

It is therefore the responsibility of the health professional to provide patients with accurate and complete information about their condition, treatment, or procedure and to inform them of what is at stake if a variety of different actions are taken. Benefits gained from accepting or not accepting treatment must be assessed in terms of the patient's own values. This also means that the health professional must discuss alternatives that the patient may see as beneficial even if the health professional disagrees.

Such was the case of Ms. Caldwell, a 38-year-old woman with a strong family history of breast cancer. Her last mammogram revealed suspicious areas in her left breast. In consultation with her physician, Dr. Rogers, leakage of blood-tinged fluid from the nipple of her breast was also noted. Dr. Rogers recommended a biopsy, but also informed Ms. Caldwell that, with her family history of cancer and because of the leakage of fluid, there was a greater possibility that a malignancy was present and suggested that a simple mastectomy be performed. The biopsy was positive, and Ms. Caldwell returned for surgery a few days later.

Ms. Caldwell was given a thorough explanation of what the surgery entailed, the risks involved, and the consequences of having a malignancy untreated. Consequently, she signed the consent for a simple mastectomy.

Ms. Caldwell's postoperative recovery was uneventful, and all appeared to be going well. Two months after her surgery, however, she returned to

Dr. Rogers's office, charging that she had not been given full information when she agreed to have the major surgery performed. She had recently read of the possibility of having a "lumpectomy" in which the entire breast is not removed. She stated that several of her friends had also reported knowing individuals who had had this procedure and were apparently doing well.

Dr. Rogers stated that the procedure would not have been appropriate for her type of breast cancer and given her age and strong family history of breast cancer, it appeared that the simple mastectomy was the most effective means for saving her life. Ms. Caldwell did not share Dr. Rogers's opinion. Her decision had been made at a time of personal stress in which she felt very vulnerable, not even thinking to ask whether there were alternatives to the mastectomy. She felt that had options been presented to her, she would not have agreed to have the mastectomy.

Ms. Caldwell's case illustrates several points. First, although she received complete information about the procedure and the risks involved, Dr. Rogers did not provide her with information regarding possible alternatives. Dr. Rogers did not discuss any other options with Ms. Caldwell because of the belief that a mastectomy was the most effective way to cure breast cancer in her case. Dr. Rogers's judgment of what treatment was most effective was based on the assumption that Ms. Caldwell would consider cure more important than amputation of her breast. Even if the mastectomy were to be more effective in treating Ms. Caldwell's malignancy, Dr. Rogers cannot assume that she would consider longevity to be in her best interests.

Second, Ms. Caldwell did not ask about alternatives because she was not yet aware of them. In addition, because of the stress of the news she had received, she may not have been thinking clearly enough to request information about alternatives. Withholding information about alternatives was probably not, in this case, in Ms. Caldwell's best interest.

THERAPEUTIC PRIVILEGE

Withholding information was once thought to be an acceptable practice if the health professional felt that providing the patient with full information would be detrimental to the patient (Pirakitikulr & Bursztajn, 2006). This exception to full disclosure was called *therapeutic privilege*. Under these circumstances, exception to full disclosure of information was believed to be justified under the ethical principles of beneficence (doing good) or nonmaleficence (avoid doing harm). Whether therapeutic privilege is ever legally or ethically defensible has been questioned from the standpoint that it is the patient, rather than the health professional, who is in the best position to determine what is in his or her best interest or best for his or her welfare (Johnston & Holt,

2006). Therapeutic privilege creates conflict between beneficence and patient autonomy and self-determination, and is now commonly thought of as unacceptable practice (Bostick et al., 2006).

Although there has been legal recognition of therapeutic privilege in several court cases from the standpoint that under certain circumstances it is viewed as protecting patients' well-being, common thought is that it not ethically justified (Edwin, 2008). The postponement of full disclosure of information has been viewed by some as acceptable under certain circumstances. Examples of when full disclosure of information might be postponed would be the case of a patient so physically ill that full disclosure of information could potentially cause serious health consequences, such as an individual who is in a weakened and debilitated state after a severe heart attack, but who, in the course of hospitalization is also found to have leukemia. Although the patient would be given information at a later time, their current critical state may preclude disclosure of the second diagnosis until his or her current physical condition is stabilized. Another possible example is a case in which the patient is so emotionally unstable that he or she has impaired decision-making abilities or when there is concern that disclosure of information would cause the patient harm (Côté, 2000). Others have questioned whether patients have a right to request waiver of full disclosure, stating that they would rather not know a diagnosis or potential for poor outcome (Sirotin & Lo, 2006).

Even under these circumstances, therapeutic privilege is just that—a privilege that should not be misused. If the health professional purposefully withholds information from a patient because of fear that, with full information, the patient would not accept treatment the health professional feels is needed, the health professional has violated the ethical principles of autonomy, beneficence, and nonmaleficence (Edwin, 2008). Such is the case of a person who, after having an abnormal stress test, is told that a cardiac catheterization is indicated. Fearful that the patient would refuse to have the catheterization if risks of the procedure were outlined, the health professional may not address the risks involved or may at least minimize them. In this instance, the purpose of withholding information would be not to protect the patient from harm but rather to coerce him or her into a procedure deemed to be in the patient's best interest by the health professional. Withholding information for this reason prevents patients from making a truly informed consent about whether or not to undergo the procedure. Failure to disclose information is a violation of the patient's right to informed choice.

In rare instances where therapeutic privilege is exercised, health professionals should document that the patient's susceptibility to harm from receiving the information is above the norm, or that the patient is incapable of making a truly informed choice at that time because of psychological or other factors related to competency. When this occurs, factual evidence to support the health professional's use of therapeutic privilege is crucial. In addition, professionals may want to seek a second opinion confirming their observation. This second opinion should also be documented on the patient's chart.

In cases in which patients waive their right to information, the health professional should ascertain that the patient has full understanding of the implication of their request and that their request is documented. Such might be the case of a patient who states that they do not want to know if their condition is considered terminal. In these instances, however, if the patient asks directly at a later time whether or not the illness is terminal, a truthful answer is mandated. Even in these circumstances, it should be noted that tact should prevail. Truth can, even in these instances, be presented in such a way as not to destroy the patient's hope.

The once held view that health professionals generally know what is best in promoting patients well-being has now largely been replaced by concepts of patient autonomy and shared decision making (Bostick et al., 2006). For the most part, the relationship between patient and health professional should be one of candor, since an important part of the relationship is trust, which cannot be upheld without honest and open discussion regarding the patient's condition (Edwin, 2008). Health professionals cannot assume that honest and full disclosure, even of bad news, will necessarily be harmful; often, withholding information may cause more harm than good (Buckman, 1992).

IMPLIED OR EXPLICIT CONSENT

Disclosing information to patients that enables them to make their own healthcare decisions is the basis of patient teaching as well as the basis of the legal doctrine of informed consent. It is hardly feasible, however, that health professionals will obtain written or even verbal consent from patients every time they interact with them. Obviously, patients do not give written consent every time they visit an ambulatory care or receive an injection in the hospital.

Patients' consent may be either implied or explicit. *Implied consent* is a type of consent that is inferred from the patient's actions. For example, it is assumed that when a patient makes an appointment to be seen by a physician for a specific physical problem, he or she is authorizing the physician to do an examination in order to arrive at a diagnosis and prescribe appropriate treatment. Under these circumstances, no specific written or oral consent is necessary. The underlying principle is based on the voluntary and active nature of the patient's action with the understanding that in seeking medical advice, an exam will ensue.

Implied consent is limited, however, to situations in which the patient is aware of what may be reasonably expected under specific circumstances. Any additional treatment or procedure that is not obvious at the time the patient submitted to the original examination or procedure is not warranted without further consent. For instance, a patient who seeks advice from a physician because of an earache may reasonably expect the physician to examine the ear. If it is found, however, that a more serious procedure is indicated, such as a myringotomy, the procedure should not be performed without providing the patient with additional information and without the patient's explicit informed consent.

Implied consent applies to situations in which procedures are noninvasive, routine, without significant risk, or when the patient has the ability to voluntarily withdraw from the procedure or circumstance. For instance, in the previous example, a patient seeking advice from a physician because of an earache may expect to receive some sort of medication to treat the ear. Given that the patient receives adequate information about the medication prescribed, he or she is able to choose whether to have the prescription filled and the degree to which the recommendations will be followed. Patients would not be expected to sign a consent form stating that they understand the treatment recommendations and any associated risks.

When a procedure imposes additional risk, the patient's *explicit consent* must be obtained. As a part of explicit consent, the patient must be made aware of inherent risks as well as alternatives to the treatment or procedure that may be available. Explicit consent requires more than the assumption that, because the patients sought advice, they also agree to submit to additional procedures. Explicit consent is obtained whenever:

1. A procedure is invasive.
2. Anesthesia is used.
3. A nonsurgical procedure is to be performed in which there is more than slight risk to the patient, such as an arteriogram.
4. A procedure involving radiation, cobalt, or electric shock is to be performed.
5. The procedure or treatment to which the patient is to be exposed is experimental.

In general, patients' consent is limited to the procedures described to them when their consent was given. At times, however, health professionals do not know which additional procedures may be needed until after the original procedure is performed. Under these circumstances, generally, another consent from the patient or someone authorized to give consent on the patient's behalf must be obtained. For example, if the patient has given consent to have an appendectomy, but during surgery it is discovered that the patient also has a malignancy of the colon that requires removal of the bowel and subsequent colostomy, consent for the additional procedure would need to be obtained from the patient or another authorized person.

Some general exceptions to this rule may apply if the patient consents to reasonable steps to correct a condition, leaving the exact choice of procedure to the health professional. For example, a patient may undergo surgery for cancer in which the extensiveness of the malignancy is unknown. Consequently, the exact procedure required in order to remedy the condition may also not be known. Under these circumstances, the patient's informed consent may reflect authorization for the proposed procedure, but also authorization for the health professional to perform additional reasonable procedures if deemed necessary. Another exception to obtaining the patient's explicit consent prior to performing a procedure would be in the case of an emergency in which the patient's life would be in jeopardy if the procedure were not performed but obtaining the patient's informed consent is not feasible because he or she is unconscious and no family members or guardians are available to act in the patient's stead.

Patients have the right, when giving informed consent, to specify whether there are particular procedures they do not wish to have performed. The case of Mr. Burnham provides an example. Mr. Burnham sought advice from a physician when he discovered a lump in his neck. Upon examination, and because of Mr. Burnham's strong family history of cancer, the physician, Dr. Simmons, suggested a biopsy. Results of the biopsy confirmed that the tumor was malignant. Dr. Simmons discussed options and alternatives for treatment with Mr. Burnham, one of which was radical surgery, which would result in neck dissection and removal of the larynx. Mr. Burnham consented to surgery, but only for removal of the tumor. He stated that under no circumstances did he want to have the larynx removed. After ascertaining that Mr. Burnham fully understood the implications of his decision, Dr. Simmons was obligated to respect Mr. Burnham's decision. Consequently the tumor was removed, but the larynx was left intact.

Patients also have the right to know who will perform a procedure or treatment. If, for example, Mrs. Dean gives her expressed consent that Dr. Flynn will perform her gallbladder surgery, she has a right to expect that Dr. Flynn will indeed be the surgeon. Dr. Flynn is not at liberty to ask one of his colleagues to perform the surgery in his stead without Mrs. Dean's prior consent and knowledge.

Patients' expressed verbal or written consent should be based on as complete and accurate information as possible regarding what the procedure will involve and specific consequences that can be expected. It is the responsibility of the health professional, when obtaining informed consent, to ensure that the patient has a clear and accurate understanding of what will occur and what he or she can reasonably expect as consequences, including risks.

WHO OBTAINS CONSENT

In general, it is the obligation and responsibility of the health professional performing the procedure to provide information to the patient and to obtain his or her informed consent. Although the health professional may delegate obtaining informed consent to another appropriate person, the health professional performing the procedure remains liable for the patient's understanding of the procedure he or she is to undergo and the subsequent consequences of that procedure. This is based on the principle that only the person performing the procedure has the expertise needed to provide the patient with an explanation sufficient enough to enable him or her to make an informed decision. This expertise of information includes not only the procedure itself and its purpose, but also risks, consequences, and available alternatives.

Therefore, although other health professionals may be involved in teaching about various procedures before they are performed, the health professional carrying out the procedure is ultimately responsible for providing the patient with a sufficient explanation of the procedure in understandable terms before the consent is considered to be valid. Consequently, although another appropriate person may be delegated to obtain the patient's signature on an informed consent form, the responsibility for determining that the patient understands the procedure and is aware of risks and alternatives remains with the health professional performing it. If there are indications that the patient does not understand the procedure or that the consent is not truly informed, a person delegated to obtain the patient's signature is responsible for immediately notifying the health professional who is to perform the procedure. If the patient confides that he or she did not actually understand the explanation or that he or she has changed his or her mind, it is imperative that the health professional performing the procedure is informed and that the observation is documented in the patient's record. In instances when another health professional discovers that the patient does not clearly understand the nature of the procedure or all its risks or consequences, the health professional performing the procedure should be notified and has the responsibility for clarifying information for the patient.

CONCEPTS OF COMPETENCE FOR INFORMED CONSENT

The term competence refers to patients' abilities to make rational, informed decisions. Patients who are competent have the right to decide whether or not they will follow medical advice and treatment recommendations. When there is doubt about the patient's competence to make an informed decision, informed consent cannot be considered to be valid.

Competence is a legal concept that can be formally determined only through legal proceedings. Health professionals cannot, on their own, make decisions regarding patients' competence to make an informed choice. Assumptions about patient's level of competence may or may not be valid. Competence must be assessed in the context of the specific situation. Competence to make an informed decision about treatment or care may not necessarily be correlated with competence for decisions about other matters. For example, an individual with a psychiatric diagnosis may be incompetent to manage his or her own financial matters but may be capable of refusing medication that causes untoward side effects. An individual with mild dementia may be incapable of driving a car but may be capable of refusing an invasive diagnostic procedure.

There are several key elements involved in competence that determine whether the patient is truly able to give informed consent. First is the patient's ability to understand the information presented. This means not only the ability to remember the information but also the ability to understand the meaning of what is told and the patient's role in the decision.

Second, the patient must be able to communicate his or her choices. In other words, even if the patient is able to understand the information presented, if he or she is unable to indicate a choice or maintain a consistent choice, competence may be called into question. This does not mean that if the patient has reasonable justification, the patient cannot change his or her mind.

Third, the patient must be able to understand the situation and the consequences of various choices that are presented. For example, some patients may have the ability to regurgitate information they have been presented and outline choices as well as risks and benefits without having full understanding of what the implications of the information and consequently their choices would have. Patients must have the ability, realistically, to assess each option and the consequences of that option and take into account their own values when weighing the risks and benefits of each option.

Last, the patient must demonstrate the ability to reach a decision by some logical process. In other words, the patient must demonstrate the ability to weigh risks and benefits according to his or her own values and according to some reasoning process, so that the patient is able to give some reasonable justification for the decision made.

ASSESSING PATIENTS' ABILITY TO GIVE CONSENT

As previously noted, competence is a legal concept. Competence and informed consent are intricately connected (Rich, 2005). Because of increased litigation, issues of competence when obtaining informed consent have gained attention. When obtaining informed consent, the health professional must be able to evaluate whether or not the patient has the ability to make an informed decision. The initial assessment may be conducted by the health professional;

however, if in conducting the assessment the patient's competence is called into question, the health professional may wish to consult with another professional who is well versed in mental status evaluations and competence determinations.

The first step in assessing patients' ability to give informed consent is to determine that they are alert and aware enough to receive the information presented. Obviously, if the patient is unconscious, delirious, or experiencing severe dementia, florid psychosis, or severe intellectual disability, he or she may not be capable of rational decision making or giving truly informed consent. In instances when the patient's mental status is in question, a brief mental status examination that evaluates the individual's orientation, memory, attention, and concentration can be a useful initial screening of the patient's ability to comprehend information.

In some instances, although patients may have full cognitive ability, severe anxiety or depression may interfere with their ability to make a rational decision. In these instances, the health professional may consult with other professionals trained in treating the underlying emotional problem. When time is crucial, the health professional may need to consult with other professionals regarding when, how, and by whom informed consent may best be obtained.

When assessing the patient's ability to make an informed decision, the health professional must also make sure that all information was clearly communicated to the patient. In some instances, the patient's inability to relate specific aspects of the information may be the result of poor communication on the part of the individual providing the patient with information rather than on the patient's inability to comprehend it. If the health professional is assured that the information has been presented completely and clearly, one of the best ways to assess the patient's understanding of the information is to ask the patient to repeat, in his or her own words, what he or she was told. Likewise, when evaluating whether or not the patient is able to make an informed choice, it is important to determine if the decision was made according to logical reasoning. If, for example, the patient gives a reason such as, "If I don't follow your advice, all the doctors and nurses will be mad, and I will have no one to take care of me," or, "I made the decision after the man on the television told me to do it," it would appear that the decision was not based on logical evaluation of the information, and the patient's ability to make a truly informed decision should probably be questioned.

Health professionals should remember that patients' refusal to accept the recommendation or treatment does not necessarily mean they are incompetent or unable to give informed consent. More important than the decision is the process by which it was made. Informed consent should be underscored by patients' understanding of the information, risks and benefits, and consequences of their decisions as well as other options and alternatives that are open to them.

CONSENT FROM SPECIAL PATIENTS

Informed consent is based on the patient's ability to understand procedures, consequences, and risks and then to make a decision of whether or not to submit to the procedure after receiving all relevant information. It goes without saying, of course, that although most patients may have the capacity to make their own informed decisions, some patients present special difficulties when obtaining consent. Examples of special groups of patients are minors, those persons who are incapacitated because of symptoms of psychiatric disability, individuals with severe intellectual disability, or those who are under the influence of drugs or alcohol. These groups, in general, require special consideration and generally require the consent of someone other than themselves for a procedure to be performed.

Laws differ from state to state regarding the minor's ability to give consent to a variety of procedures. In most instances, the health professional should seek to obtain consent from parents or another person authorized to give substitute consent. Emergency procedures that are necessary to prevent loss of life or permanent impairment may be considered exceptions to this rule, although there must also be sufficient documentation to prove that an emergency situation does indeed exist.

In some states, the ability of minors to give consent is based on their age, maturity, and ability to understand the consequences of their decision. Some states recognize minors as capable of giving valid consent if they have taken on the roles and responsibilities of adults. In this case, they are considered emancipated. Factors used to indicate that a minor is emancipated include lack of dependency on parents for support, proof of marriage, or, in some instances, having become a parent.

In some instances, an individual other than the patient may be responsible for giving informed consent. These circumstances include instances in which the person to be treated is unconscious; is under the influence of substances that affect reason, such as drugs or alcohol; or has been declared mentally incompetent by a court because of psychiatric disability, intellectual disability, or mental deterioration as a result of organic processes or injury. In these cases, consent may be obtained from the next of kin or from another person authorized to act on behalf of the patient. Exceptions, as with minors, generally apply in emergency treatment, when the individual's welfare or safety is at risk and substitute consent from an authorized individual cannot be obtained.

If the patient has been declared legally incompetent and a legal guardian has been appointed, then the guardian is authorized to give consent for the patient. When the patient is not legally declared incompetent but is not able to make informed decisions, as in the case of an individual who is unconscious, for example, the situation may not be as clear-cut. In general, under these circumstances, the nearest relative may give consent. If the patient has a spouse, then the spouse would be authorized to give consent for the individual. It should be recognized, however, that the right of one spouse to give consent for the other extends only in those circumstances when consent may not be deferred until the patient can give consent.

Under some circumstances, consent of a spouse may be an issue even when the patient is capable of making an informed decision. Such is the case when procedures may affect the marital relationship, such as in instances of sterilization or abortion. Although laws may vary from state to state, in general, if the spouse is competent, the power to consent to procedures still rests with the patient on whom the procedure is to be performed.

It should be noted that different states have different laws about informed consent of special populations. Health professionals should check on the regulations of their individual states and keep abreast of changes that occur periodically with new court rulings.

USE OF CONSENT FORMS

When the patient gives consent to have a procedure performed, there must be some means of documenting that he or she was provided with adequate information on which to base the decision and that he or she did give consent. Although verbal consent can be binding, such consents may be difficult to prove if the matter is ever brought to court. Consequently, written forms to document patients' consent are commonly used.

Informed consent forms are only a means of documentation and in no way take the place of interpersonal communication in explaining a procedure to a patient. Even a form that is written in great detail in the simplest of terms is useless if the patient does not understand it, cannot read it, or is not given the opportunity to ask questions.

In the past, consent forms were broad in nature rather than addressing the specifics of individual procedures. Such broad statements as, "I hereby consent to surgery and to have whatever organs that are diseased or deemed by the surgeon in need of removal to be excised," although leaving considerable latitude to the physician in carrying out surgery, are also extremely ambiguous in terms of the patient and what he or she can expect as a result of surgery. There is no evidence that the patient has been told the possible consequences or risks of surgery or has even been given the option to specify which organs he or she may object to having removed.

The consent form must document that the patient's consent has been informed. In order for the patient's consent to be valid, he or she must be provided with information about diagnosis, the procedure and purpose of the treatment or procedure proposed, risks and consequences of having or not having the proposed treatment or procedure, and alternatives that may be available. All information must be provided to patients in terms they understand. Therefore, if the informed consent form does not reflect that adequate information has been provided to the patient and that he or she fully understands the explanation, the form cannot be considered valid documentation of informed consent. Even if adequate explanation has been given, a form that contains less than sufficient information or that contains information in technical terms does not fulfill its purpose. The consent form should reflect the explanation the patient has received.

COMMUNICATION IN INFORMED CONSENT

Informed consent, although a legal duty of the health professional, involves much more than a duty. Informed consent becomes a vital part of the relationship between patient and health professional in which facts, concerns, and alternatives are openly discussed, and through which the patient actively participates in the decision-making process about his or her care.

The key to effective informed consent, like other forms of patient teaching, is effective communication between patient and health professional in which individual patient needs and concerns are identified and addressed. This requires information exchange between patient and professional in which there is a continuing flow of two-way communication.

Through two-way communication, health professionals are able to provide patients with information that is best suited to their individual needs in order to assist them to make a rational decision based on benefits that can be expected from the procedure compared to the risks and other options that might be available. Obviously, to inform the patient, some technical aspects of the procedure must be discussed. The technical aspects of the procedure should, however, be free of jargon and put in terms the patient can understand.

Patients vary in their degree of understanding of terminology and technical terms. Words have different meanings to various individuals. Although health professionals may attempt to be clear and honest in explanations, they may still fail to convey information in a way that leads patients to an actual understanding of their condition or treatment. To be confident of patients' understanding of the information, health professionals may ask patients to interpret the explanation given. In this way, the health professional can be assured that the information was received the way it was intended, and that the patient has all the facts necessary to make an informed decision.

Although it is important to provide patients with sufficient information in order to make an informed decision, providing them with too much information can be cumbersome and time-consuming, and can actually impede patients' decision-making process. Only information that is pertinent to the patient's decision making, which does not include every inconsequential detail that may confuse more than enhance the patient's ability to make a decision, need be given. At times, it may be difficult for the health professional to determine how much detail is enough and how much is too much. The amount of detail is more easily determined if the professional considers the purpose of informed consent and that, in order to give rational consent, the patient must be reasonably informed of benefits, consequences, risks, and alternatives. For example, if the patient is receiving an explanation about upcoming surgery, in addition to giving information about the specific procedure to be performed, the health professional may also note that all surgery contains a certain degree of risk. Not every possible risk or complication of surgery, in general, need be addressed as long as the patient recognizes the serious nature of surgery and the risks that are more likely to pose a potential problem in a particular case.

When providing patients with information in preparation for a procedure that requires consent, health professionals should remember that their own attitudes and feelings can also influence patients' decisions. Nonverbal cues that indicate disapproval or hesitance about a procedure or alternative in question can bias the patient's perception of the verbal meaning of the explanation provided. Patients should be able to base their decision on facts and unbiased information, not on information that has been biased by the values and attitudes of the health professional who is presenting the information.

Other aspects of the communication in obtaining informed consent are the timing of the explanation and the amount of time the professional devotes to providing the patient with information. As in other patient teaching situations, if the patient is uncomfortable, distraught, or in some other way preoccupied, information provided may not be incorporated by the patient. Although it is not always possible to find an ideal time when the patient is free of pain or concern, it is obvious that some times are better than others. All efforts should be made to give patients explanations when they are most likely to be receptive and when information will have a greater chance of having the most meaning and will provide a basis for truly informed consent.

If at all possible, patients should be given some time to think about the information and to weigh benefits and risks before making a decision. Providing patients with information and then immediately requesting that they make a decision may create undue pressure, and may affect the extent to which the consent was actually informed.

When providing patients with information, health professionals should not rush, should provide it in an atmosphere as free of distraction as possible, and should allow sufficient time for answering questions and addressing concerns. The health professional should be accessible to the patient, both physically and through conveying a sense of approachability, so that the patient feels free to ask questions and discuss concerns. If the patient feels intimidated by the health professional or does not feel the health professional is willing to take time to answer questions, he or she may not seek nor receive all the information needed in order to make an informed choice.

FAMILY INVOLVEMENT IN INFORMED CONSENT

Informed consent remains an individual decision. However, most individuals also live in a social or family group on whom their decisions have an impact. When making decisions of whether or not to consent to a procedure, many patients weigh the risks and benefits not only in terms of themselves but also in terms of what their decisions may mean to their families.

The influence of family or social group cannot be discounted in the informed consent process any more than it can be discounted in any other form of patient teaching. It must also be remembered that the term "family" might be defined broadly to include not only relatives but also other persons to whom the patient feels close and who have special concern for the patient and his or her well-being. Patients often make decisions based on how having the procedure or not will affect their own lives and the social groups in which they live. Consequently, there are no standard rules that apply to everyone, even when conditions or procedures appear the same. Take, for example, two patients receiving information about treatment for the same type of cancer, both at the same advanced stage. Mrs. Hiu refused further treatment, including chemotherapy, stating that she was concerned about the added burden and strain such treatment would have on her family, since the potential for cure or remission at this stage was slight. Although the prognosis for cure or remission was the same for a second patient, Mrs. Boyd, she consented to additional treatment even though she had a clear understanding of what the procedure would involve. Mrs. Boyd had two small children and felt that even if the treatment extended her life for only a few weeks, the extra time with her children was well worth the discomfort and strain. In both instances, the patients' families were major considerations in their decisions.

Families can provide additional support and encouragement to patients if they are involved in the decision-making process. Health professionals may occasionally feel that involving the family causes too much confusion and that diversity of opinion may actually impede the patient's ability to make a decision. Each patient's situation, of course, is different, and at times, family involvement may not be advantageous or even desired by the patient.

In many instances, directly involving the family can enhance communication between the patient and the health professional as well as providing the patient with a sounding board on which to discuss pros and cons. Family members may also help clarify information that the patient may otherwise be hesitant to question or that the patient may have difficulty understanding. Including the family may also facilitate discussion between family members that can be beneficial throughout the course of the patient's illness or treatment. Family members who also have an understanding of the procedure the patient has undergone are in a better position to offer support as well as to assist the patient in follow-up care that may be required.

Although family involvement in helping the patient to make an informed decision about care and treatment can enhance communication between patient and health professional, and may even enhance the patient's course through the condition and treatment, it must also be emphasized that some families provide more hindrance than help. In some situations, the patient may specifically not want family members involved. Except for the special patient problems mentioned earlier, the patient maintains the right to make his or her own informed choice without input from other individuals. The decision of whether or not to involve family members, then, may best be discussed with the patient in advance. Even if the family is insistent on being involved in the decision-making process, it is the responsibility of the health professional to make it clear to the family that, ultimately, it is the patient who has the right to the information that will help yield an informed decision.

INFORMED CONSENT IN RESEARCH

Just as the health professional must obtain patients' informed consent prior to performing a procedure, so must informed consent be obtained before patients participate as research subjects. Just as patients have the right to refuse treatment, they also have the right to refuse to participate in research. Four elements for patients are included in informed consent for research (Burns & Grove, 2007):

1. Receipt of explanation of essential study information
2. Comprehension of the information
3. Competence to give consent
4. Voluntary consent

Specifically, these elements must include (US Department of Health and Human Services, 2005):

1. Identification and credentials of researcher
2. How subjects are to be selected
3. Purpose of the study
4. Procedures to which the patient will be exposed during the research
5. Potential risks of participation
6. Potential benefits of participation
7. Whether or not the individual will be compensated for their participation
8. Whether or not there will be alternative procedures
9. Assurance of anonymity or confidentiality
10. Right to refuse to participate without penalty
11. Offer to answer individual questions
12. Access to study results

To truly give informed consent, individuals must have been able to understand the elements of discussion of the above points and must understand the implications (Jorgensen et al., 2009). Consequently, patient teaching about the study must be conducted in terms the patient can understand and in the context of the circumstances of individual (Nieswiadomy, 2008; Yap et al., 2009). A key element of informed consent to research is that the individual has the right to refuse to participate as well as a right to withdraw from participation at any time (Sumner, 2007). Effective patient teaching about research, just as effective teaching about other issues of health care, can be measured by the degree to which the patient is able to make his or her own truly informed decision (Lin, Yeh, & Chen, 2009; Pattinson, 2009).

REFERENCES

Bostick, N. A., Sade, R., McMahon, J. W., & Benjamin, R. (2006) Report of the American Medical Association Council on Ethical and Judicial Affairs: Withholding information from patients: Rethinking the propriety of "therapeutic privilege." *Journal of Clinical Ethics, 17*(4), 302–306.

Buckman, R. (1992). *How to break bad news: A guide for health care professionals.* Baltimore: John Hopkins University Press.

Burns, N., & Grove, S. K. (2007). *Understanding nursing research: Building an evidence based practice* (4th ed.). St. Louis: Saunders.

Canterbury v. Spence, 464 F 2d. 772 (C.C. Cir. 1972).

Côté, A. (2000). Telling the truth? Disclosure and therapeutic privilege and intersexuality in children. *Health Law Journal, 8*, 199–216.

Dickey, S. B. (2006). Informed consent: Ethical issues. In V. D. Lachman (Ed.). *Applied ethics in nursing* (pp. 25–38). New York: Springer.

Edwin, A. (2008). Don't lie but don't tell the whole truth: The therapeutic privilege - Is it ever justified? *Ghana Medical Journal, 42*(4), 156–161.

Johnston, C., & Holt, G. (2006). The legal and ethical implications of therapeutic privilege - Is it ever justified to withhold treatment information from a competent patient? *Clinical Ethics, 1*, 146–151.

Jorgensen, K. J., Brodersen, J., Hartling, O. J., Nielsen, M., & Gotzsche, P. C. (2009). Informed choice requires information about both benefits and harms. *Journal of Medical Ethics, 35*(4), 268–269.

Koch, K. A. (1992). Patient Self-Determination Act. *Journal of the Florida Medical Association, 79*(4), 240–243.

Lin, M., Yeh, L., & Chen, C. (2009). Patient involvement in medical decision making. *Journal of Nursing, 56*(3), 83–87.

Miola, J. (2009). Informed consent and the rise of autonomy. *British Journal of Nursing, 18*(8), 504, 506.

Natanson v. Kline, 186 Kan. 393, 409–10, 350 p. 2Nd 1093, 1106; rehearing denied, 187 Kan. 186, 354p. 2D 670 (1960).

Nieswiadomy, R. M. (2008). *Foundations of nursing research* (5th ed.). Upper Saddle River, NJ: Pearson/Prentice Hall.

Pattinson, S. D. (2009). Consent and informational responsibility. *Journal of Medical Ethics, 35*(3), 176–179.

Pera, S. (2005). Ethical principles and rules in moral decision-making and professional-patient relationships. In S. A. Pera & S. van Tonder (Eds.). *Ethics in health care* (2nd ed., pp. 46–55). Landsowne: Juta & Co.

Pirakitikulr, D., & Bursztajn, H. J. (2006). The Grand Inquisitor's choice: Comment on the CEJA report on withholding information from patients. *Journal of Clinical Ethics, 17*(4), 307–311.

President's Commission for the Study of Ethical Problems in Medicine and Biomedical and Behavioral Research. (1982). *Making health care decisions: The ethical and legal implications of informed consent in the patient-practitioner relationship.* Washington, DC: Superintendent of Documents, US Code Annot US 1982: Title 42, Section 300V.

Rich, K. (2005). Ethics in psychiatric and mental health nursing. In J. Butts & K. Rich. *Nursing ethics: Across the curriculum and into practice* (pp. 147–173). Sudbury, MA: Jones and Bartlett.

Sirotin, N., & Lo, B. (2006). The end of therapeutic privilege? *Journal of Clinical Ethics, 17*(4), 312–316.

Sumner, J. (2007). Ethics and nursing research. In Boswell, C., & Cannon, S. *Introduction to nursing research: Incorporating evidence-based practice* (pp. 47–74). Sudbury, MA; Jones and Bartlett.

US Department of Health and Human Services. (2005). Protection of human subjects. Code of Federal Regulation Title 45 Part 46. Retrieved August 4, 2009, from http://ohsr.od.nih.gov/guidelines/45cfr46.html

Yap, T. Y., Yamokoski, A., Noll, R. Drotar, D., Zyzanski, S., & Kodish, E. D. (2009). A physician-directed intervention: Teaching and measuring better informed consent. *Academic Medicine, 84*(8), 1036–1042.

CHAPTER 16

Instructional Aids in Patient Teaching: Used or Abused

A number of new products ranging from written instructional aids to computer applications have been introduced in recent years to be used in patient teaching. Instructional aids can be powerful tools that can enhance patient teaching; however, as with any innovative technique, there is also the potential for misuse and abuse. Use of instructional aids in patient teaching can become a fad, to the extent that more attention is given to obtaining and promoting instructional aids than is given to the quality of the teaching interaction. Instructional aids may be thought to be obligatory for effective patient teaching without consideration of the quality of the material used. Instructional aids, if used, should supplement patient teaching by the health professional—not replace it. Health professionals may become so preoccupied with use of instructional aids that they forget that their relationship with the patient is one of the most important factors in effective patient teaching, and that the overall goal of patient teaching is not to bombard patients with information, but rather to enable them to make more informed decisions.

Placing extreme value on instructional aids can lead to dehumanization of the relationship between the patient and health professional, which is debilitating if patient teaching is to be effective. Before using instructional aids, health professionals should examine not only the materials, but also their own motivation for their use. In some instances, health professionals may be anxious and inexperienced in patient teaching, and consequently may use instructional aids excessively as a substitute for active presentation of information. In other instances, health professionals may rationalize that because of limited time, they still have done an adequate job of patient teaching because they have provided the patient with a number of patient education materials.

Not only can misuse of instructional aids lead to poor patient teaching results, sometimes misuse can be traumatic. Some materials that use graphic representation of concepts may be used by health professionals to "shock" the patient into adherence. Such examples would be slides of mutilated bodies in an attempt to coerce patients into using safety belts in cars. Another example may be showing pictures of diseased or cancerous lungs to a patient who smokes. There has been little empirical evidence that shows that the shock value of such methods is effective in motivating patients to adhere with recommendations. In fact, in some instances, the shock is so great that it tends to have the paradoxical effect. Use of any instructional aid should be considered in the context of the primary purpose of patient teaching: to provide patients with information based on their individual needs and that enables them to make informed choices in accordance with their own goals. Instructional aids in the form of DVDs or audiocassettes, movies, pamphlets, books, and fact sheets are available on a wide variety of topics—ranging from prevention and health maintenance to information that is disease-specific or that focuses on certain treatments or procedures. The abundance of instructional aids, although helpful in providing numerous sources and types of materials from which to choose, can also be overwhelming. Health professionals may have difficultly determining which instructional aids are the most suitable, which are of the best quality, and how instructional aids are most appropriately used.

There are a number of misconceptions about instructional aids: Patients learn best when they are exposed to many educational resources, costly or elaborate educational materials are more beneficial than those developed by health professionals themselves, or the "packaging" of the materials is equal to the quality of the information inside.

As with most other procedures or technology, instructional aids can be useful if used appropriately. If they are not used appropriately, instructional aids can be costly as well as ineffective in patient teaching. An important skill in patient teaching is the ability of the health professional to evaluate instructional aids and choose those that are most beneficial under specific circumstances.

ASSESSING CONTENT OF INSTRUCTIONAL AIDS

Even if instructional aids are well organized and attractive in presentation, of most importance is the quality of information contained within. Health professionals may be swayed by the appearance of the written material and fail to carefully evaluate its content. Since the purpose of using written instructional aids is to enhance or reinforce patients' understanding, it is crucial that the information contained within the instructional aid is consistent with and complementary to the information the health professional has provided.

Health professionals should be familiar with the content of all instructional aids before distributing them to patients. Information and illustrations should be factual and accurate. Health professionals should continue to check written instructional aids on a regular basis, so that any materials that require updates or that no longer accurately represent current views are identified and changed. Periodic checks of instructional aids help ensure that information in the handouts is still consistent with the verbal explanation provided by the health professional and still represents information that the health professional wants to emphasize.

Information presented in the instructional aid should be presented in an objective way, with no major distortions. Although the health professional may be tempted to choose or to develop instructional aids that present only one side of controversial issues, or that address only positive aspects of a treatment or procedure, it is important to remember that the purpose of the instructional aid is to enhance patient teaching, with the ultimate goal of enabling patients to make informed choices based on facts, not bias. Therefore, if all relevant information is not presented by the instructional aid or if information presented in the aid is distorted so patients receive biased information, they have not been provided with adequate facts on which to make an informed choice about the degree to which they will adhere with recommendations. As with verbal communication, information contained in the instructional aids should be objective, factual, and current.

Written instructional aids can serve as reminders or reinforcers of information provided to patients by health professionals. If the content of the instructional aid does not accurately reflect the content of the patient teaching session, however, it is of little value. For example, a nurse may teach a patient about the use of hormone replacement therapy after menopause to help prevent osteoporosis and, during the teaching session, explain the advantages and disadvantages of hormone replacement therapy as well as potential risks. However, if the nurse then gives the patient a handout that only contains positive information, with none of the potential problems or risks, the patient may forget the information provided verbally and depend solely on the written materials to make her decision. If the patient later experiences complications because of hormone replacement therapy, even though the nurse verbally discussed the possibility of complications, the patient may feel she was not aware of all the facts before making her decision. Likewise, avoiding negative aspects of a condition or treatment or slanting material in an instructional aid to one viewpoint can cause health professionals to lose credibility if patients later discover that the information in the instructional aid was not entirely accurate.

In assessing instructional aids, health professionals should evaluate whether the breadth and scope of the information is sufficient for the purpose intended, and whether more or less detail is needed to accomplish the objectives of patient teaching. Sometimes instructional aids can provide so much detail that the patient is overwhelmed with information. Patients may not be prepared to absorb all the information presented in the instructional aid, especially if it is more detailed than the personal explanation given by the health professional. In this case, the instructional aid may do more harm than good. Patients may become confused rather than gaining increased understanding, or may become anxious or overly concerned because they are overwhelmed by the information provided. For example, consider the following case. A pharmacist, Ms. Anderson was anxious to supplement verbal information provided to Ms. Leber, a patient by her physician. Ms. Anderson made sure Ms. Leber was given the drug insert accompanying the medication. Although Ms. Anderson discussed the major side effects with Ms. Leber, she did not realize that Ms. Leber, when reading the drug insert, might be alarmed by the number of additional side effects mentioned in the insert. Ms. Leber became so apprehensive about taking the medication after reading the long list of potential side effects that she discontinued the medication of her own volition. If the drug insert was to be useful, the pharmacist, Ms. Anderson should have underlined key side effects, explaining that there was little probability that the others listed would develop.

Health professionals should also be aware of messages that instructional aids convey that may not be directly related to the accuracy of information but rather to the views of the manufacturers or producers of the materials. Although these views may not be those of the health professional, patients receiving instructional aids may interpret the information as representative of the views of the health professional. For instance, in an effort to be supportive and encouraging, instructional aids may be written in an overly optimistic way. Patients may interpret the tone of the information in the instructional aid as an indication that any concerns, fears, and anxiety they may be experiencing are negative attributes rather than a natural part of adjustment or adaptation to their condition or treatment. Other instructional aids may portray unrealistic images of situations to which patients may be exposed. For example, a written aid describing breastfeeding may contain factual information but may be presented in such a way that unless the patient is able to breastfeed with absolutely no problems, the patient is made to feel inadequate because she has not been able to achieve the standard that was implied by the information in the instructional aid. If the patient does not want to breastfeed or, if for some reason she is unable to do so, she may experience guilt and may be reluctant to discuss her feelings with the physician or nurse because she assumes that the instructional aid reflects their feelings as well. In assessing instructional aids, it is important to be alert to value orientations presented in the teaching materials and to determine the extent to which they reflect the values or views of the health professional and/or health facility. Unless the two are congruent, the instructional aid can hinder the effectiveness of patient teaching.

USING INSTRUCTIONAL AIDS

Keeping patients informed may be viewed by some health professionals as requiring more time than they have to spend. In other instances, health professionals may feel insecure about their ability to teach patients effectively or may feel they have inadequate patient teaching skills. They may equate information with education, believing that the more information the patient is given, the more "educated" he or she will be.

Any of these views may lead to misuse of instructional aids. Misuse of instructional aids can result in needless financial expenditure and less than desired results. Dr. Anderson serves as an example. After completing his medical residency, Dr. Anderson set up a solo practice in a small rural community near the town where he grew up. He remembered lectures he had heard in medical school about the importance of patient teaching and the importance of keeping patients informed about their condition and treatment. Eager to offer the most up-to-date and quality medical care, he began planning how he could implement a patient education program in his practice. Although he believed patients should be provided with information, he was also concerned that being in solo practice would require more time than he had available. He was concerned that if he took the time to provide patients with all the information he thought they needed, the number of patients he could see each day would be severely limited.

In addition, although he had heard some lectures about patient teaching, there was no instruction during medical school or his residency that helped him build skills and confidence in patient teaching. As a consequence, Dr. Anderson felt somewhat unsure of his ability to teach patients effectively. He had begun to receive numerous advertisements through the Internet that promoted a variety of instructional aids for patient education. In addition, he visited a number of vendor display booths at medical conferences and talked with numerous sales representatives about instructional aids available for a comprehensive patient education program.

After reviewing advertisements and talking with the sales representatives, Dr. Anderson bought a number of DVDs on a variety of illnesses and prevention topics, computer programs that could be used for patient teaching, and numerous pamphlets and brochures that addressed aspects of prevention and a variety of chronic and acute illnesses. Dr. Anderson asked the nurse, Ms. Lucas, to index the instructional aids and file them in a way that all materials would be easily retrievable. He also directed Ms. Lucas to distribute pamphlets to appropriate patients on a routine basis. For instance, he specified that all pre-natal patients were to receive the pamphlet on preparation for childbirth, all patients requesting birth control were to receive the pamphlet on choosing birth control methods, all patients with hypertension were to be given informa-tion on how to control hypertension, and all patients with elevated cholesterol were to be given a pamphlet on how cholesterol could be lowered. In addition, Dr. Anderson asked that patients with the diagnosis of diabetes be shown a DVD about it. Women having a regular physical examination were expected to view the DVD on breast self-examination. For other patients interested in specific topics, he offered them the opportunity to use the special computer program that he had purchased.

Feeling confident that he had developed a comprehensive patient educa-tion program for his teaching education program, Dr. Anderson spent very little time conducting individual patient teaching with his patients about their conditions or treatments, assuming that most of their teaching needs could be taken care of by the instructional aids he provided. Ms. Lucas was the only other person in the office besides the receptionist and, likewise, had little extra time to spend with patients. Involvement in patient teaching from Ms. Lucas's standpoint became a matter mainly of organizing instructional aids, distribut-ing pamphlets and brochures to designated patients, starting the DVD player, and helping patients use the computerized patient education program on the topic of their choice.

After some time, Dr. Anderson became concerned when Ms. Lucas reported that many patients were not viewing the DVDs or using the computer program, saying they could not afford the extra time. In addition, many of the pamphlets and brochures distributed to patients were found lying in the examining room or waiting room, seemingly untouched. Dr. Anderson became further dismayed that patients seemed no more prone to follow recommendations after receiving the additional materials than before. They actually seemed to have no clearer understanding of their condition and treatment than the patients he had worked with previously who had had no exposure to instructional aids at all.

Somewhat exasperated by the whole experience, Dr. Anderson discussed the matter with a physician friend in private practice in a nearby town. Dr. Ander-son was surprised to hear that his friend, although an advocate of patient edu-cation, had actually spent little money on instructional aids. His friend had, however, been very selective about the materials that were purchased. In addi-tion, Dr. Anderson's friend appeared to have more patient cooperation and rap-port while still seeing as many patients per day as Dr. Anderson.

Through discussion of the issue with his friend, Dr. Anderson discovered that his friend used the instructional aids to supplement patient teaching he or his nurse provided, not to act as the sole source of information. Although supplying patients with abundant information in the form of instructional aids, Dr. Anderson conducted little patient teaching himself, nor did he encourage Ms. Lucas to become involved in direct patient teaching. Patients had begun to interpret Dr. Anderson's approach to patient teaching as cold and impersonal. Also, many of the instructional aids were reported by some as difficult to read or as being poorly written. Others stated that although they were offered the opportunity to use computerized teaching programs, they found them to be of little value because they did not know how to use the computer. The materials were not achieving the results Dr. Anderson had anticipated. Luckily, rather than viewing patient education as generally not worth the effort, Dr. Arnold realized that he had been equating information and instructional aids with patient teaching, rather than seeing them as tools which could be used to supplement, reinforce, and enhance patient teaching.

Dr. Anderson, although well meaning, had misconceptions not only about the role of instructional aids in patient teaching, but also about the process of patient teaching itself. The most important ingredients in patient teaching are a trusting and collaborative relationship between patient and health professional and patient teaching that is geared to the individual patient's needs and circumstances. Without this relationship, and without tailoring patient teaching to meet the patient's needs, instructional aids—no matter how elaborate or comprehensive—have little chance of being effective in reaching the goals that patient teaching is designed to accomplish.

After talking with his friend, Dr. Anderson returned to his office. He and Ms. Lucas discussed alterations that needed to be made in the strategy for how instructional aids were used for patient teaching. Together, they carefully read and reviewed all the instructional aids, discarding the materials that were poorly written or designed, that contained incomplete or inaccurate information, or that contradicted information contained in other sources. Dr. Anderson began to spend more time talking with patients and encouraged Ms. Lucas to engage patients in discussion, assessing their understanding of information after they had used an instructional aid. During this time, Ms. Lucas had the opportunity to answer questions or to address patients' concerns.

Implementation of the new plan for using instructional aids changed Dr. Anderson's approach to patient teaching. Now when a woman came to his office for a physical exam, he explained the importance of regular breast self-examination and, while performing the exam, demonstrated to the patient how the exam should be performed at home. The DVD on breast exam was viewed by women while they were waiting, thus serving as preparation for the instruction and demonstration Dr. Anderson was to provide. This approach appeared to cause little inconvenience and required little extra time on the part of Dr. Anderson.

When women requested advice on contraception, Dr. Anderson discussed various methods, along with advantages and disadvantages of each, and provided patients with a brochure on contraception that reiterated different methods. When giving them the written instructional aid, he preceded it with a statement such as, "This brochure contains much of the information I've discussed with you. Sometimes hearing so much information all at once can be confusing, and it can be difficult to make a decision. I'd like for you to take the brochure home where you'll have time to look it over at your leisure and think about which method you feel might work best for you. When you've decided or if you have questions or would like more information, make another appointment with me and we will discuss it further." Using the brochure in this way offered a review of the instruction Dr. Anderson had given and helped the patient assess the information at her own pace.

When patients were diagnosed as hypertensive, Dr. Anderson would briefly explain their condition and then say, "Hypertension can be controlled, but it requires understanding and cooperation on your part. Because I feel it's so important for you to understand your condition so you can really work to control it, I'd like for you to view a DVD about hypertension. After you've seen the DVD, Ms. Lucas can answer questions you may have and then escort you back to my office where we'll talk more about how to treat your hypertension."

After viewing the DVD and engaging in further discussion with Ms. Lucas and Dr. Anderson, the patient was given the handout on hypertension. The handout reinforced what Ms. Lucas and Dr. Anderson had said and the information contained in the DVD. By using a variety of teaching methods and instructional aids, patient learning and understanding can be enhanced through repetition and reinforcement of information and emphasis of important points.

When Dr. Anderson had a patient who had been newly diagnosed with diabetes, he explained the patient's condition and treatment, and arranged for the patient to come for a separate office visit to view the DVD on diabetes. After the patient viewed the DVD, Ms. Lucas spent time discussing various aspects of the patient's condition, assessing his or her reaction, answering his or her questions and addressing his or her concerns, and reinforcing and clarifying points covered in the DVD and by Dr. Anderson. At subsequent visits, Ms. Lucas assessed whether the patient had problems or concerns regarding his or her condition or in following recommendations, and if problems were identified, worked with the patient to resolve them. In addition, Ms. Lucas made additional supplemental instructional aids available to the patient as needed.

Dr. Anderson's situation was in the outpatient setting. The same principles regarding use of instructional aids apply regardless of the setting in which patient teaching takes place or who is conducting the teaching. Instructional aids are valuable only to the extent that they facilitate communication between the patient and health professional. This is accomplished when the instructional aid offers an accurate description of the information discussed at the teaching session and is written or produced at a level that the patient can understand. Choosing the appropriate instructional aid for each individual patient is an important skill for health professionals to learn in order to facilitate patient teaching. However, skill in assessing and/or developing materials to be used is just as important.

Instructional aids are most likely to be effective if patients view them as an extension of the health professional, not as a replacement for contact with them. Instructional aids should be used to supplement information the health professional has provided the patient. Patients frequently forget much of the information they have been given. Providing patients with instructional materials they can take home enables them to review and clarify information discussed during patient teaching with the health professional and helps to reinforce points that were emphasized during the teaching interaction. Visual aids can be helpful in illustrating points and increasing understanding of concepts. The saying, "A picture is worth a thousand words," is true in patient teaching as well, especially for patients who are unfamiliar with certain concepts or various anatomical terms. The use of models or pictures can be beneficial in helping patients conceptualize various aspects of their condition or treatment. Audiovisual aids such as DVDs can help supplement information given by the health professional or can provide a mechanism to stimulate discussion. For patients who are computer literate, computerized instructional aids, especially if they are interactive, can help patients become actively involved in learning.

No matter what type of instructional aid is used in patient teaching, it will be more useful if health professionals have taken the time to select the material carefully themselves. Information contained within instructional aids should be consistent with that presented by the health professional, reinforcing the professional's teaching, not confusing it. Instructional aids should also be geared to the needs and level of the individual patient. Therefore, the same instructional aids are not appropriate for all patients.

Just as health professionals are responsible for the accuracy of information they give a patient verbally, so are they responsible for the content of the instructional aids they use. Consequently, health professionals should be as careful in choosing types of instructional aids as they are in delivering information to the patient orally. Appropriate use of instructional aids requires skill to ensure that their use facilitates communication between patient and health professional rather than hindering it. The following points should be considered when utilizing instructional aids.

- Use instructional aids to reinforce and illustrate information, not to replace interaction with the health professional.
- Evaluate the content of instructional aids before using them.
- Make sure information contained within instructional aids is consistent with the oral information presented.
- Tailor the type of instructional aid to each patient.

WRITTEN INSTRUCTIONAL AIDS

Written instructional aids can enhance patient teaching effectiveness if used appropriately. Written instructional aids can have many uses, depending on the situation and the associated goals of patient teaching. For example, written aids can be used as a preliminary source of information in preparation for more comprehensive patient teaching. Or, in other instances, written instructional aids may be used to answer frequently asked questions or to address common concerns. In still other instances, written instructional aids may be used to stimulate questions or to reinforce information. In each instance, providing the patient with written information makes more time available for the health professional to provide in-depth coverage of information or to elaborate on patients' concerns. Written instructional aids may be given to patients before health professionals give instructions about a procedure or test. The information contained within the instructional aid thus provides the patient with a general outline of what will be covered and prepares them for the information they will receive. Although providing the patient with instructional aids prior to patient teaching can be helpful, it can also have certain pitfalls:

- Potential patient misinterpretation of the material contained within the instructional aid, which may in turn affect their receptiveness and understanding of further teaching.
- Increase in patient anxiety before teaching takes place
- Over reliance by the health professional on the patient's absorption of the material before patient teaching.
- Reluctance of patients to ask questions because they believe the health professional expected them to gain most of the information from the instructional aid.
- Lack of personal interaction and communication on initial contact, thus potentially affecting the degree of rapport developed between patient and health professional.

Written instructional aids may also be used to reinforce information provided by the health professional or to help the patient remember complex information provided in the teaching session. A pharmacist, for example, may give the patient a written instruction sheet that emphasizes important points about the prescribed medication. Or, after explaining exercises to a patient with low back pain, a physical therapist may give the patient a pamphlet illustrating the exercises.

Another use of written instructional aids is to increase patients' understanding of their condition or treatment by providing more detailed information. For instance, a dietitian who has conducted patient teaching with a patient with celiac disease about their diet may provide the patient with a comprehensive booklet on celiac disease and diet that the patient can study in more detail at home. Another example would be that of a nurse who has instructed a patient on ostotomy care and then provides the patient with a book called *Life with an Ostotomy* that can be shared with his or her family and friends.

Written instructional aids can be used with patients to stimulate thought and ideas or they can be used to facilitate attitude change. As an example, a physician may not only spend considerable time teaching patients about their condition and treatment but also feel strongly about prevention. Although the physician may not take additional time with every patient to talk about health promotion and prevention, the seed can still be planted by having written materials in the waiting room or examining room or by including such materials with the patient's bill.

Obviously, it is not practical for most health facilities to have written instructional aids for every condition or situation for which the health professional may be conducting patient teaching. Likewise, written aids may be more useful for patients than others. Consequently, before ordering, developing, or using written instructional aids, it is important that the health professional has a general idea of what the aid is expected to accomplish and in what situations the use of such aids might be most worthwhile.

Written instructional aids are most practical for conditions or situations that are most common in the health professional's practice or in the health facility. Investing in materials that will seldom be used wastes time and money. For example, even though the health professional identifies an excellent written instructional aid on pheochromocytoma, if, in the past, only one patient with that diagnosis has been seen in the health facility, having large quantities of a written instructional aid on the subject is probably not cost-effective. Having written instructional aids available for conditions seen frequently is a better use of resources.

Choosing Written Aids

A variety of printed instructional aids is commercially available. In some instances, health professionals may find it more beneficial to develop materials themselves.

The source of the aid chosen is dependent on the resources available—in terms of money, time, and interest—and on the particular nature of the objectives the instructional aid is to meet. For example, the physician reviewing commercially prepared materials for use when teaching prenatal patients in the clinic may not find one instructional aid that alone covers all the information he or she feels is important to emphasize. Therefore, the physician may elect to develop his or her own written handout. Thus, the physician is assured that all the information considered important is covered in one comprehensive handout and that the information reflects his or her own personal recommendations.

In other instances, health professionals may find that commercially available written instructional aids cover the information comprehensively and that there is no need to develop further materials. At times, health professionals may not have the time or expertise to develop materials and may feel that commercially available materials can be of the same benefit. For example, a nurse involved in teaching diabetic patients on the inpatient unit may find that developing written instructional aids to illustrate or emphasize points would be a needless expenditure of time when commercially prepared instructional aids are already available and have been used with relative success.

Financial resources may also be a determinant of the types of written instructional aids used. Although it may seem that, in the long run, instructional aids developed by the health professional are cheaper, the time invested in developing the aid, printing costs, or photocopying costs must be considered. Commercially prepared written instructional aids are frequently less expensive if purchased in large quantities. Many excellent written instructional aids may also be obtained free of charge from local sources, such as health advocacy groups, associations specific to a particular condition, public health departments, or other government offices. Although when choosing written instructional aids to be used in patient teaching cost must be considered, of more importance is the extent to which the instructional aid helps to meet the goal of patient teaching. Before incorporating any instructional aid into patient teaching, the health professional should scrutinize the aid carefully. All information contained in the instructional aid should be accurate, current, and appropriate to the reading level and culture of the patients to whom they will be distributed.

By remembering that the purpose of using instructional aids is to supplement patient teaching rather than supplant it, the health professional will be guided in determining the types and amount of written instructional aids needed. Depending too much on written instructional aids for patient teaching not only reduces the effectiveness of patient teaching, but causes needless expenditure of time and money spent in ordering or developing materials that do little to achieve patient teaching goals.

Not all written instructional aids are of the same quality, and more expensive materials do not necessarily mean that they are the best. In addition, the successful use of written instructional aids in one healthcare setting does not mean that the same instructional aid will be equally effective in another facility. The type of written instructional aid chosen should be based on the patient population served by the health facility, the conditions that occur most frequently, and the goals and objectives that patient teaching is to accomplish. The number of written instructional aids possessed by health professionals or health facilities is not nearly as important as the quality and applicability of the instructional aid to the specific population served.

Assessing Readability of Written Instructional Aids

Before a written instructional aid can be effective, the patient must be able to read, understand, and remember the information within it. The effectiveness of a printed instructional aid depends to a great extent on how it is written and organized. Information should be structured and presented in a logical way that patients are able to follow. Subheadings separating major content areas are frequently helpful in separating material into "bite-sized" pieces so that the information can be put into the proper perspective. Subheadings also help patients identify areas they may want to review or clarify.

In general, information contained in written instructional aids should be presented in an appropriate sequence, starting with simple concepts and moving to the more complex. Basic concepts should be introduced first so they serve as building blocks for more complicated ideas. For example, providing a patient with a handout on diabetes that begins with a detailed description of insulin-producing cells in the pancreas, rather than beginning with more basic information about diabetes in general, may do more to confuse the patient than to increase his or her understanding of the condition.

Although goals or objectives of the written instructional aid may not be stated explicitly as part of the content, there should be implicit objectives that are easily inferred from the material. Learning outcomes that are to be met through use of the material should be clear. For example, is the information contained in the written instructional aid geared toward increasing the patient's knowledge of the condition or treatment? Or is it directed toward helping the patient achieve a specific skill? Is the information within the instructional aid directed toward only providing a general overview of a subject or are there specific details regarding the subject that the instructional aid is designed to address? The types of outcomes expected from use of the instructional aid can be inferred from the content of the aid, repetition of important ideas for emphasis, or the general level of detail presented. Are the objectives inferred in the written instructional aid congruent with the objectives of patient teaching with a specific patient? For example, if the objective of patient teaching is specifically to help the patient learn steps involved in administration of insulin with the anticipated outcome that the patient will be able to successfully administer his or her own insulin, then an instructional aid which only provides information about different types of insulin will be ineffective in reinforcing the objectives that the teaching session was originally designed to accomplish. A better choice of written instructional aid, in this situation, would be one that reviews the points discussed, provides cues for carrying out each step involved in insulin administration, and outlines each of the steps involved.

Sentence structure, style, and word use are also important considerations when assessing printed instructional aids. The reading level should be appropriate for the audience. For example, written instructional aids used at an inner-city clinic may be quite different from those used at a university health service. Although it may be tempting to use written instructional aids that use slang terms appropriate to various cultures or subcultures, it is important to remember that such terms may date otherwise useful materials as well as having the potential to cause resentment if the health professional does not belong to the patient's culture or subculture. In most cases, written instructional aids that use these terms should be avoided.

In general, no matter where written instructional aids are used, they will be more effective if sentences are short and simple, using common words rather than medical jargon. If one of the objectives of patient teaching with a particular patient is to acquaint him or her with specific medical terms, medical terminology that is interspersed throughout the handout should be explained in lay terms placed in parentheses after the medical term. Health professionals should remember that at times even nonclinical words may cause confusion. Depending on the reading level of the patient, such words as "predispose" or "incapacitate" may not be clearly understood by some patients or they may be misinterpreted. In evaluating written instructional aids for use in patient teaching, especially for situations in which the patient population comes from all walks of life or consists of many different age groups, written materials most likely to be understood by the majority are probably also the most practical and the most likely to be effective.

The length of the instructional aid should also be considered. Although a written aid that is longer may seem more comprehensive, patients may not take time to read it. Generally, the longer and more complicated the written aid, the less likely patients are to read or understand it. Written instructional aids are of little use if the patient discards the material before reading it because of its length.

The technical quality of the printed material is also important. Health professionals should assess print size and contrast and determine if the materials are easily readable by patients who may have problems with vision. This is especially important in situations when patient teaching is conducted with older adults. Written instructional aids with larger print, more ample spacing, high contrast such as black on white, and on a matte finish rather than glossy to avoid glare are generally easier to read (Mayer & Villaire, 2007). Printed materials should be appealing visually so that they attract patients' attention and potentially motivate patients to read them.

Illustrations and diagrams can help to catch the patient's eye as well as illustrate points. Illustrations can be helpful if a patient has difficulty visualizing a procedure or anatomical part. Just as language contained within the aid should be simple, so should illustrations. For example, a detailed, anatomically correct diagram of the heart may not be nearly as effective for teaching a patient about placement of a pacemaker as a simple line drawing. Illustrations can also make written material more interesting; however, pictorial representations may also convey messages that can interfere with the effectiveness of the handout. For example, some illustrations may be offensive to different groups or other illustrations may be perceived by the patient as treating lightly issues that to them are serious. Humor must also be viewed within patients' frame of reference. In these instances, illustrations can defeat the purpose of using the instructional aid. Illustrations are most effective when they are tasteful and are sensitive to patients' concerns.

In general, the tone of the written instructional aid should be personal and informal and should make patients feel as if the content of the handout is a personal extension of the health professional rather than a mass-produced general handout impersonally supplied to every patient. The more readable the instructional aid is, the more likely the patient is to take the time to read it and incorporate the information it contains.

USE OF AUDIOVISUAL AIDS

In an age of automation and technology, it is not surprising that use of audiovisual aids to assist in patient teaching has gained increasing popularity. These audiovisual aids take the form of DVDs, CDs, PowerPoint slides, photographs, computerized programs, or closed-circuit television. As with written materials, the effectiveness of audiovisual aids is dependent on the accuracy and completeness of the information contained within them. Before incorporating audiovisual aids into patient teaching, health professionals should review and evaluate their content and presentation. Health professionals also need to review their objectives for patient teaching and determine whether or not using the audiovisual aid is the most effective way of reaching those objectives.

Although there has been a proliferation of commercially produced audiovisual aids, there is no evidence that using these aids will drastically increase patient adherence. Use of visual aids can supply an additional means of communication through representing concepts that may be difficult to communicate through words alone. This might be especially true of procedures, such as dialysis or various types of surgical procedures. Audiovisual aids may be useful in patient teaching to increase patient understanding when it is not possible for the patient to observe an actual situation or to observe a demonstration of a particular situation, such as showing prenatal patients a film on childbirth to prepare them for their delivery room experience.

Use of audiovisual aids in patient teaching has its merits; however, there are also a variety of factors health professionals should consider before incorporating them as a major portion of the teaching interaction. First, audiovisual aids can be costly. DVDs or CDs are usually available either for purchase or for rent, but at considerable expense. Use of audiovisual aids also requires special equipment, such as a DVD and/or CD player, computer, or a video monitor. If not already available, the purchase of special equipment can take up all or most of the patient education budget, leaving little money for software that might be needed. Health professionals should also check to see if audiovisual aids can be used with all types of equipment or if purchase of special equipment is also needed.

Commercially prepared audiovisual aids may not be appropriate for the patient population with whom the health professional is working, or audiovisual aids may not address specific issues that the health professional wants to emphasize. The personal development of DVDs or CDs, while perhaps better suiting the patient population and goals, also requires considerable time and expertise, as well as resources and equipment to produce the aid.

Audiovisual aids, like written instructional aids, can become outdated quickly. However, because of the expense of purchasing the audiovisual aid, it may not be possible to replace it as easily as written instructional aids. Even if content remains up-to-date, visual portrayal of people or environments in the audiovisual aid may seem irrelevant to present-day circumstances. Hairstyles, clothing, or specific situations within the film may date it and detract from its credibility despite the accuracy of the information it presents. Patients viewing the audiovisual aid may become more absorbed in noticing the differences in styles than in absorbing the information the aid was meant to confer. In addition, patients may automatically assume that because the visual presentation is dated, the content is also dated and not to be taken seriously. Obviously, audiovisual aids using cartoon characters do not have the same properties of change with regard to time. Cartoon representations may, however, not be the most effective or appropriate way to present information for a variety of conditions, and may in fact insult some patients who feel they are being talked down to or that their condition is being taken less than seriously.

The danger of using any type of instructional aid in patient teaching lies in substituting the aid for personal contact. The temptation may be even greater with audiovisual aids, which may appear to be more personal and comprehensive than written aids. Use of audiovisual aids will be most effective as a patient teaching tool if they are used as a supplement to patient teaching provided by the health professional. Use of such aids will be more cost-effective if they are chosen carefully and if the number of patients with a particular condition is sufficient to warrant purchase of the audiovisual aid. Effective use of audiovisual aids requires resources in terms of time, money, and equipment as well as effective coordination. The checklist in Table 16-1 (see Table 16-1 toward the end of this chapter) can be applied to audiovisual aids as well as printed material. Health professionals should not lose sight of the fact that one of the most important components of effective patient teaching is the relationship between the patient and health professional.

PRESENTING INSTRUCTIONAL AIDS

The manner in which an instructional aid is used can be as important, if not more so, than the instructional aid itself. Printed or audiovisual aids alone are not strong motivators. Without personal contact with the health professional, instructional aids are of little benefit in patient teaching. If patients feel that health professionals are using instructional aids to avoid questions or to avoid additional contact, receptivity to the aid and the information it contains will not be nearly as great. Consider the following examples of appropriate and inappropriate presentations of an instructional aid.

> *Patient*: "I did have some additional questions about Johnnie's asthma. What can we do at home to minimize his attacks?"
> *Inappropriate Response*: "Here's a pamphlet that will explain it all. Johnnie should make a follow-up appointment for his asthma in a week."
> *Appropriate Response*: "Why don't you take this pamphlet home with you and read it over at your leisure? It points out a variety of things that might be helpful. When you come back next week for Johnnie's follow-up visit, we'll discuss some of the points covered in it and answer any questions you might have about it."

The health professional in the second example communicated interest in continuing discussion of the material and the patient's questions. In addition, because of how the material was presented, patients may be more motivated to take the time to read the pamphlet and incorporate the information within it.

As with most patient teaching, timing is also important in the presentation of instructional aids. If the patient is anxious or upset, he or she will probably be no more receptive to instructional aids than to any other method of patient teaching at that time. The health professional who gives an instructional aid at this point risks having the patient misinterpret the action as a demonstration of noncaring or aloofness. Consider the following examples.

Patient: (crying) "The doctor just told me that I'm going to have to have surgery. Although he says it's a fairly routine procedure, I've always been frightened of the thought of anesthesia and of not being in control."
Inappropriate Response: "The procedure is as routine as the doctor says. Here's a pamphlet that explains the procedure in detail, so you'll have a more realistic idea of what to expect"
Appropriate Response: "I know you're frightened. Can you tell me a little more about your fears?"

In the first example, the health professional communicated a lack of sensitivity and concern. Not only will the information in the pamphlet probably not be read, but the relationship between the patient and the health professional has probably also been weakened. The pamphlet may more appropriately be given to the patient at another time, after initial fears and concerns have been addressed.

Instructional aids should be an extension of interaction between health professionals and patients rather than a replacement. The health professional who is uncomfortable talking with patients about various situations or who uses instructional aids to avoid certain situations will probably find that the aid will not accomplish the desired results. Even though the health professional may feel that providing patients with information contained within the instructional aid is better than providing them with no information at all, providing information in this way may do more to hinder reaching the objectives of patient teaching than to help it. The following clinic situation illustrates this point.

Dr. Joyner had encouraged her nurse, Ms. Maris, to develop a structured plan for teaching adolescents about sexuality. Being rather shy in nature, Ms. Maris reviewed a variety of pamphlets and audiovisual aids on sexuality and selected those that were felt to be the most appropriate for the adolescents in Dr. Joyner's practice. Dr. Joyner also reviewed the aids and agreed that they conveyed the information she felt was important.

As part of their regular physical exam for school, all adolescents in Dr. Joyner's practice were first referred to Ms. Maris for teaching on sexuality. Ms. Maris placed each adolescent in a room that had been established as a patient education resource center, turned on the DVD, and left the room. After the adolescents viewed the DVD, Ms. Maris provided them with several pamphlets on sexuality and took them to the exam room to wait for Dr. Joyner. The adolescents were given no opportunity to ask Ms. Maris questions, nor did Ms. Maris attempt to engage in discussion or to elaborate on points illustrated in the DVD or in the pamphlets.

Ms. Maris, in her avoidance of discussion with adolescents, communicated discomfort and embarrassment with the information presented. This in turn caused the adolescents embarrassment. Using audiovisual aids and pamphlets in place of discussion also communicated that questions and further discussion with Ms. Maris or Dr. Joyner were to be avoided. Consequently, the adolescents rarely brought up questions with Dr. Joyner during their exams. Dr. Joyner, assuming that the teens had had their questions answered by Ms. Maris after they viewed the DVD, took little time to ask if they had any questions or to discuss the topic of sexuality further.

The DVD and pamphlets could have been useful instructional aids had they been used to "break the ice" and to stimulate questions or discussion. By being available for and open to questions or by encouraging the adolescents to discuss their concerns, both Dr. Joyner and Ms. Maris could have increased the effectiveness of patient teaching greatly.

DEVELOPING INSTRUCTIONAL AIDS

Although many excellent instructional aids are available, health professionals may want to develop instructional aids that most closely align with their own philosophy or their own patient population, or in some instances they may want to use a combination of commercially prepared and custom designed instructional aids. When developing instructional aids, health professionals should first determine which aids are better developed and which are better obtained commercially to best fit the goal of the patient teaching. Whether health professionals develop their own instructional aids or use those commercially available depends on these factors:

- Is there money available for purchase of commercial aids, and how does the cost compare to developing them in house?
- Are sufficient time, interest, expertise, and resources available for development of instructional aids?

Once the health professional has answered these questions, priorities for purchase or development of materials can be established. When developing instructional aids, whether written, audio, or visual, certain preliminary steps should be taken.

First, an individual with interest and expertise should be identified to supervise the project. In some instances, individuals may be interested in developing instructional aids but may not have the technical skills needed. In this case, outside resources may be needed to assist with printing or layout of written materials or producing audiovisual aids. Many computer graphic programs are now available that can be used by someone with computer expertise to prepare professional looking products (Baker, 1991). PowerPoint slides can be a relatively inexpensive way of visually portraying a concept or outlining steps to be followed in procedures. Likewise, portable video cameras now readily available make it possible for health professionals to produce products of high quality if they are well planned and executed.

The degree to which the project supervisor is directly related in the production of instructional aids is a matter of interest and expertise. Whether directly involved in production or not, the project supervisor should first choose a committee to establish and prioritize instructional aids to be developed. In reaching these conclusions, the committee should first ask these questions:

- What are the most common conditions or most common information needs in the particular patient population served?
- Are there commercial materials available that would adequately meet those needs and that could be covered in the existing budget?

When the committee has identified those conditions for which no suitable commercial instructional aids are available, and consequently what materials need to be developed, the conditions should be prioritized according to need. After prioritization, the committee should then address which type of instructional aid would best convey the information. In some instances, pamphlets or brochures might be best; in others, audiovisual aids may be needed.

When the conditions have been prioritized and the type of instructional aid needed for each area determined, the committee should then decide what resources are needed for the development of the materials. For instance, is a computer with appropriate graphics or desktop publishing capabilities available for producing written materials? If so, is there someone available with the time and computer skills needed to produce the materials? Is there a need to allocate money for commercial printing? Is audiovisual equipment available, or does production of audiovisual aids require an outside contract or consultation?

After resources needed for production of instructional aids have been identified, costs associated with those resources should be established and a budget prepared for funding. In some cases, the cost of instructional aids is fully funded by the facility in which they are to be used. In other instances, cost may be absorbed in patient billing.

PLANNING INSTRUCTIONAL AIDS

For either written or audiovisual instructional aids to be useful and effective, certain basic steps must first be taken. First, the health professional should determine what specific knowledge, skills, attitudes, or behavior changes the instructional aid will be designed to help patients achieve. Specifically listing these behaviors and translating them into objectives before the materials are developed helps maintain focus. Being as specific and behaviorally oriented as possible provides a means for observable, testable outcomes that can assist in the evaluation of the effectiveness of the instructional aids. For instance, a knowledge objective that reads, "The patient will understand potential complications associated with diabetes," is vague and difficult to measure, whereas an objective that reads, "The patient will be able to list at least five possible complications of diabetes," provides a more concise view of what is to be accomplished and can be measured.

After behaviors have been identified and objectives written, health professionals should decide what information is essential in order for patients to achieve the objectives. Listing topics or categories of information relevant to the stated objectives prevents inclusion of superfluous information that could confuse patients. For example, a long description of research leading to the consensus that a particular treatment is now state of the art may not be essential to include in the instructional aid if the main objective of patient teaching is to teach the patient specific skills so he or she will be able to carry out the treatment recommendation.

The next step is to determine how the material is best organized. An outline of the sequence in which the information is to be presented should be developed. The outline will help to clarify thinking, will make sure material appears in a logical sequence, and will prevent extraneous information from being included. A general rule in organizing content is to progress from general to specific, ending with and emphasizing the most important points.

Planning Written Instructional Aids

After completing the steps above, health professionals should decide how the material should look visually. It should be attractive, drawing the patient's interest, and it should be easy to use. The extent to which graphics or illustrations are used will depend on the type of information contained, the type of population for which it is designed, and the talent and resources available.

The reading level to which the material is written will depend on the characteristics of the majority of the patient population for whom the material is designed (see Chapter 10 for assessment of reading level). Larger print is generally easier for most people to read and is less intimidating. For the most part, to increase ease of reading, fancy type or script should be avoided.

In most instances, technical terms and jargon should be avoided, and short sentences should be used as much as possible. Generally, material should be written in a conversational style. As much as possible, the material is usually best written directly to the patient, such as, "When first getting up in the morning you should . . ." rather than, "When a patient gets up in the morning he or she should. . . ." The flow of information should sound natural and clear, and words should be used consistently. For instance, if using the term "high blood pressure" in a handout, it should not be alternated with the term hypertension or vice versa. The term that is used should be used consistently.

As much as possible, each paragraph should contain a single idea. Presenting more than one concept in a paragraph can be confusing and interfere with patient understanding of the main point. Using subheadings can help provide a broad overview for patients regarding specific areas to be covered in the handout as well as provide easy reference for patients if they would like to return to a specific section for review.

If illustrations or graphics are to be used in written materials, health professionals should make sure that they add to the content, not distract from it. Illustrations or graphics can help to reduce the amount of writing or explanation needed. They can be used to illustrate key points, or they can be used to draw patients' interest to the material. When using illustrations, health professionals should determine what they are intending to accomplish and then develop the illustrations accordingly. In most instances, simple illustrations are better than more complex ones. Although colored illustrations can be eye-catching, a simple black-and-white line illustration can be just as helpful for getting a point across and can be less expensive. The illustration should not have to be studied by patients in order to grasp the concept it is attempting to portray. Each illustration should be in close proximity to the written idea it is to reinforce so patients do not have to search the material in order to find the illustration. It may be helpful if illustrations are accompanied by captions that relate to the text; however, if captions are used, they should be kept brief and to the point. When writing captions, health professionals should concentrate on the exact concept the illustration is designed to convey.

Planning Audiovisual Instructional Aids

Audiovisual instructional aids can provide an excellent source of supplemental teaching for patients and can reinforce information as well as prepare patients for information to be given in more detail by the health professional. Examples of audiovisual aids are photographs, PowerPoint slides, CDs, DVDs, computerized programs, and closed-circuit television.

Although audiovisual aids can be time-consuming to produce, the advantage of their use is that they are more personal and can be tailored to the views and standards of the health professional or health facility producing them. In addition, they can be made for the specific type and level of patient population for which they are to be used.

Regardless of the type of audiovisual aid the health professional produces, the same steps should be taken as for developing written materials. That is, specific objectives that the audiovisual aid is to accomplish must be established, essential information to be contained within the audiovisual aid must be determined, and an orderly, logical sequence for presentation of material must be developed. Likewise, although the message is spoken or visually transmitted in this instance, rather than written, the understandability of the audiovisual material should be established, just as the readability of written material must be determined. If a script is used, such as for CDs or DVDs, the same readability formula used for written instructional aids should be utilized. In the case of PowerPoint slides or photographs, the health professional may want to test the materials and ask the opinion of a sample of patients who are representative of the population for whom the materials were developed.

PowerPoint Slides and Photographs

PowerPoint slides and photographs may be used in isolation or with other audiovisual presentations. In some instances, health professionals may use photographs arranged in a loose-leaf binder to supplement patient teaching. Color and lighting are crucial as are good focus and clarity of the slide or photograph. In other instances, PowerPoint slides or photographs may be incorporated into a DVD presentation to illustrate or demonstrate specific points.

Good PowerPoint slides and photographs can be produced easily and with relatively little effort if time is spent in planning. Again, health professionals should have a good idea of what the visual content contained within the PowerPoint or photograph is to convey. Visual content should be kept as simple as possible, with distracting backgrounds and extraneous visual images avoided as much as possible. Health professionals should attempt to avoid introducing too much information in one PowerPoint slide or photograph. As much as possible, each PowerPoint slide should be used to convey one idea.

Using a combination of PowerPoint slides and audio can be an effective way of reinforcing or enhancing patient teaching previously provided by the health professional. The advantage is that the production can be given to the patient to view at home, or the patient can view the production in the healthcare facility. Use of PowerPoint with audio, however, assumes that there is someone available with expertise to produce it, that there is a computer available for patient use, and that patients are comfortable with computer use.

CDs and DVDs

Both CDs and DVDs developed for use in patient teaching require the same steps discussed previously. The advantage of CDs or DVDs is that patients can use them at their convenience. In some instances, the health professional may make them available to patients on loan so they can review them at home as well. If resources permit, professional actors or speakers can be used; however, the voice or visual image of the health professional adds a personal aspect that may enhance the effectiveness of the audiovisual aid.

As with written instructional aids, the message should be kept simple. When developing CDs or DVDs, health professionals should avoid using jargon and technical terms and should avoid complex sentences and multisyllabic words. The speaker should speak in a slow, clear, and distinct manner, and avoid speaking in monotone while also avoiding being overly dramatic. Inflections appropriate to the information being presented should be used.

Whether developing CDs or DVDs, a specific script should be developed. It is important to keep in mind that patients' attention span is limited. The script should be long enough to convey the message, but not so long that patients lose interest. The goal is to provide patients with essential information in a timeframe that they will be maximally receptive. Therefore, during script development, specific timelines for each section of the audiovisual aid should be predetermined. This also helps health professionals avoid spending too much time, for example, on the introduction, so that there is insufficient time left for the key points of the message.

In the case of DVDs, cue cards may be used to help the actor/speaker cover the material in an orderly sequence so nothing is left out. If other scenes or illustrations are to be used on a DVD, the health professional should look at the script and outline specifically what scene, action, or illustration would best fit at specific points of the script.

One technique that may be useful when developing CDs or DVDs is the use of dialogue to convey the message. For instance, an audiovisual aid to be used for teaching about acquired immunodeficiency syndrome (AIDS) prevention may use a dialogue between patient and health professional as follows.

> *Patient*: "I've been reading a lot about AIDS lately. It's pretty scary, but since I don't use intravenous, or IV, drugs, I guess I don't have to worry."
> *Physician*: "That's only one way people can get infected with human immunodeficiency virus, or HIV, the organism that causes AIDS. But there are other ways as well."
> *Patient*: "You mean it's not just IV drugs? How else could you get it?"
> *Physician*: "The virus is contained within all body fluids; therefore, although it's in the blood, it's also contained in the semen. Consequently, sexual contact with a person infected with HIV can also lead to infection."

Whether producing CDs or DVDs, high-quality materials that will produce high-quality recordings should be used. In either instance, the sound quality should be tested before making the audiovisual aid. The actor/speaker should make sure they are speaking directly into the microphone and not turning away from it, which creates fluctuations in sound. Background noises should be avoided.

If DVDs are produced, lighting should be considered. If lighting is not adequate, then supplemental lighting may be needed. When developing DVDs, health professionals should consider the use of other visual aids within the DVD to add interest, rather than merely speaking directly into the camera for the duration of the message. For instance, introduction of pictures or illustrations inserted at the appropriate time can help to illustrate specific points covered in the DVD as well as maintain patients' attention.

If editing of the DVD is possible, different scenes or other outside illustrations may be used as part of the DVD. However, editing may not be possible because it requires fairly sophisticated equipment and expertise that are not always available to the health professional.

DEVELOPING A PATIENT EDUCATION NEWSLETTER

Patient education newsletters are a way to communicate general health information to patients who may not come in contact with the health professional on a regular basis (Aukerman, 1991). Although perhaps most beneficial in an outpatient setting where there is a specific patient population, many inpatient facilities have also developed newsletters that are distributed to the community at large.

Newsletters can be used to convey information about specific conditions, nutrition, safety, or prevention, as well as the availability of specific patient education programs or resources. In addition, newsletters enable health professionals to address specific health issues that may be receiving considerable attention in the media, but for which all the facts are not always presented.

Newsletter production also follows many of the same development steps as those discussed earlier for written materials. The layout of the newsletter should be attractive and easy to read. Print should be at least letter quality. Many computer programs now available can produce professional-looking copies. In the event that a computer or expertise to use computer programs is not available, professional printing may be considered an option and may be less expensive in bulk than for smaller numbers. The size of the newsletter and format will depend on the resources available.

How the distribution of the newsletter is handled will depend on the facility producing it and the resources available. For example, if there is no money in the budget for mailing, the newsletter may be placed in the waiting room of the health facility, if it is possible to use bulk mailing, newsletters may be mailed to a specific patient population or to the community at large. In some instances, a copy of the newsletter may be included in regular patient mailings, such as with monthly billing statements.

There are a number of advantages to producing a customized newsletter. Not only does it enable health professionals to communicate important health information to patients who may otherwise not receive it, the newsletter may also stimulate patients to contact their health professional with questions they otherwise may not have asked.

COMPUTER USE IN PATIENT TEACHING

A variety of patient education software is now available for use in inpatient and outpatient facilities. Programs that offer a number of print-on-demand patient education products can cut down on the need for storing, filing, and reordering patient education brochures, pamphlets, or other information sources. Many of these programs have been tested for readability and acceptability to patients, many of whom use computers at home and are already used to this type of technology (Deye et al., 1997).

Some programs enable health professionals to customize and personalize information presented. Computer programs may also be available in several languages and may be able to be adjusted for print size, making it easier for older patients or patients with visual disability to read. Patient education software programs are usually purchased at an initial price, which then includes periodic updates for a minimal fee.

As with other patient education materials, health professionals should assess accuracy, usability, and cost when making decisions about the extent to which patient education software can be used effectively. Evaluation of the content of the educational material as well as whether the range of topics is sufficient for the patient population served are considerations, just as they would be with other types of instructional aids. Health professionals should determine whether information is appropriate for the patient population in terms of acceptability and readability and whether it meets the patient teaching goals to be accomplished. Cost effectiveness may also be an issue. Are there hidden costs to keep the system running or updated? Will additional equipment be needed? Health professionals should make sure that software packages are compatible with their hardware, operating system, and storage capacity and that everyone using the system has the appropriate skills for efficient use.

Computerized instructional aids, if carefully chosen and evaluated, can serve as an excellent reinforcement of patient teaching provided by the health professional. Most important, however, is recognition by the health professional that nothing can replace the interpersonal interaction between patient and health professional in which the patient's individual needs and concerns are addressed face-to-face.

USING THE INTERNET

Patients gain health information from many sources. The Internet has become an increasingly important source of health information for patients and can either complement or complicate patient teaching effectiveness. Information sources vary from national health and disease organizations, to pharmaceutical companies, to consumer groups. The type of information available also varies, from information about specific disease and treatment to prevention and alternative health practices.

Health information gained over the Internet can be a major influence in patients' decisions about treatment (Fox & Rainie, 2000), and consequently can have a major impact on patient adherence. Although health professionals may not always have control over the type of information patients access on the Internet, it is important to be aware of patients' use of this type of information and to help patients become educated consumers of health-related information they glean from the Internet.

The appeal of Internet information for patients is easy and private access to information. Unfortunately, depending on the information source, information may be incomplete, inaccurate, or generally deficient in presenting facts patients may need to make decisions about their health and health care (Beredjiklian et al., 2000).

The quality of information gained by patients on the Internet is dependent upon search engines used and links provided. Web sites differ in quality, depending on whether they are from commercial organizations, government agencies, or nonprofit educational organizations. Some Web sites, for example, are designed as advertisements to encourage users to purchase products, use services, or participate in research programs. Others present a viewpoint based on the philosophy of the organization sponsoring the Web site.

Accuracy of information can also vary, as well as the extent to which complete information about a condition, treatment, or adverse of treatment or nontreatment are presented (Berland et al., 2001; Griffiths & Christensen, 2000; Jiang, 2000; Soot, Moneta, & Edwards, 1999). Patients using information from Web sites as a basis for medical decision making may have deficient information on which to act. Usefulness of information gained from the Internet also depends on readability, how easily the information can be understood, and how it is interpreted by the user.

Health professionals should ask patients whether they use the Internet as a health information source. Providing guidance to patients who use the Internet can help health professionals ensure that information will be a helpful supplement rather than a barrier to patient teaching efforts and subsequently to patient adherence. Being open to the information patients find on the Internet as well as being noncritical or judgmental of its use will decrease the likelihood that patients will use the Internet as a substitute for consultation with the health professional. Patients should be encouraged to bring questions or concerns about information they have read on the Internet to the health professional's attention rather than changing treatment on their own.

Patients should be cautioned to check information sources to assure that information is unbiased and not being presented in such a way as to sell a product or idea. Patients should be taught how to assess credibility of agencies or organizations sponsoring the Web site and to check for references and timeliness of information presented.

USING INSTRUCTIONAL AIDS EFFECTIVELY

Instructional aids should not be used without verbal instruction. Patients should be told why they are viewing a DVD or PowerPoint presentation or why they are being given a pamphlet or brochure. They should also be told how they are to use the information contained in it. Does the aid supply additional information? Does it review the information presented verbally? Is the information in the aid to provide cues to patients to help them perform skills discussed? Patients will take the instructional aid more seriously if health professionals take time to point out major areas in the pamphlet that are of particular importance.

Table 16-1   Checklist for Choosing Instructional Aids

1. Is information contained within the instructional aid, including illustrations and/or graphics, accurate and up-to-date?

2. Will illustrations and/or graphics contained within the instructional aid add to patients' understanding of the information?

3. Is information appropriate to breadth and scope?

4. Is information appropriate for the intended audience?

5. Is information organized in a way that is logical and easy for the patient to follow?

6. Does information address issues that are of general concern to most patients with the condition?

7. Is information consistent with the philosophy of the health institution/health professional using the teaching aid?

8. For written instructional aids, is the reading level appropriate for the intended audience?

9. Does the instructional aid avoid the use of jargon?

10. Is the technical quality of the instructional aid adequate?

11. Has the instructional aid been developed by a credible source?

12. Is the instructional aid practical in terms of cost, accessibility, and usability?

13. Could the same objective be reached just as well without use of the instructional aid?

Instructional aids, in and of themselves, are useless if not presented within the context of the total process of patient teaching. Instructional aids should enhance progress toward the general objective of patient teaching in a particular area. Instructional aids should be appropriate to the patient, the situation, and the particular problem. General guidelines for choosing instructional aids are listed in Table 16-1.

Instructional aids should be appropriate to the patient, the situation, and the particular problem. Most important, teaching aids should enhance communication with health professionals, not replace it.

REFERENCES

Aukerman, G. F. (1991). Developing a patient education newsletter. *Journal of Family Practice*, *33*(3), 304–305.

Baker, G. C. (1991). Writing easily read patient education handouts: A computerized approach. *Seminars in Dermatology*, *10*(2), 102–106.

Beredjiklian, P. K., Bozentka, D. J., Steinberg, D. R., & Bernstein, J. (2000). Evaluating the source and content of orthopaedic information on the Internet. The case of carpal tunnel syndrome. *Journal of Bone and Joint Surgery, 82,* 1540–1543.

Berland, G. K., Elliott, M. N., Morales, L. S., Algazy, J. I., Kravitz, R. L., Broder, M. S., et al. (2001). Health information on the Internet: Accessibility, quality, and readability in English and Spanish. *Journal of the American Medical Association, 285*(20), 2612–2621.

Deye, D. L., Kahn, G., Jimison, H. B., Renner, J. H., & Wenner, A. R. (1997). How computers enrich patient education. *Patient Care,* Feb 15, 88–113.

Fox, S., & Rainie, L. (2000). *The online health care revolution: How the Web helps Americans take better care of themselves.* Washington, DC: Pew Charitable Trusts.

Griffiths, K. M., & Christensen, H. (2000). Quality of web based information on treatment of depression: Cross sectional survey. *British Medical Journal, 321,* 1511–1515.

Jiang, Y. L. (2000). Quality evaluation of orthodontic information on the World Wide Web. *American Journal of Orthodontics and Dentofacial Orthopedics, 118,* 4–9.

Mayer, G. G., & Villaire, M. (2007). *Health literacy in primary care: A clinician's guide.* New York: Springer.

Soot, L. C., Moneta, G. L., & Edwards, J. M. (1999). Vascular surgery and the Internet: A poor source of patient oriented information. *Journal of Vascular Surgery, 30,* 84–91.

CHAPTER 17

Research and Evaluation in Patient Teaching and Patient Adherence

IMPORTANCE OF RESEARCH AND EVALUATION IN PATIENT TEACHING AND PATIENT EDUCATION

Few would argue the importance of patient teaching in patient care. Until recently, conducting patient teaching was based on common sense, experience, and trial and error. As the concept of patient teaching has evolved, however, there has been increasing emphasis on accountability. Does patient teaching bring about positive health outcomes? Are some approaches to patient teaching more effective than others? Do the benefits of patient teaching outweigh the cost in terms of time and resources? Research and evaluation as a way of testing and validating effectiveness of patient teaching interventions has, consequently, grown in importance.

To strengthen and enhance the quality of patient teaching and patient education programs, research and evaluation are essential. Results from well-designed studies can help health professionals make rational choices among alternative patient teaching approaches and materials, validate various patient teaching interventions, and build a stable foundation of effective patient teaching practice. Well-planned and well-executed research provides the basis from which conclusions regarding patient teaching can be drawn. Sound research acts as a safeguard against proliferation of patient teaching practices that may be fashionable or faddish, but ineffective.

Well-designed research and evaluation are necessary not only to enhance the quality of patient teaching but also to increase its credibility and, in some instances, its potential for survival. Although lip service is given to the importance of patient teaching in the provision of quality health care, the extent of support, both financial and otherwise, is often contingent on evidence of cost-effectiveness. There has been a recent upswing by the patient education industry in the development of new materials, equipment, and other innovations that are marketed as tools to increase quality of patient teaching and which aim to increase patient teaching effectiveness. Decisions regarding which, if any, of these products should be purchased or implemented should be based on research that has demonstrated effectiveness. Too often, health professionals are caught up in enthusiasm and are influenced by the popularity of products. Hence, they are overwhelmed by the availability of patient teaching materials and rush out to purchase products and implement their use without first ascertaining their effectiveness. If benefit of product use has not been shown to justify the cost, when budgetary decisions are made, and especially when financial cutbacks are necessary, patient teaching may be viewed as a luxury rather than a necessity. As a result, resources for patient teaching may be the first targeted for reduction or, in some cases, eliminated.

Some research studies have been conducted regarding the effectiveness of different types of patient teaching interventions and their impact on patient adherence, with varying results. There is a dearth of studies, however, that are well controlled and randomized. Likewise, there have been studies that demonstrate positive outcomes related to patient teaching activities designed to increase patient adherence. Fewer studies, however, demonstrate the extent to which patient teaching can actually improve patients' health status. Controversy also exists regarding the extent to which adherence should be a goal of patient teaching. Should a major goal of patient teaching be increasing patient adherence, or should the goal be increasing patients' ability to make their own informed choices about the extent to which they will follow recommendations? Research and evaluation are essential for strengthening and enhancing patient teaching and for contributing to increased understanding of the phenomenon of patient adherence. While much valuable information already exists as the result of patient teaching and patient adherence research, the majority of this research has been conducted in academic or industrial settings. Researchers conducting such studies may have an interest in patient teaching and patient adherence and may even have expertise in research and evaluation methodology, but they may have little direct involvement with patient teaching and patient adherence issues in practice. Research and evaluation of various materials, methods, and programs are most relevant when built on the experiences and perceptions of those individuals most involved with patient teaching on a day-to-day basis. These health professionals are in the best position to identify specific patient teaching problems, recognize patient adherence issues, help establish research priorities, set goals, collect and analyze data, and assist in interpreting conclusions. Many health professionals, however, have not been trained in research and may be intimidated by the concept. Not all research has to be complicated to be valuable. The most elegant research and the most important findings can come from simple projects that have been well designed, well planned, and well executed.

It is important for health professionals to remember that the quality of research findings is directly related to the quality of research design, attention directed to implementation of research protocol, objective analysis of data, and careful interpretation of data (Polit & Beck, 2006). This is true whether health professionals are conducting research or evaluation as single investigators or in collaboration with experts in research methods, whether conducting research to test a hypothesis or theory or simply evaluating a specific method or material, whether conducting a study in their own setting or cooperating with a variety of individuals in other settings, or whether merely being a consumer of findings from other researchers. The importance of good research and evaluation techniques cannot be overemphasized. Planning is essential to both good research and evaluation.

DEFINING RESEARCH AND EVALUATION

Research and evaluation are often used synonymously. Although both may use many of the same procedures, they are two separate processes, with different purposes. Research, purely defined, is oriented toward the development of theory, with the purpose of searching for new knowledge or establishing facts or principles. In health care, research is often conducted with the goal of translation of findings into methods to improve patient care. Evaluation, on the other hand, is directed toward appraising or judging worth, or judging the degree to which a program, process, or material has met its predetermined goal (Eldridge, 2007). Inherent in evaluation is judgment of value, or degree to which it can be judged as good or bad. Research remains objective by reporting facts but making no value judgment related to the facts (Rich, 2009). Research frequently involves manipulation of variables, whereas evaluation does not.

As an illustration, consider the following problem. A rural health clinic had identified a low rate of screening mammography utilization by women over the age of 50. The nurse, Ms. Dunn, designed a research project to study the problem. Ms. Dunn hypothesized that the low usage was related to lack of physician encouragement and patient teaching related to mammography. In reviewing other research that had been conducted, she noted that findings from previous studies appeared to indicate that more active physician involvement in giving recommendations was correlated with the likelihood that the patient would follow through with the recommendations provided. She therefore hypothesized that patients who received more encouragement and patient teaching about mammography from their physicians would have greater likelihood of obtaining mammography than patients who did not. To study the problem, she divided patients into two groups. One group would be given specific information about mammography from the physician according to a specific protocol, and the second group would not. After collecting and analyzing the data, she found that her hypothesis had been correct. Those women who had received the information from their physicians were twice as likely to have obtained a mammogram as those who did not.

Now consider the same problem, but with an evaluation focus developed by a nurse, Ms. Janesky. In this situation, Ms. Janesky designed a specific program to increase women's use of screening mammography. The program consisted of developing a brochure that explained the importance of mammography after the age of 50 and addressed common concerns that women may have about mammography. She also developed a videotape that demonstrated the procedure of mammography that women were to view while waiting to see their physician. After implementing the program for a specified time, Ms. Janesky evaluated women's perceptions of the brochure and videotape, evaluated their attitudes about mammography before and after receiving the brochure and viewing the videotape, and evaluated the number of women who had received a mammogram after being exposed to the patient education program. She found that although women evaluated both the brochure and videotape positively, the number of women who actually had a mammography after participating in the program had not increased. She concluded that the program was not effective, and the program was discontinued.

In the first case, Ms. Dunn conducted research. She formulated a hypothesis based on findings of other research, manipulated the amount of patient education groups of women would receive, made a comparison of the two groups, and after analyzing the data, reported findings objectively, making no judgment regarding the merit of the innovation.

Ms. Janesky, on the other hand, had developed a program with specific goals. She evaluated data related to the effectiveness of the program in meeting the stated goals, using the outcome as a basis for deciding whether or not the program should still exist. In this situation, when looking at other ways to increase usage of mammography, she may consider Ms. Dunn's findings when designing a patient teaching innovation, but her evaluation will always revolve around how successful the program was in meeting its predetermined goals.

Whether conducting research or evaluation, an organized, systematic approach should be used. For both research and evaluation, a specific problem must first be identified. In the case above, the problem was the same: low mammography usage in women over the age of 50. Ms. Dunn developed her hypothesis based on the problem and developed a research protocol to study it. Ms. Janesky developed a patient education program with specific goals of what it was to accomplish. It is these goals on which the evaluation is based. Both instances had a period of implementation when, in Ms. Dunn's case, the study was carried out and, in Ms. Janesky's case, the program was implemented. At the end of a specified time, both analyzed the data and reached conclusions based on their analyses.

Both research and evaluation are needed in patient education. Both require careful planning and a clear-cut statement of exactly what is to be examined or evaluated. A brief description of the steps within the process of research and evaluation is discussed below.

STEPS IN PROGRAM EVALUATION

Before evaluation can be conducted, a program, a course of study, or materials must first be developed and implemented. Although it is not the purpose of this chapter to discuss program development, program planning and evaluation should always be integrated functions. Thorough program planning leads to logically linked and expected outcomes. The term evaluation implies systematically planning and implementing activities carried out as part of the program and measuring the effects or outcomes resulting from those activities. Evaluation, then, is a way of determining the degree to which previously determined goals or objectives of the program were reached.

The first step in program planning, essential to comprehensive evaluation, is to conduct a needs assessment. The needs assessment should identify the major needs the program is designed to address. Too often, there is little relationship between needs being measured and activities being carried out as a part of a specific program. Unless specific needs to be met are linked with specific activities designed to meet those needs, evaluation of the extent to which the program was successful in meeting those needs cannot be effectively measured. A need can be defined as the difference between what is and what should be. It is from needs that program goals and, consequently, measurable objectives are developed. It should be noted that evaluation is dependent on the clarity and observable, measurable goals and objectives that the program is designed to accomplish. The more clear, observable, and measurable the goals and objectives, the easier the task of evaluation.

Assessing individual patient needs was discussed in previous chapters. Although some of the steps and principles are the same, assessing needs on which to build a specific patient education program is somewhat different. Needs assessment at a program level requires input from more people in the planning process. Determining needs at the program level can be best illustrated by example. Ms. Janes was a nurse practitioner working with three physicians in a satellite clinic outside a large city. Although all practitioners at the clinic provided one-to-one patient teaching to their individual patients,

Ms. Janes had begun to feel that patients could also benefit from a more formalized and structured patient education program. She arranged a meeting
for the medical staff and asked them to list what they perceived to be the
greatest patient needs in their particular patient population with regard to
patient education. It is important to note that Ms. Janes focused on patient-
oriented needs rather than on preferences of individual healthcare providers.
After a list of needs had been established, Ms. Janes asked the staff to order
the needs as high, moderate, or low importance. This was important because
it was unlikely that equal resources could or would be given to ease all identified needs at once.

Ms. Janes and the staff decided to begin with only the area that was designated as the highest priority. The staff then determined goals for the program and, from the goals, developed measurable objectives. Then they needed
to design the program based on the stated goals and objectives. Key issues
involved questions such as:

- What is needed to reach the stated objectives?
- Who will be responsible for carrying out or facilitating various parts of
  the program?
- What financial and other type of resources are available?
- Which type of budget needs to be established in order to implement and
  maintain the program?
- Which criteria will be used to judge program effectiveness?

It should be noted that the most effective patient education program is
based on and responsive to patients' actual needs. When formulating programs, having patient input as well is important to achieve a more realistic
view. Health professionals' perceptions of patient need are not always the same
as patients'. In Ms. Janes's case, in addition to assessing and prioritizing needs
as identified by the clinic staff, she may also have polled a selected sample of
patients to assess their needs and priorities (sample selection is addressed
later in the chapter.)

The second step important to planning and subsequent evaluation is development of goals and objectives. Program goals and objectives should be based
on the identified needs and should be stated in terms of desired outcomes. As
discussed previously, specifically stated goals and objectives that are measurable are crucial to evaluation. When developing goals and objectives, there
should be a logical relationship between goals, objectives, resources, and activities by which the goals and objectives are to be accomplished.

Although goals can be somewhat idealistic, serving as an ideal to strive
for, objectives should be reasonable, realistic, and attainable. For example, if Dr. Farris develops a patient education program for hypertension, an

idealistic goal may be, "All complications of hypertension will be prevented in the patient population." However, since the likelihood of reaching this goal is remote, objectives should reflect a more realistic view of what the program is to accomplish. In writing program objectives, Dr. Farris should make sure that the true mission of the program is reflected. In other words, although he may list as an objective, "Patients will list the complications of hypertension," Dr. Farris's real objective in implementing the program is probably not limited to patients regurgitating facts but rather incorporating the facts into their lives so that their hypertension may be better controlled, thus striving for the goal of reducing complications. Consequently, an objective of the patient education program in hypertension may be, "At least 80% of patients with a diagnosis of hypertension who participate in the patient education program will maintain a blood pressure below 140/90." In the same context, the objectives should be clear and readily measurable. An objective that states, "Patients participating in the patient education program on hypertension will understand the potential complications of hypertension" lacks both clarity and measurability. If an objective relating to patients' knowledge of complications is to be written, a more precise, measurable objective might be, "Patients participating in the patient education program on hypertension will be able to list five complications associated with hypertension."

It should be noted that program evaluation may have several different focuses. Using the program described previously as an example:

- Did the program make a difference? For instance, did patients participating in the program develop few complications? Did patients attending the program show greater adherence to recommendations, such as engaging in a regular exercise program, lowering blood cholesterol, losing weight, and adhering to medication instructions?
- Was the program cost-effective? Did resources expended result in desirable outcomes? Was the benefit worth the cost? Cost/benefit can be measured either in actual program costs (e.g., materials, personnel time) or in terms of more global cost versus outcomes (e.g., cost of hospitalizations, days lost from work).
- Are there changes that need to be made to make the program more effective? For example, if the program was planned for six sessions, but patients stopped coming after two, what might be done to encourage fuller participation?

Program evaluation can be conducted in two phases. These two phases are called formative and summative evaluation. The first phase, formative evaluation, is a means of obtaining feedback about the program and how well it is making progress toward its stated objective. This type of evaluation takes place during program implementation, enabling midcourse corrections or refinements, if necessary, to better achieve the stated objectives or to keep the program in line with its original design. This type of evaluation focuses not only on the results of the program activity, but on the activities themselves. For example, in Dr. Farris's hypertension program, he may find that didactic sessions and video sessions are equally effective in relaying information, but that patients prefer the personal interaction of the lecture and are more likely to continue participation in the program if this format is used.

Summative evaluation takes place at the end of the program or after its full implementation to determine the extent to which objectives were achieved. Summative evaluation information that is gathered may help health professionals make decisions about whether or not the program should be continued and about modifications to improve or maintain the program in the future. In this case, evaluation focuses not only on whether the objectives were met, but also whether the objectives were appropriate. All objectives of the program might have been met, but the objectives themselves may have been meaningless. For instance, if Dr. Farris's only objective for the program was that, "At least 80% of patients with hypertension will participate in the patient education program for hypertension," and, in summative evaluation it was found this was the case, one could theoretically declare the program to be effective. If, however, in actuality patients who participated gained no new knowledge or behavior change that increased the likelihood of their well-being, although the stated objective was met, it would be hard to judge the program as truly effective.

There are many models of program evaluation. The model chosen depends on the needs of the specific individual or facility implementing the program and the general purpose of the evaluation. For example, in some instances, the major objective and thus focus of evaluation may be patient outcomes. In other instances, evaluation may focus on the effectiveness of various materials or other patient teaching innovations. Accountability in patient teaching consists of monitoring and assessing measurable outcomes. The validity of evaluation results will, in a large part, be determined by the use of appropriate methods of measurement and the accuracy of measurement used in the evaluation process. Different processes for evaluation are used for different evaluative purposes.

Measurement of effectiveness of patient education programs is important for maintenance of program quality and for program accountability. In a broader context, of importance to the field of patient education is the study of the extent to which a successful program can be implemented in different settings with similar results. Development of an effective patient teaching program that can be demonstrated to have positive effects on patient outcomes has the greatest utility if the program is effective in other settings as well. In addition, it is important to make sure that positive outcomes are a direct result of the patient education program being evaluated and not other confounding factors. For example, if the major determining factors in achievement of the objectives of Dr. Farris's program are patient loyalty and respect for Dr. Farris and not the program itself, evaluation results could be misleading. It might be difficult to determine whether the increased attention to adherence with recommendations is a function of the patient education program, Dr. Farris's individual personality, or both. These two factors are confounded, and the effects of each cannot be determined. Many of the same procedures are used for program evaluation as for evaluation of individual teaching effectiveness. A key consideration in program development, implementation, and evaluation is that none of these elements exists in a vacuum. The social context of patient education programs includes a wide variety of people, from administration, to staff, to the initiator of the project, to patients. To blindly proceed without considering all these levels is foolhardy and limits the potential for program effectiveness. This is especially true in evaluation, and specifically when evaluation of program effectiveness may be a determining factor regarding whether or not the program will still be in existence.

Program evaluations must be conducted with an awareness and sensitivity to the political atmosphere of the program's setting. Persons directly and indirectly related to the program probably represent different levels of power, influence, and authority and have their own values and priorities regarding specific goals. Program evaluation is based on scientific principles and procedures for collecting and analyzing data. Because any program operates within a social and political context, to obtain a meaningful evaluation, the relationship between these various factors must be considered.

STEPS IN RESEARCH

As with evaluation, careful planning is central to good research. The first step to conducting research is identifying a problem to be studied. The more clearly stated the specific problem to be studied, the easier it is to develop a sound research plan, which will result in valid conclusions (Burns & Grove, 2005; Haber, 2006). An ambiguous or general research question such as, "Does patient teaching make a difference in healthcare costs?" is so general that interpretation of findings that result would be extremely difficult.

The problem selected for study should be of interest to the health professional conducting the research and should be based on a conceptual framework grounded in research findings reported in the current professional literature. A comprehensive literature review provides the researcher with deeper insights into the research topic by acquainting him or her with current thinking in the area of interest. A literature review also provides insights into various methods used by other researchers studying similar research problems and can stimulate new ideas for additional research.

Depending on the research question being investigated, the literature review may include classic studies from the past as well as studies most recently published. Research on the specific topic of interest as well as studies in related research areas may be included.

Several sources may be used to search the literature. Professional journal indexes compile listings of articles by year and generally categorize articles by topical area. Computer searches are also convenient sources for identification of articles related to specific research topics. A number of computer search engines dedicated to health-related studies are available for quick and easy identification of related topics. Bibliographies from articles obtained are also good sources for identifying additional articles related to the topic being studied. When conducting a literature review, health professionals should keep their own research topic in mind, looking for literature that relates specifically to it. Without maintaining this focus, it is easy to become overwhelmed by volumes of articles that may have minimum relevance to the research problem being investigated. The second step in the research process is to develop a clear and precise research question. Refining and narrowly defining the research question is the beginning of good research design and protocol. The best stated research question is simple, brief, and unambiguous. The research design and methods are based on the research question. Consequently, the more clearly and precisely the question can be stated, the more clearly the research design and methods can be outlined.

A common mistake made by beginning researchers is collecting data before a clear research question has been formulated, hoping that some sense can be made of the data at a later time. Another common error is taking preexisting data and attempting to develop a research problem to fit them, rather than using preexisting data to answer an already well-formulated research question. Although retrospective studies have their place in research on patient teaching and patient adherence, if existing data are used, health professionals must still have a clear idea of what specific research question will be asked and how the data will be used to answer it. Too often, existing data are used merely because they are convenient and too little thought has been put into the real purpose of analyzing the data. Again, unless there is a precise research question, a sound plan for analyzing data cannot be developed.

When the research question is clearly established, other issues regarding the feasibility of the project must be considered. Such issues relate to whether the researcher has the skills, resources, or time to carry out the research. This includes access to subjects, ability to obtain a sufficient number of subjects, administrative support, financial support, and access to programs for data analysis. Although study design is important and should be appropriate to the research question being asked, health professionals must also consider the realities of the research situation. Listing resources needed for completion of the study and assessing their availability can help health professionals assess the feasibility of the study realistically as well as help identify potential resources.

The quality of findings of research is directly related to the study design and methods used to carry out the study (Boswell, 2007). Research in patient teaching and patient adherence is applied research. Many methodological issues may not be present in research conducted under more controlled conditions, as is the case for research conducted in laboratory settings. Consequently, health professionals must also consider the setting in which research is to be conducted. Different settings present their own particular problems in conducting research (Young, 2009). Conducting research in a clinic setting may present different issues than conducting research in a hospital setting. Issues of staff cooperation, patient recruitment and availability as study subjects, and political considerations may be factors that have different ramifications in different settings. Being aware of potential problems and identifying them early can save health professionals both time and money in the long run, as well as help them to develop and maintain a sound research protocol.

Many different research designs can be used when conducting research. The research design merely refers to the plan or strategy used to study the research question. It specifically addresses selection of research subjects, measures, and procedures used. The design of a research project is dependent on the purpose of the study, the nature of the problem to be studied, the setting in which the research is to be conducted, and the resources available for the investigation. The importance of good research design cannot be overemphasized. If a study is conducted and the research design is flawed, the data will be meaningless, and no amount of statistical manipulation can repair the damage. One of the goals of good research design is the elimination of confounding effects (Nieswiadomy, 2008). Without doing this, it is difficult to determine how much of the findings are results of the variables of interest in the study and how much are because of something else. For example, Dr. Lewis conducted a research study in which he investigated the effect of his prenatal classes on infant mortality and morbidity in infants of mothers who attended the classes. The classes consisted of four different sessions. He conducted the classes for 3 years. At the end of the 3-year period, he collected follow-up information regarding outcome for infants born to women attending the classes. He compared this figure with infants born to other patients in his practice who had not attended the prenatal classes. His findings demonstrated that the rate of morbidity and mortality in infants born to parents who had attended the classes was significantly less than that in infants whose parents had not. He concluded that his prenatal classes had a significant effect on reducing infant morbidity and mortality. Dr. Lewis's conclusions were invalid, however, because he had not considered all the other factors that could also affect infant morbidity and mortality. In his particular situation, those attending the classes were, in general, well-educated, upper-middle-class individuals living in two-parent homes. A large number of the remaining prenatal patients in Dr. Lewis's practice were unwed teenagers from lower socioeconomic backgrounds. Given the difference in the two groups, it is unlikely that the prenatal classes themselves had an effect on infant mortality, but rather that age, general health, and socioeconomic status of the mothers had more of an effect.

Using another example with a different research question, suppose that Mr. Roseman, a nurse, was interested in studying whether or not viewing a DVD on how human immunodeficiency virus (HIV) is transmitted increased patients' knowledge about how HIV infection could be prevented. He showed the DVD to a group of patients selected to participate in the research, and after having them watch the DVD, administered a questionnaire he had developed to assess the patients' knowledge. This study has major flaws. First, since Mr. Roseman had not assessed the extent of patients' knowledge about HIV transmission or prevention prior to viewing the DVD, he had no way of knowing whether or not scores on the questionnaire were a reflection of knowledge gained because of the intervention. To observe changes, baseline information must be gathered against which comparisons can be made. Second, since he had developed the questionnaire but had not tested it to see how accurate and sensitive it was as an actual measurement of patient knowledge, he had no way of determining that the scores on the questionnaire were a valid measurement of patient knowledge of HIV. Last, there was no provision for comparison. In other words, how did the knowledge level of those individuals who had not viewed the DVD compare with those who had? For sound research design, precautions should be taken. Certain types of studies require a control group by which comparisons can be made. Factors other than the particular intervention being studied may also contribute to any differences found. Consequently, a group that does not receive the intervention provides a means for "controlling" for confounding factors so that a comparison can be made. Otherwise, there is nothing against which to compare effectiveness of the specific procedure. In the example used above, Mr. Roseman had no basis for comparison since he did not use a control group.

SAMPLING

Another precaution that must be taken when conducting research relates to choosing study participants. This process is called sampling. Sampling procedures are critical to a good study and to the usefulness of results (Proctor &

Allan, 2006). One of the objectives of conducting research in patient teaching is to gain information that can be applied to other settings. If, for instance, a patient education technique used in a certain setting has been found to be effective in reducing patient nonadherence, findings are of little value unless the same techniques are found to be effective in other settings as well.

The extent to which research findings in one setting can be applied to other settings is called generalizability. This is accomplished in part through proper sampling techniques. Two issues are important in sampling: (1) representativeness and (2) sample size. Although larger sample sizes tend to increase the probability of obtaining statistically significant results, perhaps even more important is the degree to which the sample is representative of the group to which generalizations can be made. In order to increase the possibility of generalization as much as possible, the sample studied should be representative of the type of patient to which conclusions regarding the study could be applied. For example, in a study of the effect of a specific patient teaching intervention on patients' adherence with treatment recommendations for rheumatoid arthritis, before reaching a valid conclusion, the health professional would have to make sure that the study sample included individuals who were representative of those with rheumatoid arthritis. Only including Caucasian women in the sample, for example, would not allow any conclusions to be drawn, except perhaps as results applied to Caucasian women. Sample size is often an issue. In the case above, although it would be ideal to study the entire population of patients with rheumatoid arthritis, this would not be feasible. Therefore, a sample of the total group is used. Health professionals need to identify the minimum sample size needed so that if significant differences between groups in the study exist, those differences can be determined. When considering sample size, precision is important, but so is cost. Larger samples are more financially costly as well as more costly in time and effort, but results are more reliable and representative. Even if resources are available for a larger sample, the number of individuals in a certain area or situation who are available to participate as subjects in a research study may be limited. When it is not possible to use a large sample, smaller samples may be used. One way of determining sample size is through the use of a power table. These are available in a number of research texts. The goal is to make the power as large as possible given the practical limitations on the sample size.

An additional problem related to sample size is the fact that some patients may drop out of the study or fail to follow through with the research protocol. At times, patients drop out of the study because of excessive demands of time or effort required in study participation. When planning the study, health professionals should consider demands on study participants and adjust the sample size to accommodate the anticipated number of patient dropouts. One way to test the effectiveness of the research plan as well as to assess the potential for dropouts is to conduct a pilot study with a small number of patients before beginning the study. This enables health professionals to test the feasibility of the research and to identify and correct any problems in the study before additional resources are used. Patients participating in the pilot study should, of course, be eliminated from selection for the major study.

Another important concept in sampling is randomization. Randomization in sampling diminishes the potential of selection bias, helping to ensure that groups are similar with respect to characteristics that may be important. Random samples are obtained in a way that ensures that every member of the population to be studied has an equal chance of being chosen for the study and that selection of each person for the study has no effect on the selection of another person in the population. For example, if the health professional was comparing the effects of computerized instruction on levels of adherence for patients with gout in his or her practice, first all patients in the practice with gout would need to be identified. Unless the total number of patients in the practice with gout was very small, the health professional would probably decide to choose a random sample of the total group. Choosing every seventh patient from the list of patients with gout is not a random sample. Most commonly, random selection may be accomplished by using a random number table. Random number tables and their method of use can be found in a variety of research texts.

In addition to random selection of study participants, random assignment of individuals into different treatment groups is also important. In the example used above, from the random sample selected, the health professional would then assign patients to one of the different groups using a random selection process. This type of randomization helps to avoid the possibility that there was bias from one particular treatment group or the other. Again, a random table could be used.

In patient education settings, randomization can be difficult. Whereas in laboratory settings, animals are easily randomly assigned to different study groups, in conducting research with patients, the task is not always as easy. Patient rights must be considered. Patients must be informed of benefits as well as risks that might be involved with their participation in the study (Burns & Grove, 2007; Wood, 2006). In addition, patients have the right to refuse participation. They cannot be coerced to participate as subjects or be placed in a specific treatment group. In patient teaching situations, random assignment and control groups may not always be possible and may not also be feasible for ethical reasons. For instance, if the health professional were interested in studying the effectiveness of two different methods of patient teaching for new diabetics, ideally patients would be randomly assigned to three different groups. Each of two groups would receive patient teaching by two different methods, and the third group would receive some intervention that was unrelated to diabetes. Obviously, in this example, it is not feasible or ethical to withhold patient teaching from a group of diabetic patients. In other situations, in addition to issues of confidentiality, it may not be possible to identify all patients within a setting who have a specific condition. Consequently, a true random sample might not be drawn.

RESEARCHER AND SUBJECT BIAS

Another issue to be considered when designing research concerns diminishing researcher and subject bias as much as possible. The degree to which this precaution is followed varies, and avoiding bias is not always possible. Ideally, neither the researcher nor the subjects should know which treatment group is which. Less ideal is when the researcher knows, but the subjects do not.

Although bias on the part of the researcher or the patient may not be intentional, it can subconsciously affect interpretation of the data by the researcher and behavior of the research subject. Patients who know they are being assigned to a specific group may feel and/or act differently compared to patients not in the group. This is even more problematic if the patient knows what the group is intended to demonstrate. For instance, take a study being conducted to see whether patients who receive detailed instructions about their treatment are more adherent to treatment than those who do not. If patients are told, "We're conducting a study to see if receiving instructions about your medication will make it more likely that you will take it as prescribed," it is possible that any increased adherence of the group may be more related to the fact that patients know they are in a study group than from the special instructions they received. In the case of researchers, there may be an unconscious tendency to project into the study or into the interpretation of the data what they expected or hoped to find so that the data are subtly shaped to meet the expected outcomes. The fact that all patients participating in research must be volunteers, rather than blind participants, also introduces some bias.

MEASUREMENT IN RESEARCH AND EVALUATION

When a research study is conducted, observations of some type take place. In order to be meaningful, these observations must be measured. Again, the validity of research or evaluation results will depend on the clarity of the definition of what is to be observed or measured and the exactness of the tool used to measure it (Schmidt & Brown, 2009; Waltz, Strickland, & Lenz, 2005). If, for example, the health professional is interested in assessing differences in patient learning about colostomy irrigation when either of two patient teaching methods are used, learning and measurement of learning must first be defined. Learning is not directly observable. Consequently, the health professional must define precisely what will be considered as learning for purposes of the study. For example, learning could be defined in terms of a score on a test, or it could be defined by direct observation of behavior, such as being able to irrigate the colostomy. In order to avoid ambiguity, these definitions should be even more precise, such as providing a cutoff score on the test, below which scores would not be considered indicative of learning, or carefully defining each step of colostomy irrigation so that learning may be defined as performance of the procedure with some percentage of accuracy. A third level of defining learning would be the extent to which the patient continues to follow the protocol accurately and consistently at home when not under the watchful eye of the health professional.

Definitions should be constructed carefully to avoid obtaining results that lead to misleading conclusions from the research or evaluation. For example, consider evaluation of a specific intervention, such as determining the effect of a computerized patient education program on patient adherence with a prescribed antihypertensive medication regimen. The health professional has defined what will be measured (medication adherence). In interpreting results, however, whether or not the procedure is concluded to be effective will depend on how the health professional defined adherence. If, for example, adherence was defined as taking the medication 10% of the time, the program may be more likely concluded to be highly effective than if the standards were set at a higher level, such as 70% or 80%.

The type of measurement depends on the research question being asked. In all instances, no matter what type of measure is used, it is crucial that the measure be as accurate and as valid as possible. Two key issues in measurement are validity and reliability. Validity refers to how accurately the instrument actually measures what it is intended to measure. Reliability refers to how consistently the instrument measures. Before an instrument or observational technique is used, some attempt should be made to assess validity and reliability. Methods for doing this may be found in a variety of research texts. When feasible, it is desirable to find an existing instrument that has had tests of reliability and validity already performed.

Some research questions are such that measurement can be done with direct observation. For example, if the outcome variable of interest were appointment keeping, measurement could be done by simply observing whether or not patients kept their appointments. When the simultaneous observation of two observers is required, attempts should be made to assess the degree of reliability of the two separate ratings. The least accurate means of measurement may be patients' self-reports. Although accuracy can be increased if the health professional approaches the patient in a nonthreatening way, for the most part, this type of measure has low credibility.

QUALITATIVE METHODS IN RESEARCH

Most health professionals, if exposed to research techniques and theories, have some understanding of empirical, experimental, or quantitative research. This type of research begins with a theoretically based hypothesis and emphasizes objectivity, prediction, and control, striving to separate the researcher and the subject so that specific values or bias of the research is eliminated as much as possible when gathering data and interpreting results (Finset, 2008). The hypothesis in quantitative research is confirmed or rejected through systematic investigation, manipulation, and analysis of some body of empirical data.

There are a number of instances, however, when experimental control is not possible and when strict experimental research design is not appropriate to study the particular question at hand. For example, Dr. Dean, who conducted patient teaching for patients undergoing chemotherapy, wanted to gain more understanding into patients' feelings and fears about chemotherapy; he would use the resulting insight to improve patient teaching. Although he could give patients a structured questionnaire, with questions developed from a variety of validated theories gleaned from the professional literature, the information would not provide him with the same depth of information regarding patients' feelings as if he talked with them directly and elicited their spontaneous remarks. In this case, use of more subjective, qualitative methods may be more appropriate.

To obtain this type of information, many behavioral and social sciences utilize an approach called qualitative research or naturalistic inquiry to study special areas of interest. Until recently, the credibility of qualitative research when applied to research issues in health care has been widely disputed. The usefulness, appropriateness, and applicability of qualitative methodology in research related to patient teaching and patient adherence is becoming more widely accepted (Stone et al., 2008).

Qualitative research differs from quantitative or experimental research not only in method but also in philosophy (Dombro, 2007). Qualitative research is based on the premise that the nature of a variety of social phenomena is markedly complex, and only by in-depth investigation and integration of information can an accurate description of the phenomena result (Liehr & LoBiondo-Wood, 2006). Rather than beginning with a theory or hypothesis as in quantitative research, theoretical categories in qualitative research are developed from the data. Rather than beginning with a specific research question, the individual using qualitative research methods formulates the research questions as the study progresses. The premise is that all human behavior must be studied within the context of the social situation and the meaning of the behavior to the individual being studied. Consequently, qualitative research is nonmanipulative and descriptive, providing vivid details rather than fitting data into predetermined, standardized categories.

Qualitative research emphasizes a more subjective approach, is more intuitive, and is based on direct and vicarious experience. Qualitative research necessitates more direct interaction between the researcher and subject so that insight can be gained subjectively without necessarily separating facts and values. In qualitative research, most data are drawn from direct communication with or observation of subjects. One of the most used devices for obtaining information is the interview, which can be used to identify relevant dimensions of the research questions of interest. Interviews can be structured so that the researcher predetermines questions or has an initial outline of the interview, or the interview can be informal, relying on the natural flow of conversation to elicit spontaneous information of relevance to the research question.

Data gathered by qualitative means are usually presented in more informal, narrative form. The researcher may present information through the use of case reports in which the opinions or responses of the subjects are described, rather than placing a numerical value on whether the majority of individuals felt strongly one way or the other.

COLLABORATION IN RESEARCH AND EVALUATION

If the health professional has limited training or experience in conducting research, using a consultant or working in collaboration with another individual with research skills and experience is desirable.

If using consultants, it is usually important to involve them in the early stages of designing the study rather than waiting until all data are collected. In some instances, consultants may request a fee. In other instances, they may be willing to work as a coinvestigator and coauthor on any manuscripts resulting from the study. In either case, it is wise at the onset of the relationship to establish the role each person will play and to outline specific responsibilities each person will have. In order to benefit most from consultants, however, health professionals should have a clear idea of what they want to accomplish with the project.

MANAGING A RESEARCH PROJECT

Even a well-designed and well-planned research project does not run itself. Almost all research or evaluation, no matter how simple, requires some coordination. Depending on the nature of the project, other staff may be used for implementation of protocol, recruitment of subjects, or collection of data. Enlisting the cooperation of these individuals is crucial to a successful study. For example, Ms. Segel, a nurse, had developed a well-designed patient education study in which recruitment of subjects was to be done by the receptionist when the patient checked in for a physician visit. She told the receptionist what to do and assumed the protocol was being carried out. After a month, however, Ms. Segel grew concerned that the number of patients recruited for the project was so low. When she checked with the receptionist to see why she thought more patients were not agreeing to participate, Ms. Segel found that the receptionist had failed to follow the recruitment protocol in most instances, resenting what she considered extra work on her part and a disruption of patient flow.

To be successful, there must be a mechanism for quality control. Data must be recorded accurately and uniformly. If a number of different people are involved in data collection or data coding, the chance for error is great. Consequently, the health professional should make certain that people assisting understand the importance of accuracy. The accuracy of data collected and accuracy of coding should be randomly checked so that any systematic errors or errors of precision can be identified and corrected.

When attempting to gain cooperation from others, it is important to approach them with respect and sensitivity. No one likes to be ordered or threatened into participation. Health professionals should take time to explain the project and its purpose to all involved and clearly outline what is expected. Health professionals should be open to questions and suggestions and demonstrate appreciation for assistance received. There should be regular communication with all individuals involved with the project and updates of the progress of the study.

SPECIFIC ISSUES IN PATIENT EDUCATION RESEARCH AND EVALUATION

Research and evaluation in patient education are means to determine the most effective way to teach patients about their condition, treatment, or to teach them how to prevent disease or complications from disease. Research and evaluation in the field of patient education also helps health professionals test and expand new ideas, test new theories, and determine the extent to which current patient education practices meet stated goals.

Research and evaluation are means by which credibility of patient education programs and accountability of patient teaching and patient education programs can be established. Several issues are problematic, however, in research, evaluation, and interpretation of data in studies related to patient teaching and patient education. The first issue relates to the variation in definition of patient teaching or patient education in various studies. Studies frequently use the terms patient teaching and patient education synonymously. Consequently, it is at times difficult to establish whether research is measuring the effectiveness of teaching interventions with individual patients, or whether it is measuring the overall effectiveness of a structured patient education program. Likewise, patient teaching and/or education can be described in a variety of ways. It can be formal or informal, conducted in a group setting or on a one-to-one basis, or consist of passive patient participation such as use of audiovisual aids or written aids, or active patient participation such as use of self-directed learning through computerized patient education programs or return demonstrations. Although each of these descriptions can be considered patient teaching, or part of a structured patient education program, techniques for each are different, each may be used separately or in combination, and each has different factors that may produce different results. Because there is no consistent definition of what constitutes patient education, there is no definitive way of interpreting results. For example, if Dr. Gephart were interested in determining whether patient teaching made a positive difference in blood pressure control of patients with hypertension, she may first survey the literature and evaluate the results. She would probably find a number of studies that used patient teaching about hypertension as a means of affecting blood pressure control but might also find it difficult to reach a conclusion. Some studies may consist of patient teaching about hypertension in a group setting, whereas others use an individualized approach. Others may test patient education materials or computer simulations about hypertension as a means of helping patients understand consequences of not following recommendations. Some studies may use a combination of patient teaching approaches. Comparisons between such different approaches cannot be made categorically. Each intervention has different variables that could influence results. For instance, the dynamic of a group setting is different from that of a health professional and patient on a one-to-one basis. Passive approaches, such as giving patients written materials to read, have a different impact than more active patient participation, which would occur in computer simulations. Consequently, although Dr. Gephart may find evidence in the literature that indicates that one form of patient teaching has been shown to be more effective than another, she would have difficulty finding definite proof that patient teaching per se made a positive difference in blood pressure control.

Another issue involves the wide variation of topics addressed by patient education. Patient teaching can be directed toward primary prevention such as immunization or secondary prevention such as reduction of risk of heart disease through helping patients learn about lowering cholesterol. Although both are topics addressing prevention, variables contained in each topic present different issues that could affect patient teaching effectiveness. Patient teaching may also be directed toward tertiary goals, such as controlling progress, symptoms, or complications of disease.

Another problem regarding interpretation of results of research and evaluation in patient teaching and patient education relates to defining outcome. What do outcomes describe? Are outcomes directed toward describing effectiveness of overall patient education programs in terms of cost-effectiveness, efficiency, or patient satisfaction, or are outcomes directed toward effectiveness of specific teaching interventions. Outcomes can be individual patient behaviors, perceptions, or subjective status and may be viewed from the perspective of the patient, the health professional, or the organization. They may be viewed in terms of improvement or decline, or in terms of the degree of improvement or decline from a previous assessment (Moorehead et al., 2008).

In the same context, outcomes for both patient teaching and patient education are sometimes described in terms of "learning"; however, this term can also be ambiguous. Learning may be broadly defined. Learning may be defined as knowledge acquisition, changes in attitudes, skill acquisition, or behavior change. In patient teaching, the outcome and ultimate learning goal may be defined as increased adherence to recommendations that ultimately leads to positive health outcomes. In other instances, the ultimate goal and outcome may be patients' choices to follow or not to follow recommendations based on their own values and informed consent. In each of these cases, patient teaching effectiveness is determined by specific outcomes as defined by the health professional conducting the research.

A third problem in interpreting results from research and evaluation in patient education relates to the inconsistency of methods used to assess patient teaching and patient teaching effectiveness, and whether measurement relates to a patient teaching interaction, or to the broader concept of patient education. In some instances, effectiveness has been assessed through patients' written or oral responses to questions developed by the health professional or some other source. In other instances, direct observation of patient skill in performing a task or of other behavior has been used as a method of assessment. In each of these instances, there may be inconsistent definitions of what constituted a "successful" or "effective" intervention. For example, must the patient score 100% of items on a questionnaire correctly in order for the intervention to be considered effective, or is the difference in the score prior to the intervention and after the intervention the method of measurement used? If the method of assessment is patient adherence, how is adherence measured? Is the health professional able to observe patients' behavior directly, such as in appointment keeping, or must the health professional rely on patients' self-reports? Can patients' health status be used as a reliable assessment of the success or effectiveness of a patient teaching intervention? Not only are methods of assessing patient teaching effectiveness often inconsistent, there are also problems related to timing of measurements. Although a specific patient teaching intervention may be found to be effective in the immediate period following the intervention, would the same benefits be present if measured longitudinally? Another problem relates to the practicality of patient education programs or patient teaching interventions that are tested and/or evaluated. Even if a specific patient teaching intervention is shown to be effective in a particular setting, if its complexity and cost would preclude its subsequent implementation in a wider number of settings, then the findings are of little benefit.

In research and evaluation, the patient teaching intervention, as well as outcomes in patient teaching or patient education to be measured, must be defined with precision so that results can be more accurately interpreted. Detailed explanation of research or evaluation methods used is also important so that those who wish to replicate the study or apply the intervention to their own practice may do so.

SPECIFIC ISSUES IN PATIENT ADHERENCE RESEARCH

Although considerable time and effort have been and continue to be spent studying patient adherence and variables that affect it, there is still little definitive information that would enable the health professional to ensure patient adherence in all areas for all patients. Major questions remain unanswered and warrant further research.

First, although adherence is influenced by a variety of psychological and socioeconomic variables, little is known about how these variables may be changed by treatment management. Second, even interventions that have been shown to have a positive influence over adherence in the short term may not be as effective over time. Longitudinal research should be conducted for increasing understanding of adherence to long-term treatment regimens for chronic conditions. Likewise, little is known about change in adherence rates for the same individual as a result of progressing to different life stages. Longitudinal studies of individuals could identify potential barriers to patient adherence that may be shared by a number of individuals at different stages of life. Most emphasis has been placed on studying interventions to increase adherence; however, much might also be learned from ineffective interventions by examining them closely to establish why they did not work. In addition, although there appear to be no specific demographic variables that can be used to predict adherence behavior, it may be valuable to study in more detail issues related to nonadherence in an effort to increase understanding of the concept, thereby guiding efforts to improve it.

A number of issues are also problematic in patient adherence research. As in the case of patient education, the definition of patient adherence must also be precise and unambiguous as well as appropriate to the research setting. Inconsistency of findings in patient adherence research relates to a great extent to the inconsistency in definition of the term. There are many forms and levels of adherence. If, for example, the researcher is interested in adherence with appointments, does this mean those initiated by the patient, follow-up appointments initiated by the health professional, or both? Variables that impact on patient adherence are different for each. Health professionals conducting patient adherence research must be aware of the importance of defining terms clearly so that others who wish to replicate the work or use the results in practical application will be able to do so without difficulty.

Difficulty in interpretation of research results may be related to measurement of adherence both in degree and at different levels. For example, to be considered adherent, does the patient need to follow recommendations 100% of the time, or is the standard for adherence set at a lower percentage level? What percentage of time must the patient follow recommendations to be considered adherent or nonadherent? Is the patient considered adherent if he or she follows some of the recommendations but not all of them? Is the patient considered adherent if he or she follows all the recommendations but does so incorrectly? Will follow-up of adherence be conducted? How long does the patient need to follow recommendations to be considered adherent? For instance, an intervention to increase adherence may have different results if applied to patients with acute conditions rather than chronic conditions.

Another issue in adherence research is how adherence is measured. Adherence measures must be appropriate to the research question being investigated as well as appropriate to the recommendations and the setting. Indirect measures of patient adherence, such as self-report, are probably the least costly but are also the least accurate. More direct measures, such as direct observation or results of laboratory tests, are more accurate but more costly and difficult to accomplish. For example, research on patient adherence with taking a prescribed medication may use the direct measure of blood samples to assess adherence; however, such a measure cannot be obtained for research purposes without the knowledge and permission of the patient. If the patient knows that adherence is being monitored, how much does this knowledge alone impact the degree to which the patient follows recommendations?

Consideration of ethical issues should be inherent in any research (Speziale & Carpenter, 2007). In patient adherence research, there are two relatively unique problems that must be confronted. First, if patients as research subjects are fully informed about the purpose of the study, there is a potential for biasing results. Is it ever appropriate to not fully disclose to patients the purpose of the study in order to gain more accurate information about adherence? Second, are strategies that are designed to alter patient adherence ethical to apply? Is investigation of strategies that are designed to manipulate patients into behavior appropriate, or should strategies be directed to finding the most appropriate means to help patients make informed and rational choices based on their own goals and values?

How to determine the most effective way to increase adherence causes concern for many health professionals. Given research from the past 25 years, however, it appears that one of the most effective ways to increase adherence might also be in keeping with the goals of patient education—that of formation of a partnership between patient and health professional to facilitate communication and decide upon a plan collaboratively that can help them both attain their goal: improved health status.

FUTURE DIRECTIONS FOR RESEARCH IN PATIENT EDUCATION

The proliferation of patient education materials and expansion of patient education programs attest to the belief that information about prevention, as well as about diseases and treatments used to cure and control them, is important to the provision of good health care. In this proliferation of materials and efforts to educate the patient, there is an underlying perception that patients, given factual information designed to help them, will incorporate the information into their lives. This, of course, has been shown not to be the case. The fallacy that merely providing patients with comprehensive information is sufficient to bring about significant educational impact can be best alleviated through well-designed and well-controlled research that investigates the effectiveness of a variety of different patient teaching interventions for different medical conditions. The impact patient teaching has on patient outcomes both in terms of prevention and control of disease as well as patients' health status and perceived well-being must be carefully studied and evaluated. In addition, the role patient teaching has in reducing healthcare cost as well as human cost related to illness and disability warrants further intensive investigation.

As the field of patient education grows and more technologies and methods for providing effective patient teaching are developed, it behooves both practitioners and academics to continue to search for ways to improve and maintain the quality and accountability of practices used. This is best accomplished by sound research and evaluation, the results of which are directed toward not only maintaining credibility regarding the usefulness of patient education, but also ensuring that patient teaching interventions continue to be a sound and feasible means that contribute to higher-quality health care.

REFERENCES

Boswell, C. (2007). Data collection. In C. Boswell & S. Cannon (Eds.). *Introduction to nursing research: Incorporating evidence-based practice* (pp. 185–212). Sudbury, MA: Jones and Bartlett.

Burns, N., & Grove, S. K. (2005) *The practice of nursing research: Conduct, critique, & utilization* (5th ed.). St. Louis: Elsevier/Saunders.

Burns, N., & Grove, S. K. (2007). *Understanding nursing research: Building an evidence based practice* (4th ed). St. Louis: Saunders.

Dombro, M. (2007). Historical and philosophical foundations of qualitative research. In P. L. Munhall (Ed.), *Nursing research: A qualitative perspective* (4th ed. pp 99–142). Sudbury, MA: Jones and Bartlett.

Eldridge, J. (2007). Data analysis. In C. Boswell & S. Cannon (Eds.). *Introduction to nursing research: Incorporating evidence-based practice* (pp. 268–287). Sudbury, MA: Jones and Bartlett.

Finset, A. (2008). Qualitative methods in communication and patient education research. *Patient Education & Counseling, 73*(1), 1–2.

Haber, J. (2006). Developing research questions and hypothesis. In G. LoBiondo-Wood & J. Haber (Eds.). *Nursing research: Methods and critical appraisal for evidence-based practice* (6th ed., pp. 46–77). St. Louis: Mosby.

Liehr, P., & LoBiondo-Wood, G. (2006). Qualitative approaches to research. In G. LoBiondo-Wood & J. Haber (Eds.). *Nursing research: Methods and critical appraisal for evidence-based practice* (6th ed., pp. 148–175). St. Louis: Mosby.

Moorehead, S., Johnson, M., Maas, M. L., & Swanson, E. (Eds.). (2008). *Nursing outcomes (NOC)* (4th ed.). St. Louis: Mosby.

Nieswiadomy, R. M. (2008). *Foundations of nursing research* (5th ed.). Upper Saddle River, NJ: Pearson/Prentice Hall.

Polit, D., & Beck, C. T. (2006). *Essentials of nursing research: Methods, appraisal & utilization* (6th ed.). Philadelphia: Lippincott Williams & Wilkins.

Proctor, S., & Allan, T. (2006). Sampling. In K. Gerrish & A. Lacey (Eds.). *The research processing nursing* (5th ed., pp. 173–188). Oxford, UK: Blackwell Publishing.

Rich, K. A. (2009). Evaluating outcomes of innovations. In N. A. Schmidt & J. M. Brown (Eds.), *Evidence-based practice for nurses: Appraisal &application of research* (pp. 385–398). Sudbury, MA: Jones and Bartlett.

Schmidt, N. A., & Brown, J. M. (2009). What is evidence based practice? In N. A. Schmidt & J. M. Brown (Eds.), *Evidence-based practice for nurses: Appraisal &application of research* (pp. 3–32). Sudbury, MA: Jones and Bartlett.

Speziale, H. J. S., & Carpenter, D. R. (2007). *Qualitative research in nursing: Advancing humanistic imperative.* Philadelphia: Lippincott Williams & Wilkins.

Stone, M. A., Patel, N., Daly, H., Martin-Stacey, L., Amin, S., Carey, M., et al. (2008). Using qualitative research methods to inform the development of a modified version of a patient education module for non-English speakers with type 2 diabetes: experience from an action research project in two South Asian populations in the UK. *Diversity in Health & Social Care, 5*(3), 199–206.

Waltz, C. F., Strickland, O. L., & Lenz, E. K. (2005). *Measurement in nursing and health research* (3rd ed.). New York: Springer.

Wood, M. J., & Ross-Kerr, J. C. (2006). *Basic steps in planning nursing research: From question to proposal* (6th ed.). Sudbury, MA: Jones and Bartlett.

Young, M. (2009). Transitioning evidence to practice. In N. A. Schmidt & J. M. Brown (Eds.), *Evidence-based practice for nurses: Appraisal & application of research.* (pp. 335–362). Sudbury, MA: Jones and Bartlett.

CHAPTER 18

Building an Effective Patient Education Team: Promoting Patient-Centered Patient Teaching

PATIENT-CENTERED CARE

Quality of patient care has often been viewed objectively, referring to accuracy of diagnosis and effectiveness of treatment. However, there is increasing recognition that quality of patient care also has a subjective dimension—that of the experience of the patient. Patient-centered care has evolved as a model of health care that realigns structure and delivery of care to center around the patient while at the same time increasing both efficiency and resource use. (Deutschendorf, 2006). Patient-centered care has been defined as, "the redesign of patient care in the acute care setting so that hospital resources and personnel are organized around the patient's health care needs" (Maehling, 1995, p. 62).

Originally developed in acute care settings to make healthcare organizations more competitive and cost-effective, patient-centered care also meets the needs of patients and can be applied across the healthcare spectrum. As patient-centered care has gained popularity, more healthcare institutions are utilizing an approach to providing care that adopts the patient's perspective. A patient-centered approach has implications for many aspects of patient care, including patient teaching. As patients have become more involved in their health care and in decision making, the need for patient teaching has increased (Hansten & Jackson, 2009). The same conceptual framework that underscores patient-centered care can be applied to patient teaching in order to make it more effective.

A study that utilized focus groups of recently discharged hospital patients and their families identified seven primary dimensions of patient-centered care (Gerteis et al., 1993):

1. Respect for patients values, preference, and expressed needs
2. Coordination and negotiation of care

3. Information, communication, and education
4. Physical comfort
5. Emotional support and alleviation of fear and anxiety
6. Involvement of family and friends
7. Transition and continuity.

Results can be applied to all aspects of patient care; however, points can also be applied to patient teaching in order to make it the most effective. The approach to patient teaching should be one of respect in which individual values, preferences, and needs are considered. Patients should be provided with information that is communicated in a way they can understand. Patient teaching should be a coordinated effort in that all members of the health-care team work together to help the patient achieve his or her goals related to their health outcomes. Patient readiness to learn, in terms of physical comfort and emotional and psychological readiness should be considered. Family and friends should be included as much as possible and patient teaching should extend beyond the initial session, helping the patient transition and incorporate information into his or her daily life in the context of his or her own circumstances.

PATIENT-CENTERED PATIENT TEACHING

Although one dimension of care from the study described above specifically addresses education, emphasizing the need for information, effective patient teaching extends beyond provision of information. In addition to providing patients with information, effective patient teaching facilitates patient autonomy, self-care, and health promotion, based on patients' individual needs and circumstances. In order to be truly effective, patient teaching must incorporate other dimensions of patient-centered care as well. Dimensions mentioned above that are particularly relevant to patient teaching are (Gerteis et al., 1993):

- Patient involvement in decision making
- Respect for patients' needs for privacy, expression, and cultural values
- Integration and coordination of the healthcare team
- Emotional support and consideration of anxiety regarding clinical status, treatment, and prognosis
- Impact of illness on patients and their families and family involvement
- Consideration of financial impact
- Information, coordination, and support to assist patients in the transition from healthcare setting to home.

Patient teaching is an integrated process that occurs over minutes, hours, days, weeks, months, or years, according to the situation and the needs of the patient (Porche, 2007). The purpose of patient teaching extends beyond providing patients with new knowledge or skill. The ultimate purpose of patient teaching is to help patients participate in their own care so they can better cope with and manage their illness, prevent complications or illness from occurring, and achieve improved health outcomes in accordance with their own goals. Patients in all healthcare settings, whether in a hospital, ambulatory care setting, or extended care facility, are now expected to assume more responsibility for their own, often complicated, care when they return home. Consequently, patient teaching has become even more important to quality patient care. It should be a coordinated activity that is integrated into every part of care by every member of the healthcare team across the healthcare spectrum, so that it represents a true continuum of care (Porche, 2007). Patient teaching that is fragmented and conducted in bits and pieces, without coordination and communication between health professionals, is inefficient, ineffective, and diminishes the potential for positive outcomes (Mainous et al., 2004).

Patient teaching has been found to benefit the patient as well as the healthcare system. Not only has patient teaching been found to increase patient satisfaction and decrease anxiety (Bartlett, 1989; Devine & Cook, 1986), increase positive health outcomes (Balkrishnan, 2005; Mazzuca, 1982), and decrease rate of complications (Bartlett, 1989), it has also been found to increase adherence (Bailey et al., 1987; Balkrishnan et al., 2003), decrease rates of rehospitalization (Matthes, 1979), reduce institutional costs (Aday et al., 2004; Sokol et al., 2005), shorten lengths of hospital stay, and reduce malpractice claims (American Cancer Society, 2002). Consequently, not only can patient teaching improve quality of care, it can also save both staff and the healthcare system time and money by promoting more appropriate use of health services.

Although the importance of patient teaching and its place in health care is widely accepted, in many healthcare settings it is not sufficiently funded, not respected or promoted, and often performed ineffectively. If patient teaching is a low priority with administration and staff, the result can be lack of coordination between departments or even between health professionals, causing patient teaching to be fragmented and ineffective.

A frequent complaint of health professional is that there is too little time to teach, and that patients are often too anxious or overwhelmed to learn effectively. Some health professionals feel unconfident about their teaching skills, and may lack training in how to conduct patient teaching effectively. Even when patient teaching is promoted and encouraged in healthcare settings, health professionals may not be rewarded for their patient teaching efforts or for their success, which can decrease motivation for detailed patient teaching. In addition, even though some health professionals may have proficient teaching skills, coordination and communication between health professionals is not always present in order for patient teaching for each patient to extend through out the healthcare spectrum.

THE NEED FOR A TEAM APPROACH

Many aspects of the healthcare environment contribute to a need for change. Shortages of healthcare workers, more patients who are acutely ill but who have shorter hospital stays, frequent patient as well as staff turnover, and longer work hours all contribute to a less than ideal atmosphere for effective patient teaching. But at the same time, there is increased public scrutiny of healthcare environments and increased patient demand for more information about and participation in their own care and decision making (Hansten & Jackson, 2009; Walsh, 2003).

It is now understood that merely telling the patient what to do is insufficient. Emphasis of patient teaching is on the needs of the individual patient, tailoring the recommendations to each patient's learning needs and his or her specific circumstances at home. In addition to the expectation that patient teaching is an integral part of quality care, healthcare staff and organizations can also be held liable for patients who have not been given or who do not understand the importance of information crucial to their health and/or treatment (Center for the Advancement of Health, 2003). Although individualization, feedback, and reinforcement have been found to be the strongest predictors of patient teaching effectiveness (Mullen, Green, & Persinger, 1985), many health professionals find this difficult to accomplish in many settings.

Although problems associated with conducting quality patient teaching that not only takes time but also requires health professionals to think beyond rote information giving to all patients may seem insurmountable, the problem of lack of effectiveness is not always a result of the lack of time or need for individualization as much as it is using an inefficient process. Developing an atmosphere of collaboration and cooperation in the healthcare setting so that the responsibility for patient teaching is viewed as a team effort can remove much of the burden (Comstock et al., 2008). Every moment spent with the patient is an opportunity for patient teaching. Coordination of teaching and communication between health professionals regarding patient teaching efforts requires leadership so there is no duplication of effort and everyone is able to reinforce consistent information. Effective patient teaching requires a team.

DEFINING TEAM

Although a team is made up of a group of people, a group of people does not constitute at team. A group can be defined as people assembled together for a reason, but not necessarily to accomplish a common goal. For instance, a group of people may be assembled for a concert; however, aside from listening to the music, there is no common goal or purpose that the group is attempting to accomplish. A team, however, consists of people who are working collaboratively in order to accomplish a common goal. For instance, a sports team may work in a collaborative effort in order to win a championship. However, even though a group of people working together toward a collaborative goal might be considered a team, unless they have guided, focused efforts, they still may be ineffective in reaching their goal (Porter-O'Grady & Malloch, 2007).

Team effort for reaching patient teaching goals has many levels. For instance, at the individual patient level, a number of health professionals may work together as a team to help the individual patient gain knowledge and/or skill in order to manage his or her condition and treatment, and reach his or her chosen health goals through informed choice. A patient with diabetes with recent amputation because of complications may receive patient teaching from a physician, nurse, dietitian, physical therapist, and prosthetician, each of whom present different types of information in their patient teaching intervention, but all of whom are directing patient teaching to one patient-centered goal. When health professionals work together as a team through communication and collaboration between team members, the patient receives a coordinated teaching effort from the team. If, however, the physician, nurse, dietitian, physical therapist, and prosthetician conducted patient teaching independently and outlined their own goal for patient teaching without communication and consultation with each other, they would be acting as a group of health professionals conducting patient teaching rather than a team working toward the same goal.

Another level of team effort in patient teaching may be at a programmatic level. In this instance, members become part of a structured program that utilizes team efforts to provide consistent patient teaching to a specific patient population. For example, a stroke rehabilitation unit may form a patient education team to develop a consistent approach to and process for patient teaching, adjusting teaching to meet the individual patient's needs, but following a standard protocol to assure that each patient received consistent information. In this instance, communication and collaboration is still important among team members and would include not only information about success or deficiency of individual teaching interactions, but also decision making regarding standard information to be included in patient teaching and the process by which it is to be delivered. For example, the team may determine that, in addition to individual patient teaching, each patient would receive a standard preapproved packet of information about stroke, each patient would have the opportunity to attend a support group for patients and family members, and each patient would be given the opportunity to view a film entitled, *Life After a Stroke: What to Expect.* Working as a team, health professionals on the unit would have reviewed materials and made decisions about which materials should be used, and what other aspects of patient teaching, such as the support group, should be included.

The third level of team effort in patient teaching is at the institutional level, in which the organization as a whole adopts a commitment and philosophy regarding patient teaching and its importance. In this instance, representatives from a number of units may work together as a team to organize patient teaching initiatives for the institution and establish patient teaching protocols which then could be adjusted and individualized for each specific unit. In this instance, team effort involves creating an atmosphere in which patient-centered patient teaching is an integral and expected part of patient care throughout the institution. Regardless of the level of team activity, many of the same principles apply if the team is to be effective, and if patient-centered patient teaching is to be incorporated.

STARTING AT THE TOP

In order to be successful as an integrated and organized effort, patient teaching must have support from administration that is responsible for decision making and budgetary determinations. They must be convinced that patient teaching can make a difference in their organization and provide benefit, not only through increased patient satisfaction, but also through saving financial resources, staff time, and preventing unnecessary rehospitalizations (Bartlett, 1995). The administration must feel that there is a clear vision for the patient education program that has realistic goals and that those goals reflect the goals of their particular healthcare organization and fit into the organizational plan. Other administrative concerns are monetary. Administrators will need to see that the program has a reasonable budget and can be cost-effective.

When the administration of a healthcare agency, department, or unit is supportive of patient teaching efforts and understands the need for a collaborative team approach, implementing an effective protocol for integrating patient teaching into general patient care is much easier. In those instances, however, in which administration views a structured, organized approach to patient teaching as a nicety but one that will require too many resources, or if they view patient teaching superficially, as only distributing materials, implementing an effective patient education program is more difficult. A clear, well-thought-out plan that outlines details specifically will be needed.

DEVELOPING A PLAN

The plan for a structured patient education program that is to be presented to administration for support must clearly demonstrate how the patient education program fits into the general organization, and how the organization will benefit from it. What the program is expected to accomplish and how it is to be organized should be explained clearly and in realistic terms. Any costs associated with the program should be accurately outlined. The most effective patient education programs do not have to be costly. The plan should demonstrate how implementing the proposed patient education program can be an investment for the institution, such as in enhanced organizational image, increased patient satisfaction, increased quality of care, or actual cost savings.

Effective patient teaching is built on a philosophy of patient-centered care and coordination of efforts of a dedicated team, rather than on a large budget. Programs with expensive and elaborate patient education resources are not necessarily the best patient teaching programs, or the most effective, cost-effective, or efficient. Any items included in the budget should be justified. If there are limited resources, innovative approaches to patient teaching should be included in the plan.

The plan should indicate how the patient education program is to be organized and implemented with clear demarcation of duties and responsibilities; it should also be accountable and demonstrate how patient teaching efforts will be monitored and evaluated. An integral part of the patient education plan should outline mechanisms for regular evaluation and feedback and demonstrate how feedback and evaluation results will be used to make adjustments as indicated.

LEADERSHIP

Leadership is a pivotal part of team formation, team solidarity, and team success. A leader is an individual who has the skills and abilities to move people toward a vision (Evans, 2007). Leaders help team members develop a sense of working together in a framework of mutual trust. Leaders also coordinate activities of the team members by ensuring that team actions are understood and ensuring that new or changed information is promptly communicated to team members (Ferguson, 2008; Phillips, 2009). The degree to which a leader is able to help team members develop a commonly understood and agreed on sense of mission and purpose determines, to a large extent, the ability of the group to move forward toward those goals (Fisher & Thomas, 1996). One of the key roles of leadership when building an effective patient-centered patient education team is to prioritize and optimize patient teaching activities, focusing both on patient outcomes and larger institutional or organizational outcomes.

Leaders are facilitators. The major function of a facilitator of a group is to help the group reach consensus and reach goals by (Bruce, 2007):

- creating a clear vision of purpose and goals of the group,
- establishing active participation of group members,
- fostering commitment of individual group members, and
- building collaboration.

LEADERSHIP AND TRUST

The key component in developing effective functioning of a team is trust (Lencioni, 2002; Sullivan & Smith, 1995). Trust is built when leaders are clear about goals, open, straightforward, and realistic in what supports and barriers are present in order to achieve them, and are consistent in their approaches (Bleich & Kosiak, 2007). The goal of team building is to generate a type of "synergy" so that team members working together toward common goals have a greater overall effect than they would have as individuals working singularly (Ellis & Hartly, 2005). Creating this type of synergy requires a clear purpose of what the team is trying to accomplish so that each team member has a understanding of that purpose, is able to define and operationalize it, and attach value and meaning to it. A strong focus on the mission and purpose helps all members of the team to be motivated and committed to achieving the purpose. The purpose should reflect the common values of the institution and, consequently, members of the team. Building a team around this core of values and reinforcing how these values relate to the purpose helps to establish a firm foundation on which activities to achieve the purpose are developed.

Teams are people who come together to fulfill a common purpose, in this case patient-centered patient teaching. If a team is to be functional and work together effectively, there must be common goals and objectives that are clearly understood and endorsed by all team members. However, people must have the same objectives as well as the same understanding of what they are attempting to accomplish.

FORMING A TEAM

Teamwork is not a new concept in health care. It has long been viewed as a productive way to deliver quality patient care. Despite the emphasis on teamwork in provision of health care, teams have not always worked as functional units because of barriers between professional groups, lack of coordination and communication, and, at times, lack of commitment. In the complexity of today's healthcare system, and given the increasing demands and expectations placed on healthcare providers, it seems essential that effective teamwork become a reality rather than rhetoric (Fletcher, 2008). When teams function effectively, it is evident in the entire work atmosphere (Porter-O'Grady & Malloch, 2007).

Patient-centered patient teaching requires a team approach. To be successful, each team member must be committed to the purpose and goals established. They also must be helped to see how the purpose of the effort is consistent with values and goals of the institution (Barker, Sullivan, & Emery, 2006). Just as patients are individuals, so are health professionals with their own attitudes, prejudices, skills, and experiences. In addition, in patient education programs, team members are frequently individuals from a number of interdisciplinary professions who must work together so that patient teaching efforts can be the most effective. When team members are interdisciplinary, there must be an effort to understand the various roles and backgrounds of each discipline and how each discipline and its teaching contributes to patient teaching outcomes. Interdisciplinary teams cannot function effectively unless there is mutual trust and respect among members (Brown et al., 2003).

An important part of team building is to develop a cohesive whole in which members share the same goals while at the same time recognizing individual differences and unique contributions of each member (Barker, Sullivan, & Emery, 2006). Although not all members of the team have to have the same role or the same skill, they do need to be cohesive in their consensus of the underlying principles of the work that is to be accomplished. For example, individuals who still take a very paternalistic view of the relationship between the patient and health professional will not be as an effective member of the patient education team as would an individual who is already very patient-centered. Individuals who are uncomfortable with patients' active involvement in setting goals or who question patients' judgment and abilities to make their own decisions are not likely to show the same level of commitment for patient-centered patient teaching as individuals who readily accept patients as an integral member of the healthcare team.

Regardless of differences, it is important to have open discussion of feelings and conflicts, with thoughtful acceptance of beliefs and different opinions of others, rather than causing suppression of real views, a phenomenon that could contribute to team ineffectiveness (Davies, 2009). Even when individuals hold different views, helping them to feel part of the team is an integral part of the change process. Individuals should continue to be included in discussion and consulted throughout the process, taking their opinions into account (Chapman, 2008). When disagreements occur, it is important to attempt to respect the contributions of everyone. At times, it may be important to agree to disagree.

MAINTAINING TEAM EFFORT

All teams have a human dimension. Members of the team need to feel personal fulfillment and support, which may be no more that acknowledging and thanking individuals for their efforts (Adair, 1986). Just as patients need feedback and reinforcement in order to continue positive behaviors, so do health professionals working as part of the patient-centered patient education team.

Successful team effort is dependent on cohesiveness among members. Regardless of role, each member's performance should be a reflection of how they contribute to the mission and purpose that has been established (Porter-O'Grady & Malloch, 2007). Cohesiveness develops by increasing connections between members of the team (Clark, 2009). In order to connect, individuals need to interact. One way of building team spirit and rapport is through team meetings. Holding regular meetings of the team can (Manion & Huber, 2006):

- help the team form and consolidate an identity and solidify the group purpose,
- provide an opportunity for updates of shared knowledge regarding issues/progress,
- reinforce collective goals, and
- create a sense of commitment.

Team meetings can help team members recognize that cooperation can contribute to the success of team effort. Ongoing interactions and familiarity with one another increases the likelihood that team efforts will progress more smoothly. Meetings in which specific patient teaching issues are discussed or significant needs or problems of individual patients are reviewed and addressed by each discipline involved keeps communication open and builds cooperation and collaboration. Actively encouraging team members to help each other and to share ideas and experiences also creates a sense of community and consolidation. The more team members are helped to see that goals are worthwhile and attainable, the greater the chances are that the team will be successful and effective.

BARRIERS TO PATIENT-CENTERED PATIENT TEACHING: WHEN BUILDING A TEAM MEANS CHANGE

The benefits, including increased adherence, of involving patients in patient teaching efforts and helping them increase their understanding of care and treatment have been well-documented (Bailey et al., 1987), yet not all health-care facilities, and not all health professionals, embrace the concept of patient-centered patient teaching. Nor do they embrace the concept of an organized, coordinated patient teaching effort across all disciplines and across healthcare facilities. Barriers to building an effective patient-centered patient education team are numerous and can be rooted in the organizational bureaucracy of the institution as well as in attitudes and beliefs of health professionals.

If all team members, or all members of the organization, agree to goals and purpose of the task at hand as well as means to accomplish them, there is little stress or conflict involved. Unfortunately, in a world made up of individuals with different perceptions, values, goals, and experiences, it is inevitable that not everyone on the team or within the organization will always have consistent views. This natural occurrence has the potential for conflict either within or outside the team that can interfere with effectiveness of the group, and consequently, with the effectiveness of patient teaching.

CHANGE AND RESISTANCE

Team effort is often directed toward change. Individual team members' responses to change can either facilitate or obstruct the change process. Anticipating the responses and reactions of individuals or groups which may impede change can assist leaders to develop strategies or interventions for counteracting them.

Individuals sometimes react to the possibility of change with resistance. Individuals may feel invested in the status quo and fear that change will mean a disruption of their routine or loss of status, power, or control. Others may have concerns about the expenditure of time or energy or other resources they will need to invest because of the proposed change. In some instances, individuals may fear their own inadequacy in performing duties associated with change as a result of lack of training or skill or fear that change will decrease their perceived worth.

Resistance to change may be expressed actively, through open confrontation or aggression, or it may be expressed passively through surface acceptance but with covert undermining of implementation of proposed changes. In some instances, individuals may attempt to sabotage proposed changes by organizing others to also resist change. In still other instances, individuals may attempt to divert attention to other issues rather than the issues at hand (Huber, 2006).

For example, Dr. Paulson had practiced medicine for over 30 years and had always approached his patients in benevolent, although paternalistic, way, believing that they had neither the training nor understanding needed to be included in making decision about their own care. He prided himself in protecting them from stress by making unilateral decisions for them based on his understanding of what was best for them. When, at a staff meeting, the director of the health clinic in which he worked proposed at that a patient education committee be formed to develop a more patient-centered protocol for patient teaching, Dr. Paulson actively spoke against it and began to privately lobby against it. Dr. Paulson preferred keeping a traditional approach and felt that the proposal undermined his approach to patients. His opposition began to sabotage the proposal and threatened to interfere with its implementation.

In another situation, Ms. Adams, a nurse on the cystic fibrosis unit, became upset when the unit manager suggested that each nurse on the unit take responsibility for teaching patients and families about home care prior to discharge. Ms. Adams complained that nurses had never been expected to assume the total discharge teaching responsibility in the past and that she was far too busy to engage in that type of activity. The suggested change overwhelmed her both in terms of additional responsibility she was being given and also because of her own lack of confidence about her ability to perform the teaching task adequately.

In yet another example, Mr. McNulty, the hospital administrator, suggested the development of a patient teaching form that could be used for all disciplines conducting patient teaching so that information that had been provided to the patient as well as the patient's response and additional needs could be documented and reviewed by each discipline in order to enhance communication. Several departments in the hospital vehemently opposed the proposal, under the guise that it would precipitate confusion and potential inconsistency of information since some disciplines would be unfamiliar with content presented by others in disciplines unrelated to their own.

In each of the above examples, the responses of Dr. Paulson and Ms. Adams, as well as the opposition of departments, must be considered and dealt with if their responses are to be channeled into support. The suggestion of change may bring about a sense of loss of control or uncertainty in individuals or groups about how change will affect them. Under these circumstances, it is important to help them become comfortable with transition and change while remaining sensitive to their discomfort. Interventions may be implemented that can facilitate their willingness to participate in transition while at the same time addressing their concerns. Active and empathetic listening is essential. Providing individuals or groups with education and support as well as an opportunity to participate and become involved in the change process can promote a sense of empowerment and control that may enhance their willingness to consider change.

PUTTING TEAMWORK INTO PRACTICE

One of the major reasons for using a team approach in patient teaching is to provide a unified, consistent approach to patient teaching and to the information patients are given. Patients become confused when health professionals tell them different things. Health professionals do not always communicate well with each other. When this occurs, communication breakdown can occur, leaving patients uninformed or ill informed and affecting the quality of patient teaching as well as the positive outcomes in terms of adherence. When patients see that information is duplicated, inconsistent, or incomplete, their view of care is altered. Whether or not patients receive consistent information is dependent on how well health professionals have communicated.

Effective patient teaching consists of more than a one-time exchange of information between the patient and health professional. In order to be effective, patient teaching must be planned, organized, implemented, and evaluated so alterations and adjustments can be made if problems arise. Likewise, patient teaching must be reinforced. Consequently, everyone involved with the goal of reaching a specific patient teaching outcome should be informed.

Effective patient teaching requires a plan that outlines what needs to be done, who will do it, when it will be done, how it will be done, and how it will be evaluated. Although patient teaching may be viewed by an organization as a concept rather than a program, having a well-thought-out plan that clearly outlines expectations is important to successful and ongoing implementation. It is not enough for an organization to give lip service to patient teaching as an important part of patient care. Every member of the organization must have a clear understanding of the overall philosophy and vision of patient teaching and what that means in terms of their own specific duties and responsibilities.

MISSION, VISION, AND VALUES

A strong focus on mission and purpose helps all individuals become fully aware of the foundation on which every work activity is built. The first, and most important, part of the plan is arriving at a vision statement that reflects the mission and guides and directs behaviors and decisions. The vision statement should be realistic, attainable, credible, and attractive. The vision statement can be used to energize team members, creating a culture of commitment to values and goals of the plan. The vision statement is the foundation that provides a stimulus toward goal setting and defines expectations. The vision statement also provides a general guideline for change. When developing the vision statement, care should be taken to be sure it is relevant and as clear as possible, taking into account resources and supports available. It should focus not only on patient teaching and outcomes, but also on the role each member of the team will have in helping to attain the vision.

Planning in patient teaching means looking ahead to decide what goals or outcomes are to be accomplished and what steps need to be taken to reach them. Part of planning includes assessing what needs to be done, who will do it, when it will be done, and what methods will be used. The planning process also identifies barriers and supports that would support or interfere with reaching the desired outcomes. The plan should consist of manageable components. Whether planning an organized patient education program is at the institutional, programmatic, or individual level, a clear logical plan that clearly outlines steps involved in the process is needed. The organizational structure that will be needed for making decisions about personnel, materials, communication, activities, and resources, in order to reach the desired goal should also be included. Roles, responsibilities, and general processes for teaching and documentation should be clearly outlined so that each individual is aware of expectations of their contribution to the whole.

Implementation consists of putting the plan into action and trying out the activities. The final step is evaluating the process and outcomes. This component of the plan is ongoing. There should be continual monitoring that consists of information gathering about the effectiveness of the plan. Information gathered should then be utilized to make changes as needed. Performance and outcomes must be continually monitored and activities altered as necessary in order for the plan to remain viable and in order for the desired goals and outcomes to be reached.

REFERENCES

Adair, J. (1986). *Effective Team Building.* London: Cower.

Aday, L. A., Begley, C. E., Lairson, D. R., & Balkrishnan, R. (2004). *Evaluating the healthcare system: Effectiveness, efficiency, and equity.* Chicago, IL: Health Administration Press.

American Cancer Society. (2002). Patients report doctors do a good job at a difficult time. *CA: A Cancer Journal for Clinicians, 52,* 62–63.

Bailey, W. C., Richards, J. M., Jr., Manzella, B. A., Windsor, R. A., Brooks, C. M., & Soong, S. (1987). Promoting self-management in adults with asthma: An overview of the UAB Program. *Health Education Quarterly, 14*(3), 345–355.

Balkrishnan, R. (2005). The importance of medication adherence in improving chronic-disease related outcomes: What we know and what we need to further know. *Medical Care, 43*(6), 517–520.

Balkrishnan, R., Rajagopalan, R., Camacho, F. T., Huston, S. A., Murray, F. T., & Anderson, R. T. (2003). Predictors of medication adherence and associated health care costs in an older population with type 2 diabetes mellitus: A longitudinal cohort study. *Clinical Therapy, 25,* 2958–2971.

Barker, A. M., Sullivan, D. T., & Emery, M. J. (2007). *Leadership competencies for clinical managers: The renaissance of transformational leadership.* Sudbury, MA: Jones and Bartlett.

Bartlett, E. E. (1989) Patient education can lower costs, improve quality. *Hospitals, 63*(21), 88.

Bartlett, E. E. (1995). Cost-benefit analysis of patient education. *Patient Education and Counseling, 26,* 87–91.

Bleich, M. R., & Kosiak, C. P. (2007). Managing, Leading, and Following. In P. Yoder-Wise (Ed.), *Leading and managing in nursing* (4th ed., pp. 3–25). St. Louis, MO: Mosby/Elsevier.j

Brown, M., Ohlinger, J., Rusk, C., Delmore, P., & Ittmann, P. (2003). Implementing potentially better practices for multidisciplinary team building: Creating a neonatal intensive care unit culture of collaboration. *Pediatrics, 111*(4), 482–488.

Bruce, W. R. (2007). *More than 50 ways to build team consensus* (2nd ed.). Thousand Oaks, CA: Corwin Press.

Center for the Advancement of Health (2003) Talking the talk: Improving patient provider-communication. *Facts of Life: Issues for Health Reporters, 9*(3), 1.

Chapman, L. (2008). Effective teamwork. *Nursing Management, 15*(6), 18–21.

Clark, C. C. (2009). *Group leadership skills for nurses and health professionals* (5th ed.). New York: Springer.

Comstock, D. L., Hammer, T. R., Strentzsch, J., Cannon, K., Parsons, J., & Salazar, G. (2008). Relational-cultural theory: A framework for bridging relational, multicultural, and social justice competencies. *Journal of Counseling and Development, 86,* 279–287.

Davies, N. (2009). Build an effective team. *Nursing Standard, 23*(29), 72.

Deutschendorf, A. L. (2006). Models of care delivery. In D. L. Huber. *Leadership and nursing care management* (3rd ed., pp. 315–336). Philadelphia: Saunders.

Devine, E. C., & Cook, T. D. (1986). Clinical and cost-saving effects of psycho-educational interventions with surgical patients: A meta-analysis. *Research in Nursing and Health, 9,* 89–105.

Ellis, J. R., & Hartly, C. L. (2005). *Managing and coordinating nursing care.* Philadephia: Lippincott Williams & Wilkins.

Evans, M. L. (2007). Developing the role of a leader. In P. Yoder-Wise (Ed.), *Leading and managing in nursing* (4th ed., pp. 27–43). St. Louis, MO: Mosby/Elsevier.

Ferguson, S. L. (2008). Military nursing. TeamSTEPPS: Integrating teamwork principles into adult health/medical-surgical practice. *Medsurg Nurs, 17*(2), 122–125.

Fisher, B., & Thomas, B. (1996). *Real dream teams: Seven practices used by world-class team leaders to achieve extraordinary results.* Delray Beach, FL: St. Lucia Press.

Fletcher, M. (2008). Multi-disciplinary team working: Building and using the team. *Nuroo, 35*(12), 42–47.

Gerteis, M., Edgman-Levitan, S., Daley, J., & Delbanco, T. L. (1993). Introduction: Medicine and health from the patient's perspective. In M. Gerteis, S. Edgman-Levitan, J. Daleyy, & T. L. Delbanco (Eds.), *Through the patient's eyes: Understanding and promoting patient-centered care* (pp. 1–15). San Francisco: Jossey-Bass.

Hansten, R. I., & Jackson, J. (2009). *Clinical delegation skills: A handbook for professional practice.* Sudbury, MA: Jones and Bartlett.

Huber, D. L. (2006). Change and innovation. In D. L. Huber (Ed.). *Leadership and nursing care management* (3rd ed., pp. 805–826). Philadelphia: Saunders.

Lencioni, P. M. (2002). *The five dysfunctions of a team: A leadership fable* (pp. 341–369). San Francisco: Jossey-Bass.

Maehling, J. A. S. (1995). Process reengineering: Strategies for analysis & redesign. In S. S. Blancett & D. L. Flarey (Eds.), *Reengineering nursing and health care: The handbook for organizational transformation* (pp. 61–74). Gaithersburg, MD: Aspen.

Mainous, A. G., Kern, D., Hainer, B., Kneuper-Hall, R., Stephens, J., & Geesey, M. E. (2004). The relationship between continuity of care, trust, and stage of cancer at diagnosis. *Family Medicine, 36*, 35–39.

Manion, J., & Huber, D. L. (2006). Team building and working with effective groups. In D. L. Huber. *Leadership and nursing care management* (3rd ed., pp. 561–586). Philadelphia: Saunders.

Matthes, M. L (1979). Beyond the hospital: Diabetic day care. *American Journal of Nursing, 79*(1), 105–106.

Mazzuca, S. A. (1982). Does patient education in chronic disease have therapeutic value? *Journal of Chronic Diseases, 35*, 521–529.

Mullen, P. D., Green, L. W., & Persinger, G. S. (1985). Clinical trials of patient education for chronic conditions: A comparative meta-analysis of intervention types. *Preventive Medicine, 14*, 753–781.

Phillips, A. (2009). Realistic team building in a nurse managed clinic setting. *Internet Journal of Advanced Nursing Practice, 10*(1), 15236064. Retrieved December 23, 2009, from http://www.ispub.com/ostia/index.php?xmlFilePath=journals/ijanp/front.xml

Porche, R .A. (2007). *The Joint Commission guide to patient and family education* (2nd ed.). Oakbrook Terrace, IL: Joint Commission on Accreditation of Healthcare Organizations.

Porter-O'Grady, T., & Malloch, K. (2007). *Quantum leadership: A resource for health care innovation* (2nd ed.). Sudbury, MA: Jones and Bartlett.

Sokol, M. C., McGuigan, J. A., Verbrugge, R. R., & Epstein, R. S. (2005). Impact of medication adherence on hospitalization risk and health care cost. *Medical Care, 43*(6), 521–530.

Sullivan, D. T., & Smith, A. E. (1995). Effective team building in the emergency department. *Critical Decisions in Emergency Medicine, 9*, 153–162.

Walsh, P. (2003). We must accept that health care is a risky business. *British Medical Journal, 326*, 1333–1334.

Index

Note: Page numbers followed by "*t*" indicate tables.